KT-146-054

Essential Orthopaedics and Trauma

Fifth Edition

David J. Dandy MD MA MChir FRCS

Emeritus Consultant Orthopaedic Surgeon, Addenbrooke's Hospital, Cambridge, UK

Dennis J. Edwards MBChB, FRCS(Orth)

Consultant Orthopaedic Surgeon, Addenbrooke's Hospital, Cambridge, UK

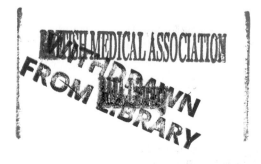

BRITISH MEDICAL ASSOCIATION
WITHDRAWN FROM LIBRARY

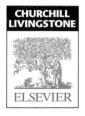

CHURCHILL LIVINGSTONE

ELSEVIER

Edinburgh   London   New York   Oxford   Philadelphia   St Louis   Sydney   Toronto   2009

CHURCHILL
LIVINGSTONE
ELSEVIER

© Longman Group UK Limited 1989, 1993 assigned to Pearson Professional Ltd 1995
© Pearson Professional 1998
© Harcourt Publishers Limited 1999
© Elsevier Science Limited 2003
© 2009, Elsevier Limited. All rights reserved.

No part of this publication may be reproduced or transmitted in any form or by any means, electronic or mechanical, including photocopying, recording, or any information storage and retrieval system, without permission in writing from the publisher. Permissions may be sought directly from Elsevier's Rights Department: phone: (+1) 215 239 3804 (US) or (+44) 1865 843830 (UK); fax: (+44) 1865 853333; e-mail: healthpermissions@elsevier.com. You may also complete your request on-line via the Elsevier website at http://www.elsevier.com/permissions.

First published 1989
Second edition 1993
Third edition 1998
Fourth edition 2003
   Reprinted 2004, 2006
Fifth edition 2009

ISBN: 978-0-443-06718-1
International Edition ISBN 978-0-443-06717-4

British Library Cataloguing in Publication Data
A catalogue record for this book is available from the British Library

Library of Congress Cataloging in Publication Data
A catalog record for this book is available from the Library of Congress

Notice

Knowledge and best practice in this field are constantly changing. As new research and experience broaden our knowledge, changes in practice, treatment and drug therapy may become necessary or appropriate. Readers are advised to check the most current information provided (i) on procedures featured or (ii) by the manufacturer of each product to be administered, to verify the recommended dose or formula, the method and duration of administration, and contraindications. It is the responsibility of the practitioner, relying on their own experience and knowledge of the patient, to make diagnoses, to determine dosages and the best treatment for each individual patient, and to take all appropriate safety precautions. To the fullest extent of the law, neither the Publisher nor the Authors assume any liability for any injury and/or damage to persons or property arising out or related to any use of the material contained in this book.

The Publisher

your source for books,
journals and multimedia
in the health sciences
www.elsevierhealth.com

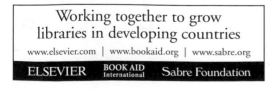

Working together to grow
libraries in developing countries

www.elsevier.com | www.bookaid.org | www.sabre.org

ELSEVIER   BOOK AID International   Sabre Foundation

The
publisher's
policy is to use
**paper manufactured
from sustainable forests**

Printed in China

www.bma.org.uk/library

Essential
Orthopaedics
and Trauma

WITHDRAWN
FROM LIBRARY

BRITISH MEDICAL ASSOCIATION

0930238

Commissioning Editor: Alison Taylor
Development Editor: Kim Benson
Project Manager: Joannah Duncan
Designer/Design Direction: Charles Gray
Illustration Manager: Bruce Hogarth

Contents

Preface
to fifth edition

Again, this edition has kept the same basic layout as previous editions. All have been, we hope, simple to read and useable as either an undergraduate or postgraduate student. Although orthopaedic surgery remains a constantly changing specialty, the essential core knowledge remains the same.

There is now more emphasis on the biological approach to chondral repair and gene therapy as well as an update of the newer methods of managing trauma cases. In particular, locking plates have changed our method of fixing juxta-articular and osteoporotic fractures.

D.E.
D.J.D.
Cambridge 2009

Acknowledgement

I remain indebted to David Dandy for his support, for his encouragement, and for allowing me to contribute to this book. He is a wonderful teacher and an even better colleague! Thank you.

D.E.

Preface
to first edition

When starting to prepare this text, we had three main objectives. The first was to write it from scratch without reference to any other texts in the hope that this would avoid the perpetuation of old errors. In doing so, we have almost certainly introduced a few new mistakes of our own which have eluded us and the reviewers. If any reader feels strongly about a point in the text, we would like them to write to us.

The second aim was to produce a text that was relevant to modern orthopaedics. Many textbooks dwell at length on the Grand Old Diseases of the past, even if they are seldom seen today. We have tried to avoid this temptation in the belief that textbooks must change just as the spectrum of disease changes, but will doubtless be criticized because important conditions have not received their customary space. We will not help the critics by listing the conditions to which we refer.

Our third aim was to allocate space in proportion to the frequency with which the conditions occur, rather than their degree of fascination. There is more, for example, on Colles' fracture than on the mucopolysaccharidoses and facts about rare conditions are reduced to the minimum essentials. It is to be hoped that examiners approve of this approach, but there is still a tendency to believe that the candidate who knows all about extreme rarities must know even more about very common conditions.

Some sections of the text may appear so basic as to be patronizing, but we make no apologies for this. There is no fact so basic that it can be left unstated. Finally, we have tried to make the text easy to read. Orthopaedic surgery is neither dull nor boring, and its textbooks should be equally enjoyable. We hope that this textbook will serve the undergraduate student well, lay a good foundation for the Fellowship examination, and be a useful manual for family practitioners, physiotherapists and nurses who work closely with orthopaedic patients.

D.J.D.
Cambridge 1989

Part | 1 |

Background knowledge

Chapter | 1 |

Introduction

History and development

Orthopaedic surgeons deal with deformity, diseases of bones and joints, and injuries to the musculoskeletal system. Because these are among the commonest things to affect humankind there must always have been orthopaedic surgeons of one kind or another, even in the most primitive communities. Wherever there was a witch doctor or medicine man dealing with illness and disease, as general practitioners and physicians do now, somewhere there would have been a 'bone setter' treating fractures and straightening limbs.

Despite these ancient origins, the word 'orthopaedic' is a recent introduction derived from the title of a book published by a French physician, Nicolas Andry, in 1741: *Orthopaedia, or, The Art of Correcting and Preventing Deformities in Children: By such Means, as may easily be put in Practice by Parents themselves, and all such as are Employed in Educating Children*.

The word itself is derived from the Greek *orthos pais* and means only 'straight child', but orthopaedic surgery has expanded from the correction of deformities in children to embrace every aspect of musculoskeletal surgery. Apart from coining the word orthopaedics, Andry also designed the symbol that has now become the worldwide logo of orthopaedic

surgery. The 'Tree of Andry' is taken from an engraving in *Orthopaedia* that showed a crooked tree tied to a stake in order to straighten it (Fig. 1.1). The fact that it is virtually impossible to straighten a crooked limb by tying it to a straight splint has not affected the popularity of the symbol, which has been adapted for many purposes (Fig. 1.2).

In some countries, the work of the bone setter was willingly carried out by physicians, and Hippocrates himself is credited with the development of a technique for reducing dislocated shoulders which stood the test of time until general anaesthesia made it easy to overcome muscle spasm. Hippocrates is also said to have treated recurrent dislocation of the shoulder by applying a flaming torch to the axilla, but this treatment has not survived.

Physicians were not always as enlightened as Hippocrates. The bone setter, who earned his living by his ability to manipulate broken limbs, was often regarded with disfavour by the established medical profession, and this was certainly true in Britain. When the Medical Act of 1858 restricted the use of the title 'Doctor' to those who had passed certain recognized examinations, bone setters were excluded and became unregistered practitioners; however, this did not stop them practising, and their success remained a source of continual irritation to the medical profession. Orthopaedic hospitals existed in London and other large cities during the middle

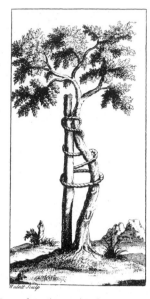

Fig. 1.1 The Tree of Andry. By kind permission of the Wellcome Institute Library, London.

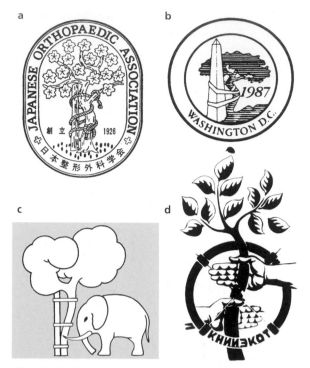

Fig. 1.2 (a) The emblem of the Japanese Orthopaedic Association. By kind permission of the Japanese Orthopaedic Association. (b) The emblem of the Eighth Combined Meeting of the Orthopaedic Associations of the English Speaking World, Washington DC, 1987. By kind permission of the American Orthopaedic Association. (c) Emblem of the Orthopaedic Department, Katholieke Universiteit, Nijmegen, by kind permission. (d) Emblem of the Kurgan Scientific Research Institute of Experimental and Clinical Orthopaedics and Traumatology, Kurgan, Russia. By kind permission of Professor G.A. Ilizarov and the Pan Union Kurgan Scientific Centre for Reconstructive Traumatology and Orthopaedics.

of the 19th century but they remained under the direction of registered medical practitioners.

The medical profession might have been denied access to the 'black arts' of the bone setters altogether if it had not been for Evan Thomas, renowned as the last of the great Welsh bone setters, who decided to put all five of his sons through medical school. One of these sons was the legendary Hugh Owen Thomas (1834–1891), who trained in Edinburgh but qualified with the London MRCS in 1857 (Fig. 1.3). It is ironic that when Hugh Owen Thomas joined his father's practice in Liverpool, they found themselves unable to work together and quickly parted.

Hugh Owen Thomas had an enormous impact on the development of orthopaedic surgery in Britain, both by his own effort and through his influence upon his nephew Robert Jones (1857–1933). Between them, Hugh Owen Thomas and Robert Jones laid the foundations of British orthopaedic surgery so successfully that it is easy to forget that less than a century ago much of its present work was carried out by practitioners regarded as charlatans by the rest of the profession.

As orthopaedic surgery became established, it attracted much the same attention from factions within the medical profession as the profession had shown the bone setters of the previous century. In 1918, 12 surgeons founded the British Orthopaedic

Association. Also in 1918, the Royal College of Surgeons in England found time in a busy schedule to 'view with mistrust and disapprobation the movement in progress to remove the treatment of conditions, always properly regarded as the main portion of the General Surgeon's work, from his hands and place it in those of "orthopaedic specialists". The general surgeons were right to be worried; they are now almost outnumbered by orthopaedic surgeons and the gap is closing fast.

Orthopaedic surgery today

Modern orthopaedic surgery has changed radically since the time of Andry, and now extends from the neonate to the elderly. The following are some of

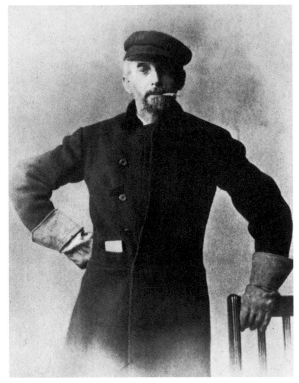

Fig. 1.3 Hugh Owen Thomas. By kind permission of the Wellcome Institute Library, London.

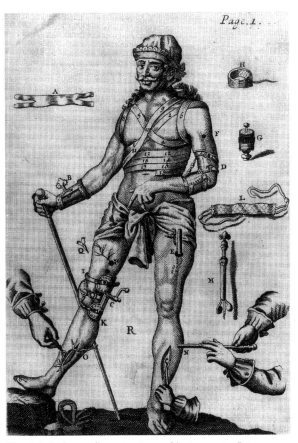

Fig. 1.4 Orthopaedic apparatus and instruments. From Cooke J (1685) *Mellificum Chirurgiae*. By kind permission of the Wellcome Institute Library, London.

the more important segments of orthopaedic surgery today.

Neonates

The orthopaedic surgeon takes care of congenital deformity. Prompt treatment of some conditions in the first few days of life can produce an almost perfect result, but treating the same condition later may be much more difficult (see 'Developmental dysplasia of the hip', p. 354).

Children

As in Andry's time, children's deformities are the province of the orthopaedic surgeon, but children's orthopaedics now presents so many unusual and difficult problems that it has become a specialty in its own right (see Ch. 21).

Trauma

Trauma has always filled much of the surgeon's time (Fig. 1.4). Today, multiple injuries, particularly road

trauma, keep many beds full and form a large part of orthopaedic practice, sometimes to the exclusion of elective orthopaedic surgery.

Sports medicine

In some countries sports medicine is a separate specialty but in the UK sports injuries fall within the scope of orthopaedics. Because the fitness of sportsmen and women attracts the interest of the public and the press, the orthopaedic surgeon can find this part of his or her work receiving special scrutiny.

Degenerative joint disease

Like trauma, degenerative joint disease occupies a great deal of orthopaedic attention. Total joint replacement, particularly of the hip and knee, is a

5

hugely successful operation which relieves pain and restores mobility to patients who would otherwise be condemned to persistent pain and restricted movement for the rest of their lives.

The elderly

Finally, there are the disorders of old age. With increasing age, the bones become progressively more brittle until they fracture with negligible trauma. All too often, fracture of the neck of the femur in an old person living alone, with little family support, creates social problems that prove insuperable and mark the start of a downhill path that leads to death.

Involvement with other specialties

No modern doctor can practise 'general' medicine in isolation from colleagues, and this is particularly true for orthopaedic surgery. The orthopaedic surgeon must therefore have a working knowledge of many other disciplines.

Rheumatologists

Rheumatologists and orthopaedic surgeons deal with the same structures and must work closely together. A working knowledge of rheumatology is essential to the orthopaedic surgeon, just as a knowledge of orthopaedics is essential to the rheumatologist. In some countries the orthopaedic surgeon doubles as the rheumatologist.

Plastic surgeons

The management of trauma involves treating extensive skin loss: close liaison with the plastic surgeons is important for making the best use of available skin. If the initial management of a wound is bad, the work of the plastic surgeons is made more difficult. This is true of not only extensive skin loss but also the suturing of seemingly simple wounds in the accident department.

Neurologists

Apparently simple 'orthopaedic' problems, such as a recurrent sprain or weakness of an arm, may be the first indication of a neurological disorder such as a spinal tumour, muscular dystrophy or

multiple sclerosis. To be able to detect the exceptional patient who has a neurological disorder and not a truly orthopaedic problem takes considerable experience.

General and thoracic surgeons

In the treatment of trauma, a good knowledge of the management of thoracic and abdominal injuries is mandatory. Much major trauma is first seen by the orthopaedic surgeon because of the damage to the limbs, and he or she must also assess the damage to the chest or abdomen (pp. 167–176).

Community services

Community services are important to orthopaedic surgeons because they are closely involved with the health services outside hospital. An elderly lady with a fractured hip, for example, cannot be sent home to fend for herself without careful consultation with both the general practitioner and the community nurses (p. 75). The orthopaedic surgeon must also know how to arrange special educational facilities for children with physical handicap and how to arrange the rehabilitation of disabled patients.

What does orthopaedic surgery achieve?

The wide range of conditions and different types of patients makes orthopaedic surgery an unusually interesting specialty which offers 'something for everybody', but there is also the satisfaction of knowing that the majority of patients can be helped. Patients with disabling arthritis are made more comfortable, deformities can be corrected or prevented; few orthopaedic patients are 'ill' in the true sense of the word, and malignant disease is rare. Trauma patients, in particular, are usually healthy individuals plucked from the community at random, quite literally by accident, and restoring them to full fitness is very rewarding.

Orthopaedic operations

From a technical point of view, orthopaedic operations require a wide range of skills and techniques. Although many of the operations involve the traditional 'wet carpentry' of bone, using hammers, chisels and drills, techniques such as joint replacement demand a sound knowledge of mechanics and materials science. Orthopaedic surgery can also include the microsurgical repair of nerves and vessels, massive spinal surgery, intricate operations on the tendons of the hand, and endoscopy, all of which require different skills. This wide variety of techniques, involving instruments ranging from the operating microscope to the traditional hammer and chisel, demands a technical ability not required by surgeons in other specialties.

Chapter | 2 |

History and clinical examination

By the end of this chapter you should be able to:

- Take an appropriate history.
- Perform a competent general clinical examination of all joints.
- Understand and use the correct orthopaedic terminology.
- Competently perform the common examinations of large joints.

Most of the 'orthopaedic' words are explained in detail the first time they appear in the text but some words, which most people will already know, are not explained. These words are printed in **bold** type when they first appear, and their meaning, together with those of obscure or ancient terms, is explained in the Glossary.

If you are uncertain about the meaning of a word, look it up in the Glossary on p. 467.

History

In most branches of medicine there is seldom any argument about the correct management once the diagnosis has been established. Orthopaedic surgery is different: the diagnosis is easy but the choice of management is difficult. The appropriate treatment varies from one patient to the next and is determined by age, sex, occupation and home circumstances, all of which must be established while the history is taken. The patient's attitude is also important and it is helpful to consider the following points while taking the history.

General aspects of a consultation

1. Why has the patient come?
2. How well motivated is the patient?
3. Does the patient have a reason (litigation, for example) not to hope for recovery?
4. Does the patient have realistic expectations of treatment?
5. Has the patient really understood what you have said?

The patient

Reason for consultation

Most patients will be looking for the relief of pain or deformity but many seek only an explanation of their condition and its likely progress. A patient with sudden pain in one joint may be worried because a relative had severe arthritis that began with pain in just one joint and the patient fears that she, too, is destined for a wheelchair. Other patients fear that their pain is the first sign of widespread cancer, particularly if a relative died with bone metastases; and parents' worries about the shape of their children's feet can be fuelled by concerned grandparents, friends or health visitors.

These patients need nothing more than a sympathetic ear, firm and authoritative reassurance, and a careful explanation of the condition and its prognosis. To treat the symptoms energetically will only increase the patient's anxiety.

Motivation

Motivation is very important. Many orthopaedic operations demand hard work and complete cooperation from the patient in the postoperative period. If the patient gives the impression of being unable or unwilling to take an active part in the rehabilitation process, there is unlikely to be a good result from operation, however well it is done. To detect such people before operation is difficult, but only too easy after operation.

Litigation

When symptoms are the result of a road traffic accident or an injury at work, the patient may be involved in legal action to obtain compensation. Although the great majority of patients give a perfectly honest and straightforward account of their symptoms, they cannot help becoming a little introspective if they think that compensation is related directly to the severity of symptoms. Most people involved in litigation will say so, but if this is not mentioned and patients begin the history with the exact date when the symptoms began, they should be asked specifically about impending litigation. A clear and careful record of the symptoms is essential in these patients and may be a little more difficult than usual to obtain.

Patients' expectations

Sensible patients understand that no operation is painless and that all leave a permanent scar, but some expect the impossible. Athletes cannot accept that declining performance is due to age, and patients with gross osteoarthritis expect a perfect cure. If treatment is offered to patients with unrealistic expectations they are bound to be disappointed,

and are sometimes even vengeful. It is as well to recognize such people before any definitive treatment is suggested.

Does the patient understand?

No matter how thorough the explanation of the condition or proposed operation, it is unlikely that the patient will remember everything that has been said. Some understand more than others but a few do not remember a word. Because close cooperation between patient and doctor is particularly important in orthopaedic surgery, special attention must be given to ensuring that the patient understands as clearly as possible exactly what the treatment involves.

Specific questions

Apart from general impressions of the patient's attitude, specific questions must be asked, both to establish the diagnosis and to select management. Social and occupational histories are vital because the impact of symptoms on lifestyle varies from one patient to the next. It is essential to have detailed information about the patient's occupation and home circumstances before any treatment is suggested.

Specific questions

1. *Symptoms.* Record them as precisely as possible.
2. *Occupation.* Find out the exact nature of the patient's work.
3. *Impact of treatment.* How will it affect the patient's work, life, leisure, etc.?
4. *Home circumstances.* Are the stairs at home easy to climb? How far away are the shops? Is there any help in the house?

Symptoms

Pain, deformity, swelling and loss of movement in a joint are the commonest complaints in an orthopaedic clinic. The duration, manner of onset (sudden or gradual) and variability of the symptoms must all be established. If there is a joint swelling, is it related to use of the limb? If so, does it begin during the activity, or the next day? These are the same straightforward questions needed in any clinical history except that, when asking about pain, special attention should be paid to referred pain, a classic pitfall for the unwary. The commonest example is pain in the knee caused by disease at the hip.

Occupation

Find out not only the name of the patient's job but also exactly what it involves. One driver may spend the entire day sitting behind the steering wheel but another will have to load and unload the vehicle, which entails a great deal of heavy physical work. A lathe operator who stands for most of the day could not work with a painful foot but could manage with a stiff knee, while a motor mechanic could tolerate a painful foot but a stiff knee would make it impossible to work in tight corners or under vehicles. The loss of the terminal phalanx of the ring finger would be of little consequence to a labourer, but disastrous to a musician.

Impact of treatment

Treatment always disturbs the patient's life, sometimes seriously. To suggest an operation that would make a self-employed tradesman unable to work for 2 or 3 months needs careful thought. Timing is also important: to be rendered unfit during the harvest could bring financial ruin to a single-handed arable farmer for whom the quietest period of the year is at Christmas; on the other hand, shopkeepers need to be at their fittest during the Christmas period and, except in a tourist centre, would probably choose August for operation.

Home circumstances

Knowledge of the home circumstances is vital when dealing with the elderly. Problems are inevitable if the patient cannot climb stairs and the only lavatory is on the top floor. If the patient cannot walk out of the house, who will do the shopping?

These mundane details have no bearing on the diagnosis or the operations that are technically possible but they have everything to do with selecting the right treatment for the individual patient.

Clinical examination

Approaching the patient

Every clinical examination should be conducted carefully, confidently and without hurting the patient needlessly, which is difficult when muscles are tight or rigid. The patient must be encouraged to relax. If an injured, perhaps broken limb is to be put into the hands of a stranger, the patient must have complete confidence in the person carrying out the examination.

The simplest and best way of obtaining the patient's full confidence is to conduct the examination calmly, methodically and without fumbling. The patient can easily tell (as can an examiner) if a doctor or student is doing something for the first time. Only practice brings confidence.

Routine of examination

The established routine for clinical examination in orthopaedic surgery is as follows:

Routine for clinical examination	
Inspection	**Listen** to what the patient tells you.
Palpation	**Look** at the area.
	Feel gently for swelling, painful areas, temperature changes and tenderness. Measure limb length and girth.
Movement	**Move** the limb to assess the range of motion. Active movement is observed first, then passive.
Stressing	**Strain** the ligaments to look for abnormal movements.
	Radiographs are useful but do not replace any part of the clinical examination.

Note: Examine painful areas last!

Take heed of that final note – in practice there is much to be said for leaving the most painful manoeuvre until last, even if this means breaking the routine of examination. In particular, do not start the examination by leaping to the most painful area, prodding it and making the patient jump; to begin the examination thus usually marks the end of cooperation. There is also much to be said for examining any available radiographs before examining the patient, especially if there is a fracture.

Children, particularly between the ages of 1 and 3 years, must be approached with caution. It is virtually impossible to derive any useful information by examining a screaming and struggling child, but there are several ways to overcome this problem.

First, do not overwhelm the child with attention as soon as he or she enters the consulting room. A quiet talk with the parents will give the child time to appraise the doctor and decide that there is no threat.

Second, children do not like to be laid flat on an examination couch; if any part of the examination can be conducted with the child sitting on the mother's knee, so much the better.

Third, children do not like strangers examining their bodies but they rather enjoy strangers admiring their clothes, and this vanity can be exploited. To look carefully at a child's shoes, for example, gives the opportunity to put the hip, knee and ankle through a full range of movement, assess limb length and muscle tone and look for deformities.

Finally, if a child does have to be stripped and laid flat on the couch, leave that until last.

Inspection

Much information can be gained simply from looking at the patient as a whole rather than concentrating on details; a slow, careful inspection of the painful area can give more information than palpation and manipulation combined. The area must be fully exposed and properly prepared: a shoulder cannot be examined through a shirt or a knee through trousers.

When examining a limb, always compare the two and ask yourself the following questions:

1. Is one limb straighter or shorter than the other?
2. Are the joints swollen?
3. Is there muscle wasting?
4. Are there any scars and, if so, are they surgical or traumatic?

Examining a limb

- Deformity?
- Shortening?
- Swelling?
- Wasting?
- Scars?

Measurement is part of inspection. To measure the distance between bony points, choose fixed points that are easily recognizable, such as the medial malleolus or anterior superior iliac spine, rather than variable points, such as the umbilicus or the centre of the patella. When applying the end of the tape, run the finger past the bony point and bring the tape

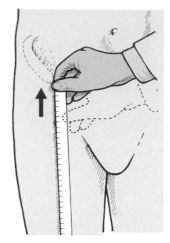

Fig. 2.1 Measuring the distance from a bony point. Move the hand just past the bony point and then back up to it.

back up to it (Fig. 2.1). This reduces the error caused by overlying soft tissue.

When measuring limb girth, be sure that the measurements are reproducible and that the point of measurement is recorded, e.g. the narrowest part of the ankle, the widest part of the calf, or the thigh at a measured distance above the tibial tubercle.

Palpation

There is a strange temptation to start palpation by poking the painful area, but this should always be deferred until last. A hand laid gently on the affected area will detect abnormal warmth, and gentle pressure will identify soft tissue swelling or a joint effusion.

Firmer pressure will locate swellings and tender areas, and show whether the patient is apprehensive when the area is touched. Apprehension is significant, particularly if the joint is unstable, as in patients with recurrent dislocation of the patella.

Sensibility. Sensibility is examined in the usual way, but with a special effort to try to relate the pattern of abnormal sensibility to anatomical structures, such as the distribution of a cutaneous nerve or dermatome (see Ch. 3).

Movement

Always compare the range of movement with the opposite limb. This is essential because there is a wide variation in the 'normal' range of movement.

Check the range of active movement by asking the patient to move the limb. The passive range can then be measured to see how far the joint will move, detect a lag or find which part of the range is painful.

The quality of movement is also important. Is the movement free, or stiff? Smooth or noisy? Does the joint feel loose and unstable? Is it sound? These are subjective assessments and judgement only comes with experience.

Range of movement. The movement in a joint is always measured from 0°, every joint being at 0° when the body is in the anatomical position (Fig. 2.2). This convention is now almost universal but there are still a few who refer to the straight joint as being at 180° instead of 0°, and this causes untold confusion.

In most joints, flexion/extension are in the sagittal plane and **abduction/adduction**, which represent movements away from and towards the midline of the body, in the coronal plane. Abduction and adduction of the toes and fingers are measured from the second toe and the middle finger (Fig. 2.3).

Rotation occurs about the long axis of a structure and **circumduction** is movement of a limb in a circular direction.

The only slight exceptions to these rules are for the thumb, the movements of which are in a plane facing about 30° forward from the coronal plane. Flexion and extension, abduction and adduction of

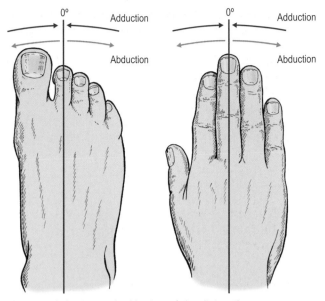

Fig. 2.3 Abduction and adduction of the digits. The toes are adducted to the second toe and the fingers to the middle finger.

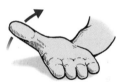

Fig. 2.4 Movement of the thumb in the direction of the arrow is adduction.

the thumb are all measured relative to this plane (Fig. 2.4).

Stressing, straining and strength

Ligaments. Ligamentous instability, which is difficult to assess, is detected by stressing the ligaments and looking for excess movement.

Muscle power. Muscle weakness must be looked for and recorded. The muscle power is graded according to the MRC (Medical Research Council) scale, which recognizes six grades of muscle power (0, 1, 2, 3, 4, 5 – do not forget 0):

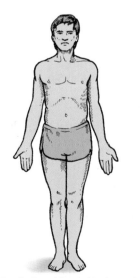

Fig. 2.2 The anatomical position with the palms facing forwards and thumbs outwards.

Six grades of muscle power

Grade 0 – no power.

Grade 1 – a flicker of movement only.

Grade 2 – enough power to move a joint with gravity eliminated.

Grade 3 – enough power to move a limb against gravity.

Grade 4 – more than 3 but less than 5 – enough power to move a limb against active resistance. This is a wide range of muscle power and is sometimes divided into 4, 4+ and 4++.

Grade 5 – full and normal muscle power.

This may sound complicated but it can be simplified by remembering that 0 is complete absence of power and 5 is normal, and the difference between 2 and 3 is the ability to move the limb against gravity.

Examination of individual areas

Every area must be examined carefully according to a routine but the important parts of the examination vary from area to area. This section sets out the things which should be looked for particularly carefully but this does not mean that the rest of the examination is unnecessary.

Cervical spine

Inspection

Although deformity of the cervical spine is unusual, always look at the head and neck as a whole before palpating or assessing movement. Patients with cervical **spondylosis**, for example, may have a 'poke' neck, and deformities of the cervical spine are seen in the Klippel–Feil syndrome (p. 447) and a few other conditions. Check also that the patient can support the head without difficulty – instability of the cervical spine can be easily missed in a recumbent patient.

Palpation

Midline tenderness over the supraspinous ligament is found after injuries to the neck, such as a sprain or whiplash injury. A defect is sometimes felt in the supraspinous ligament following a major spinal injury, and is a serious finding (p. 152). Tenderness and spasm of the paraspinal muscles extending down to the trapezius are found in cervical spondylosis.

Movement

Movement of the neck cannot be assessed in degrees like a simple synovial joint; it is expressed as a percentage or fraction of the usual range, e.g. two-thirds normal, half normal, 50% normal (Fig. 2.5). The

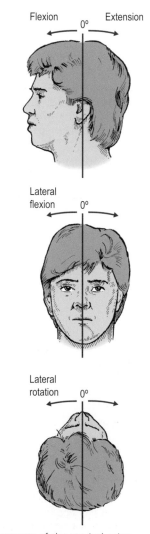

Fig. 2.5 Movements of the cervical spine.

patient can be examined sitting down, to eliminate compensatory movements in the thoracic and lumbar spine. The following movements are recorded:

- Flexion – 'look downwards'.
- Extension – 'look upwards'.
- Lateral rotation – 'look over your shoulder'.
- Lateral flexion – 'lean your head sideways'.

The combined range of flexion and extension is about 110°. Flexion and extension are best seen from beside the patient, and the lateral movements from behind.

Stressing the cervical spine is not helpful.

Thoracic spine

Inspection

Deformities of the thoracic spine are important.

Scoliosis usually develops during adolescence but also occurs in early childhood. The rib 'hump' is demonstrated by standing behind the patient and asking them to bend forward with the hands held together (Figs 2.6 and 2.7).

Kyphosis is best seen from the side (Fig. 2.8). An even, regular and rounded kyphosis is seen in Scheuermann's disease and is of little significance, but a sharp angular bump like a knuckle may indicate collapse of a vertebra, nowadays most often due

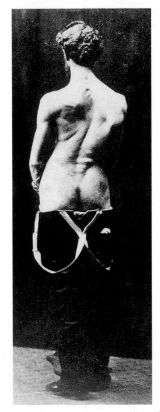

Fig. 2.7 Thoracic scoliosis. From Sayre LA (1877) *Spinal Disease and Spinal Curvature*. By kind permission of the Wellcome Institute Library, London.

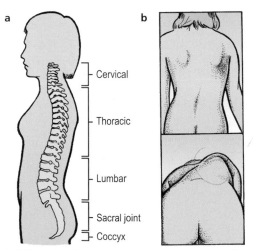

Fig. 2.6 The spine: (a) the successive lordosis and kyphosis of the cervical, thoracic, lumbar and sacral regions; (b) scoliosis can be seen with the patient standing but is more marked when the patient leans forward.

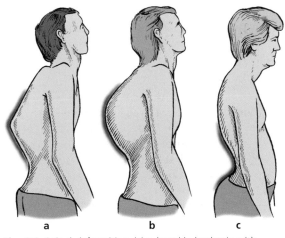

Fig. 2.8 Spinal deformities: (a) a knuckle kyphosis with gibbus; (b) rounded kyphosis; (c) exaggerated lordosis.

15

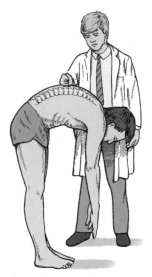

Fig. 2.9 Testing for tenderness of the lumbar vertebra by gentle percussion of the vertebral spine with the spine flexed.

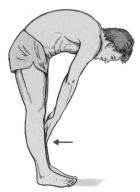

Fig. 2.10 Movement of the lumbar spine. Movement can be recorded by noting how far the fingers can reach, e.g. fingertips to knees, mid-tibia, ankles, etc.

to a tumour or a pathological fracture in porotic bone but in the past usually due to tuberculosis. Such a lump is called a gibbus. The opposite of a kyphosis, a **lordosis**, may also be seen, but is rarely a serious problem.

Palpation

Tenderness can be elicited by gently percussing, tapping the spinous processes with the patient leaning forward (Fig. 2.9). Tenderness in the midline at the thoracolumbar junction may be due to collapse of the T12 or L1 vertebra. In an elderly patient this is usually caused by osteoporosis, sometimes following a surprisingly trivial injury. In the younger patient, more force – such as a fall from scaffolding – is needed, but the physical signs are the same as in the elderly.

Movement

There is little movement in the thoracic spine. Stressing is not applicable.

Lumbar spine

Inspection

Look for deformities, particularly scoliosis with the patient leaning forward. This is best done when movement is examined.

Palpation

Tenderness at the lumbosacral junction may be caused by a simple ligament strain, but if there is a step at the lumbosacral junction, **spondylolisthesis** is likely (p. 457).

Movement

The commonest abnormality in the lumbar spine is a loss of movement. Osteoarthritis is the most common problem in the older patient but prolapsed intervertebral discs and ankylosing spondylitis also present with pain and loss of movement in the lumbar spine.

Movement can be recorded either as a percentage or fraction of normal, as with the cervical spine, or by noting how far the patient can reach. Forward flexion can be recorded as 'fingertips to the knees', 'fingertips to the ankles', etc. (Fig. 2.10), and lateral flexion as the distance of the fingers from the fibular head. This is quick and easy but has the disadvantage that stiffness of the hips also restricts motion. An alternative is to measure the amount of movement, using a tape measure. This is more reliable and takes a little longer.

The pattern of flexion and extension is also important. Generalized stiffness and loss of the normal lumbar curvature in the elderly patient are often due to osteoarthritis. Asymmetrical flexion with spasm of the paraspinal muscles may indicate a disc prolapse or a structural scoliosis, and a painful catch as the spine is straightened from the flexed position suggests mechanical instability or a muscle strain.

Root involvement. Prolapse of an intervertebral disc usually involves a neurological deficit and at least

90% of disc lesions occur at the L4–5 or L5–S1 levels. The fifth lumbar and the first sacral roots are therefore most often involved, and examination of these roots is an essential part of the examination of the lumbar spine.

Remember that because the ankle jerk is supplied by a single root (S1), it is usually either normal or absent altogether, while the knee jerk, supplied by three roots (L3, 4 and 5), may be only slightly diminished. A 'slightly diminished ankle jerk' is probably an incorrect finding, and the commonest cause of a 'completely absent knee jerk' is poor examination technique. A crude test for the power of dorsiflexion and plantar flexion is to ask the patient to walk on heels and toes, respectively.

Check also for perianal anaesthesia, which is rare but a sure sign of a cauda equina lesion that needs urgent action.

Straight leg raising. A prolapsed disc will press upon a nerve root, stretch it and cause pain. Lifting the leg straight increases the tension and reproduces the pain. Several tests based on this phenomenon are available (Fig. 2.11). Conversely, if the range of straight leg raising is normal, a disc prolapse is unlikely.

Chest

Inspection

Apart from pectus carinatum, pectus excavatum and scoliosis, there is little to be found on examination of the chest.

Palpation

Localized tenderness of the ribs may be the only sign of a broken rib or metastasis.

Movement

Restriction of chest expansion to less than 5 cm may be the first objective sign of ankylosing spondylitis.

Stressing

'Springing' the ribs (Fig. 2.12) is a useful screening test for fracture of the ribs.

Shoulder

Inspection

Look for an abnormal contour. In a dislocated shoulder the humeral head is less prominent than normal and the tip of the acromion can be joined to the lateral epicondyle with a straight line (Fig. 2.13). A similar appearance is seen in patients with a paralysed deltoid, whose shoulders have a characteristic square outline but with the humeral head in the correct position. Look also for swelling around the shoulder, wasting of the supraspinatus, and a step at the acromioclavicular joint. Be sure to inspect the shoulder from the front, side and back. If this is not done a posterior dislocation may be missed.

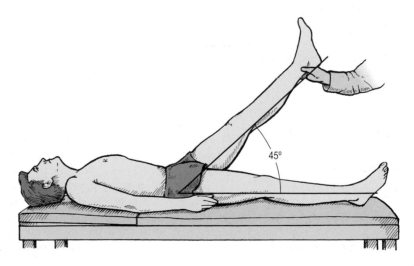

Fig. 2.11 Straight leg raising. The angle between the leg and the couch is recorded. The end point is reached when the patient experiences pain or moves the pelvis.

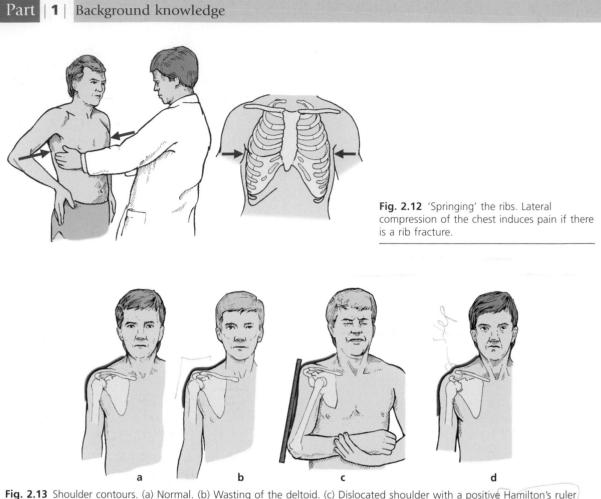

Fig. 2.12 'Springing' the ribs. Lateral compression of the chest induces pain if there is a rib fracture.

a   b   c   d

Fig. 2.13 Shoulder contours. (a) Normal. (b) Wasting of the deltoid. (c) Dislocated shoulder with a positive Hamilton's ruler sign. A ruler will touch both the acromion and the lateral epicondyle. (d) Acromioclavicular separation. There is a step at the acromioclavicular joint.

Palpation

There is tenderness at the tip of the acromion in patients with supraspinatus tendinitis, and the acromioclavicular joint is tender if it is abnormal. Tenderness in the biceps groove at the front of the shoulder indicates bicipital tendinitis.

Movement

Movement of the glenohumeral joint must be distinguished from scapulothoracic movement, which can disguise stiffness at the shoulder joint, as movement of the lumbar spine can disguise stiffness at the hip. Look at the rhythm of movement by standing behind the patient and looking at the way the shoulder girdle moves as a whole, comparing one side with the other.

Scapulothoracic movement can be almost completely eliminated by holding the palm downwards (Fig. 2.14). When the full range of glenohumeral abduction has been reached, the patient can turn the palm upwards and complete abduction by rotating the scapulothoracic joint. Holding the palm downwards prevents this final range of movement.

Forward flexion is examined with the palm facing medially, and must also be separated from scapulothoracic movement. This and other shoulder movements are measured in degrees. Flexion of the shoulder with the arm abducted is called horizontal flexion and is recorded separately.

Rotation is measured with the elbows flexed and tucked into the waist. Extension can also be measured but is less important than abduction and rotation.

separately. A full range of active movement may be impossible if there is inflammation of the supraspinatus tendon because it is accompanied by a painful arc of movement between 30 and 120°. In these patients, a full range of passive movement is possible but active movement is limited because active contraction of the supraspinatus presses the painful tendon against bone.

Check also the function of serratus anterior by asking the patient to push against the examiner's hand, or a wall. Winging of the scapula indicates weakness of serratus anterior muscle.

The rotator cuff can be assessed by resisted contraction of the cuff muscles.

Stressing

Stressing the shoulder is often useful. Unstable shoulders make the patient apprehensive when they are put into abduction and external rotation, and anteroposterior movement of the humeral head is helpful in the assessment of capsular lesions and osteoarthrosis.

Abnormal movement can be detected at the acromioclavicular joint and osteophytes here cause pain on abduction and external rotation.

Acromioclavicular joint

Try to separate the shoulder and the acromioclavicular joint in your mind when examining the shoulder area. The acromioclavicular joint causes different problems from the shoulder joint.

Inspection

Look for a step at the acromioclavicular joint when the arm is hanging. There is much variation between one individual and another and the other side must be used for comparison.

Palpation

The acromioclavicular joint may be tender and there may be osteophytes around it. If the joint is disrupted the acromion can be lifted back to its normal position. To do this put one hand on the clavicle and lift the elbow with the other. The acromion will rise to meet the clavicle.

Look also for abnormal backward and forward movement between the acromion and the end of the clavicle.

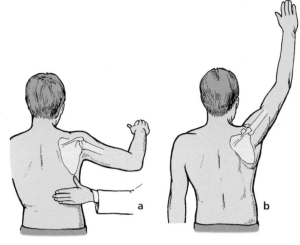

Fig. 2.14 Scapulothoracic versus glenohumeral movement: (a) pure glenohumeral movement with the palm facing downwards will lift the shoulder only to 90°. In order to elevate the arm completely (b) the scapula must rotate.

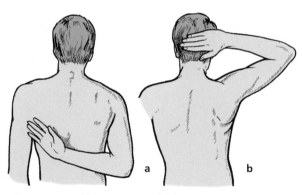

Fig. 2.15 Shoulder movement: (a) full internal rotation and extension; (b) full external rotation and abduction.

Most movements at the shoulder involve composite movements of the whole shoulder girdle. A useful test of overall shoulder function is to ask the patient to put the hand behind the head and then behind the back (Fig. 2.15). For a woman, this is equivalent to combing hair and fastening a bra. The first movement requires external rotation and full abduction; the second requires full internal rotation and extension.

The difference between active and passive motion is very important and the two must be examined

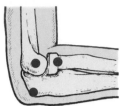

Fig. 2.17 Bony points around the elbow. The lateral epicondyle, radial head and olecranon are marked.

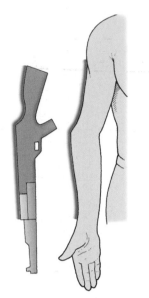

Fig. 2.16 Gunstock deformity of the elbow, often due to supracondylar fracture.

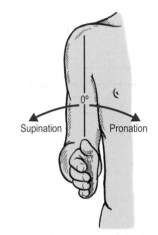

Fig. 2.18 Pronation and supination of the forearm.

Elbow

Inspection

Apart from abnormalities of growth resulting from injuries in childhood, such as a gunstock deformity from a malunited supracondylar fracture (Fig. 2.16), swelling from a joint effusion and the knobbly osteophytes of osteoarthritis, there is seldom much to find on inspection of the elbow.

Palpation

Tenderness of the lateral epicondyle is common in 'tennis elbow', the medial epicondyle in 'golfer's elbow' and the radial head in rheumatoid arthritis (Fig. 2.17).

Movement

Flexion and extension are the only movements of the elbow and are recorded in degrees. Always compare with the opposite elbow; hyperextension is common.

Pronation and supination occur about an axis that runs through the head of the radius and the lower end of the ulna (Fig. 2.18). Rest the ulnar margin of the forearm on a table and then pronate and supinate the forearm to see how this works. A pencil held in the clenched fist can be used to indicate the range of movement. The movement is complex and involves not only the two joints at the lower ends of the forearm but the muscles and interosseous membrane.

Stressing the elbow is not helpful.

Wrist

Inspection

A 'dinner fork' deformity of the wrist is seen after a Colles' fracture and is the commonest deformity at the wrist. Deformity is also seen in rheumatoid arthritis and bizarre abnormalities such as congenital absence of the radius (p. 214).

Palpation

Tenderness of the radial styloid often indicates a fracture of this bone following a minor fall. De Quervain's tenosynovitis is also a cause of tenderness in this area and can be confirmed by flexing the wrist and adducting the hand while the fingers hold the thumb, a manoeuvre which stretches the long tendons of the thumb and reproduces the patient's pain.

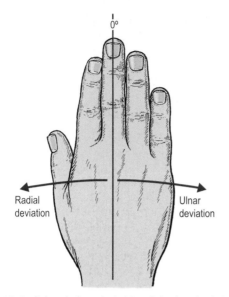

Fig. 2.19 Radial and ulnar deviation of the hand relative to the forearm.

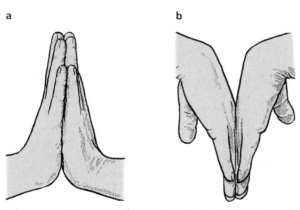

Fig. 2.20 An easy way of testing (a) extension and (b) flexion of the wrists.

Movement

Flexion, extension and **radial** and **ulnar** deviation at the wrist are measured in degrees (Fig. 2.19). Extension is easily measured by putting the hands together as if in prayer, and flexion by the opposite position (Fig. 2.20). Like the shoulder, most movements of the wrist are composite, and a general appraisal of circumduction gives an overall assessment of all the joints involved.

Stressing the wrist is seldom helpful.

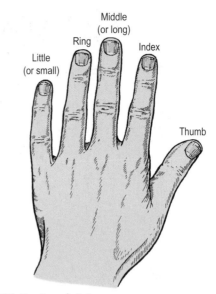

Fig. 2.21 Naming of digits.

Hand and fingers

Assessment of the hand and fingers is an enormous subject and many tests are described (see Ch. 23).

Naming digits

Digits must be named, not numbered (Fig. 2.21). The thumb is the first digit and the second digit is the first finger, unless you count from the little finger, in which case the index is the fourth finger. Confusion of this degree is unacceptable, especially when writing operating lists, where it has resulted in amputation of the wrong finger. Always use these names for the fingers:

Thumb

Index

Middle (long in America)

Ring

Little (small in America)

Americans call the middle finger the long finger and the 'little' finger the small finger to avoid confusion when dictating.

Inspection

Careful inspection for deformities (Fig. 2.22), cuts, scars and wounds is essential, as in other areas, but with special emphasis on possible damage to nerves and tendons.

21

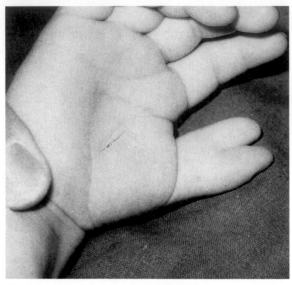

Fig. 2.22 Reduplicated thumbs in an infant.

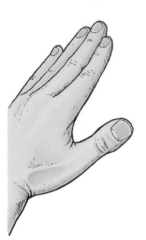

Fig. 2.23 The 'anatomical snuffbox', produced by extending the thumb with the fingers extended.

Palpation

Tenderness of the anatomical snuffbox (Fig. 2.23) indicates a possible fracture of the scaphoid; tenderness over the joints may be the first sign of rheumatoid arthritis.

Sensibility. The innervation of the hand is described on pages 42–43. An attempt should be made to fit sensory symptoms such as numbness or paraesthesiae into an anatomical distribution. Carpal tunnel syndrome due to median nerve compression at the wrist is a good example. Patients with this condition have sensory abnormalities in the distribution of the median nerve below the wrist.

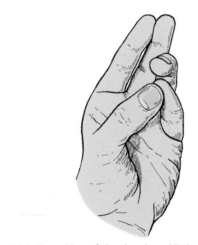

Fig. 2.24 Opposition of the thumb and little finger.

Movement

Movement of the fingers includes flexion, extension, adduction and abduction as well as **opposition** of the thumb and little finger (Fig. 2.24). Movement can be recorded in degrees (°) of motion at each joint but a more convenient way is to note the distance from the pulp of the fingertip to the palm of the hand with the finger fully flexed (Fig. 2.25).

Tendons. The function of every tendon should be tested and any difference between active and passive movement recorded. Test the flexors carefully. Flexor profundus is the only flexor attached to the distal phalanx and flexion of the distal interphalangeal joint is only possible if this tendon is intact. If the patient is asked to flex the whole finger without

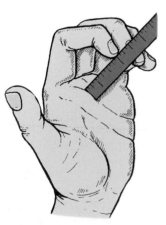

Fig. 2.25 Measuring finger movements. 'Fingertips 5 cm (2 in) from palm'.

controlling the proximal interphalangeal joint, flexor superficialis will come into play and a profundus lesion may be missed (Fig. 2.26). The flexor profundus can only be tested by holding the proximal and middle phalanges down while asking the patient to flex the finger. If the patient can flex the distal interphalangeal joint, the flexor digitorum profundus is intact (Fig. 2.26a). If this is not done, the flexor superficialis will flex the entire digit and the lesion may be missed.

The integrity of the flexor superficialis can be assessed by holding the adjoining fingers in extension (Fig. 2.26b) to eliminate the action of the flexor digitorum profundus.

Stressing

Longitudinal pressure on the fingers is a useful screening test for the mechanical integrity of the metacarpals and phalanges (Fig. 2.27). Longitudinal pressure can also be used to test the toes.

Function

Testing the function of the hand is described on page 22. Many tests exist, including the different types of grip, e.g. pinch grip, power grip, and key grip. Coordination and function may be tested with the many tests of manual dexterity.

Pelvis

Inspection

As with the chest, inspection is seldom helpful.

Palpation

Palpation may reveal tender areas over a fracture.

Movement

Unless there is a grossly unstable fracture, movement is absent in the pelvis.

Stressing

'Springing' the pelvis is an invaluable test for fractures and should be performed routinely in any patient with a crush injury of the trunk (Fig. 2.28) or possible pelvic fracture.

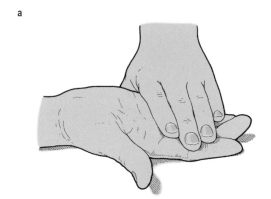

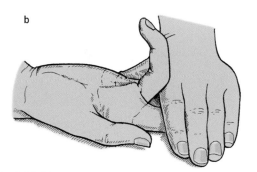

Fig. 2.26 (a) Assessing the function of the flexor digitorum profundus by holding down both the proximal and middle phalanges as the patient tries to flex the finger; (b) the flexor superficialis tendon is assessed by asking the patient to flex the finger while holding the other fingers extended.

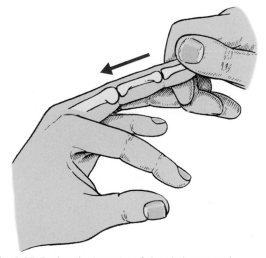

Fig. 2.27 Testing the integrity of the phalanges and metacarpals by longitudinal pressure along the finger.

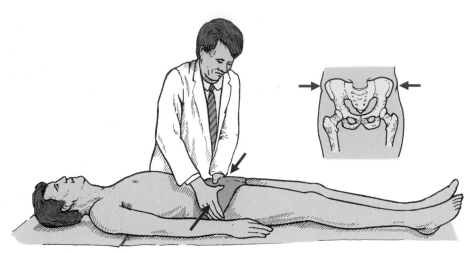

Fig. 2.28 'Springing' the pelvis. Lateral pressure on the pelvis produces pain if there is a pelvic fracture.

Hip

Examination of the hip is an essential part of ortho-paedic examination, and is best done in an orderly manner.

Inspection

Although inspection of the hip itself is seldom helpful, measurement of limb length is essential.

Real and apparent shortening. It is important to be able to measure limb length, both for clinical practice and for examination purposes. Real shortening, in which there is loss of bone length, must not be confused with apparent loss due to a deformity at the hip, in which there is no loss of bone length (Fig. 2.29).

True length is measured from the anterior superior iliac spine to the medial malleolus, and apparent length from a midline structure, such as the pubic symphysis, to the medial malleolus. The patient must be lying as straight as possible when these measurements are made.

Palpation

Feel for bony prominences and check that they are in their correct relationship. The greater trochanter lies more proximal than normal in most mechanical instabilities of the hip.

The relationship of the greater trochanter to the rest of the pelvis can be estimated by Nélaton's line, which joins the anterior superior iliac spine to the ischial tuberosity (Fig. 2.30). Run a tape between

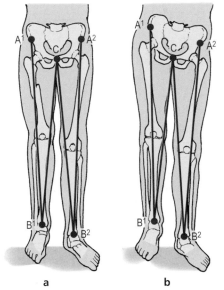

Fig. 2.29 Real (a) and apparent (b) shortening of the lower limb. In (a) A^1B^1 is shorter than A^2B^2. In (b) they are the same length. In both (a) and (b), CB^1 is shorter than CB^2.

these two points: if the tip of the greater trochanter lies proximal to the tape, the hip joint is abnormal.

Movement

Flexion, extension, abduction, adduction, external rotation and internal rotation are recorded in degrees. The movements are self-explanatory but rotation in flexion always causes confusion because,

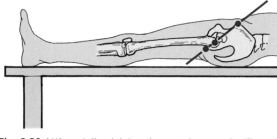

Fig. 2.30 Nélaton's line joining the anterior superior iliac spine, greater trochanter and ischial tuberosity.

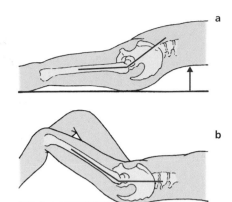

Fig. 2.32 Thomas' test. (a) If there is a fixed flexion deformity of the hip, the patient can put the leg flat on the couch by arching the back; (b) flexing the knee puts the back flat against the couch and reveals a flexion deformity.

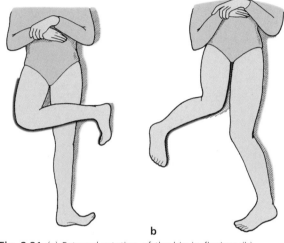

Fig. 2.31 (a) External rotation of the hip in flexion; (b) internal rotation of the hip in flexion. If this is confusing, imagine the position of the hip with the knee extended.

with both knee and hip flexed, internal rotation at the hip moves the foot outwards and vice versa. If in doubt, rotate the hip and straighten the knee to see which way the foot is pointing (Fig. 2.31).

It is sometimes difficult to distinguish movement of the hip from movement of the spine. To be sure that movement is occurring at the hip alone, rest a hand on the pelvis and note when it begins to move.

Fixed flexion deformity and Thomas' test. If the hip has a fixed flexion deformity, common in osteoarthritis, the patient will hide the deformity on the examination couch by arching the back so that the leg lies flat (Figs 2.32 and 2.33). This is partly because it is more comfortable to lie with the leg flat, and partly because the weight of the limb pulls it onto the couch. Lying in this way conceals the flexion deformity from the unwary, but it can always

be exposed by flexing the opposite hip and knee fully, so that the pelvis is brought back to its correct position and the flexion deformity exposed. This is Thomas' test and is very reliable, even if both hips are affected.

Trendelenburg test. Standing on one leg without support and with the spine vertical is only possible if the hip is stable and the muscles around it are working normally (Fig. 2.34). The Trendelenburg test is useful as an overall assessment of the function of the hip and will expose dislocations of the hip or weakness of the glutei, but beware of false negatives and trick movements.

Stressing

Stressing the hip is not helpful in itself but the following tests of function are most important.

Gait

Gait involves many joints but the hip is the most important. Gait is assessed by watching patients walk, preferably without being aware that they are being watched. The following are the most common abnormal gaits.

Antalgic (pain-relieving) hip gait. The patient leans the body over to the side of the painful hip when weight-bearing, in order to reduce the load on the hip, and takes a short stride to minimize the time that the painful limb bears weight (Fig. 2.35). The commonest cause is osteoarthritis.

Scissor gait of cerebral palsy. In a true scissor gait, adductor spasm makes the legs cross over one

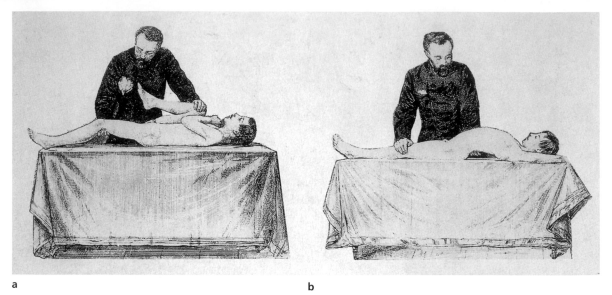

Fig. 2.33 (a), (b) H. O. Thomas performing the Thomas test. From Thomas H O (1876) *Diseases of the Hip, Knee and Ankle Joints*, T Dobbs, Liverpool. By kind permission of the Wellcome Institute Library, London.

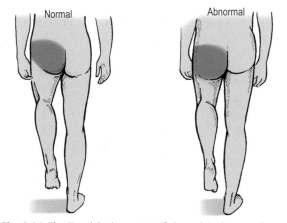

Fig. 2.34 The Trendelenburg test. If the pelvis droops when the left leg is raised, there is an abnormality of the abductors in the right hip.

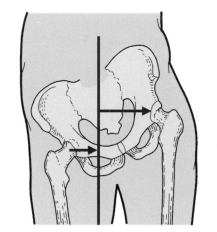

Fig. 2.35 Tilting the pelvis moves the centre of gravity nearer to the hip joint, reducing the load across the joint.

another. In less severely affected patients the thighs are internally rotated and held firmly together.

Drop foot gait. If the ankle dorsiflexors are weak because of a common peroneal palsy or a lumbar root lesion, the patient lifts the knee unusually high and puts the foot down toe first to produce a high stepping gait that is easily recognizable (Fig. 2.36).

Hemiplegic gait. The abnormal gait of hemiplegia is caused by flexor spasm on the affected side. The upper limb is usually affected as well and the abnormal posture and gait are easily identified.

Trendelenburg gait. If the hip is unstable or the abductors inadequate, the Trendelenburg sign will be positive on every step and the pelvis will tilt downwards on weight-bearing to produce a dipping or rolling gait.

Painful foot gait. Patients with painful feet walk with a typical shuffling gait to minimize sudden

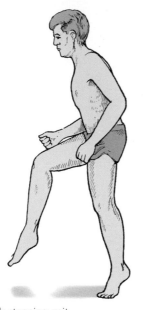

Fig. 2.36 A high stepping gait.

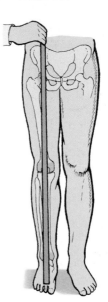

Fig. 2.37 Alignment of joints of the lower limb. The hip, knee and ankle should be one above the other.

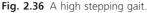

increases in load. This gait can be caused by simple problems such as a blister or a stone in the shoe. Most people are familiar with this gait from personal experience.

Other abnormal gaits result from weakness of the tibialis anterior, rupture of the tendo Achillis and choreoathetosis.

Knee

Inspection

Unlike the hip, the knee is a superficial joint and many abnormalities are easily visible.

Alignment. Look for **varus** and **valgus** deformities at the knee by asking the patient to stand. The hip, knee and ankle should lie in the same straight line and this can be checked with a tape measure (Fig. 2.37).

Effusion. A large collection of fluid in the knee is seen as a swelling above the patella but a small effusion will only fill the hollows on either side of it. A small effusion (5–10 ml) is detected by stroking the fluid into the opposite gutter of the knee and then pushing it back to the other side, when the gutter can be seen to fill (Fig. 2.38).

This test is much more sensitive than the 'patellar tap', in which fluid is pushed up into the suprapatel-lar pouch so that the patella can be bounced against the femur. This test is only positive if there is a large effusion.

Thigh circumference. The thigh circumference gives a rough indication of muscle bulk. The hamstrings and quadriceps waste rapidly if the knee is injured and thigh circumference is sometimes used as a guide to the fitness of the leg as a whole. Although undue importance is attached to this sign, it is useful to know how to measure thigh circumference accurately in order to satisfy examiners.

First, look at the two legs and see if one is thinner than the other, particularly in the region of vastus medialis. Next, mark a point on the thigh approximately 20 cm above the tibial tubercle and measure the circumference of each thigh at this level. More than 1 cm of wasting may mean that at some stage in life the patient has not used one leg as vigorously as the other one, but soft tissue swelling, joint effusion, or the callus round a fracture increase thigh circumference and make the test meaningless.

Do not talk of 'quadriceps circumference'. The hamstrings are larger than the quadriceps and contribute more to the thigh circumference. The tape cannot distinguish between them.

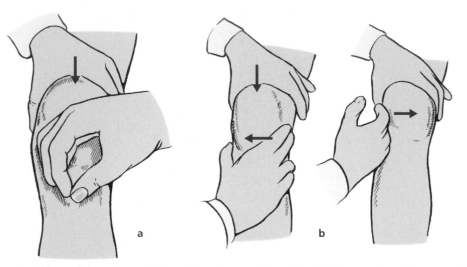

Fig. 2.38 Two methods of assessing a knee effusion: (a) patellar tap; (b) stroking fluid into and out of a parapatellar gutter.

Palpation

Jointline tenderness is a non-specific sign found in any patient with synovial irritation, including those with torn menisci, generalized synovitis and osteoarthritis.

Movement

Flexion and extension at the knee can be easily measured in degrees but the two legs must always be compared. Many knees hyperextend (back knee) and a knee which goes straight has a block to exten-sion if the other knee hyperextends. Feel for crepitus, clicks and other abnormal thuds or sounds.

Stressing

Stressing the knee will reveal abnormal mobility due either to lax ligaments or to bone collapse, and abnormal clicks and clunks from meniscal tears.

Medial ligament. Laxity of the medial ligament should be tested in full extension and slight flexion. A slight jog is always present in slight flexion and comparison of a flexed knee with a straight knee is meaningless (Fig. 2.39a).

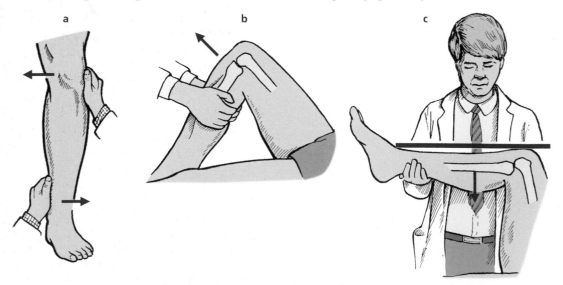
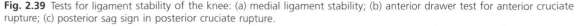

Fig. 2.39 Tests for ligament stability of the knee: (a) medial ligament stability; (b) anterior drawer test for anterior cruciate rupture; (c) posterior sag sign in posterior cruciate rupture.

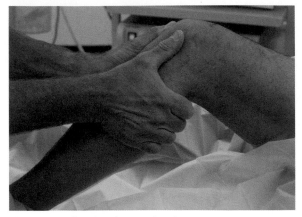

Fig. 2.40 Performing the anterior drawer test.

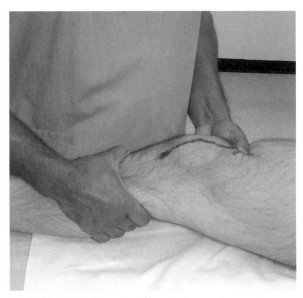

Fig. 2.41 The Lachman test for anterior cruciate rupture. The tibia is moved forwards and backwards relative to the femur in almost full extension.

Anterior cruciate. The anterior cruciate holds the tibia back relative to the femur. If the anterior cruciate is ruptured, the tibia moves anteriorly when the anterior drawer test is performed (Figs 2.39b, 2.40). The test can also be performed with greater accuracy when the knee is flexed a few degrees only. This is called the Lachman test (Fig. 2.41).

The anterior cruciate cannot be properly assessed unless the patient is fully relaxed and lying flat. If sitting up, drawing the tibia forwards will pull the patient down the bed. The hamstrings contract and relaxation becomes impossible.

The pivot shift, or jerk test, is positive if the anterior cruciate is ruptured and reproduces the collapsing that the patient experiences. The test is done by applying a valgus and internal rotational strain while pushing the proximal tibia forwards, which subluxes the lateral tibial plateau in front of the femoral condyle (Fig. 2.42). The knee is then flexed and the tibia reduces to its correct position with a sharp jerk, which the patient will recognize as reproducing the symptoms (p. 420). This is a difficult test to perform.

Posterior cruciate. The posterior cruciate holds the tibia forwards relative to the femur; if the posterior cruciate ligament is ruptured, the tibia sags posteriorly (Figs. 2.39c, 2.43). The sag is visible even if the patient is not fully relaxed because the hamstrings tend to pull the tibia backwards, exaggerating the abnormality.

Meniscal tests. A meniscal fragment can sometimes be displaced into the joint space by rotating the tibia on the femur in flexion, producing a distinct and painful click. The test can be repeated while loading the medial and lateral compartments alternately to decide which meniscus is torn (Fig. 2.44). This is McMurray's test, and must be distinguished from the click which is often felt in the normal knee when the tibia is rotated in full flexion. The meniscal click of the McMurray test is louder, more easily felt and painful.

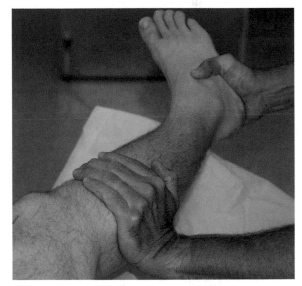

Fig. 2.42 The pivot shift test for anterior cruciate rupture. The upper end of the tibia is pushed forwards, the foot internally rotated and a valgus strain applied as the knee is flexed and extended.

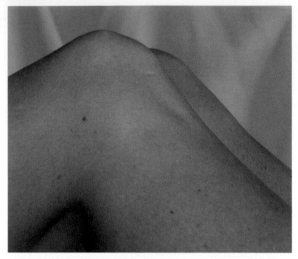

Fig. 2.43 The posterior sag sign. The tibia sags backwards in relation to the femur. A straight line drawn up the front of the nearer tibia would pass through the patella but a similar line drawn on the far tibia would pass just in front of the patella.

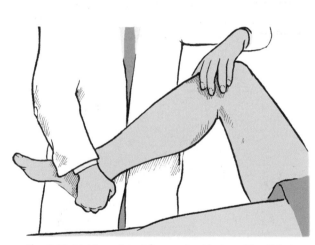

Fig. 2.44 McMurray's test for meniscal lesions. The tibia is rotated on the femur as the knee is extended from flexion.

Patellofemoral joint

Inspection

Look at the size and position of the patella. Small or high patellae are often unstable.

Palpation

Abnormalities of the patellofemoral joint cause pain around the front of the knee when it is bent under load, and the patella may be tender. If the bone is worn, crepitus will be felt when a hand is placed over the patella as the knee is flexed, and firm backward pressure of the patella against the femur causes pain.

Movement

Watch the 'flight path' of the patella as the knee flexes. Unstable patellae, particularly small high patellae, have excessive lateral movement at the start of flexion.

Stressing

If the patella is unstable, attempts to push it laterally will make the patient apprehensive – the 'apprehension' sign (Fig. 2.45).

Ankle, subtalar joint and foot

Inspection

Examine the patient standing, both wearing shoes and without shoes, and inspect the shoes for abnormal wear or stretching. The weight-bearing foot looks very different from the relaxed foot.

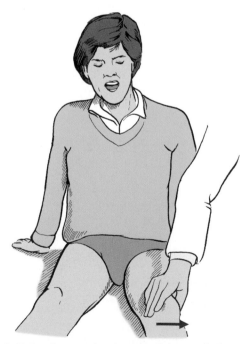

Fig. 2.45 Patellar apprehension test. If the patella is unstable, lateral pressure makes the patient apprehensive.

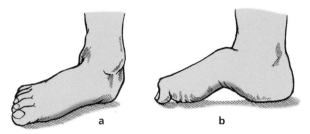

Fig. 2.46 (a) Flat foot (pes planus); (b) high arched foot (pes cavus).

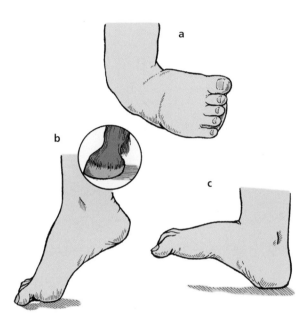

Fig. 2.47 Foot deformities: (a) equinovarus deformity; (b) equinus deformity; (c) calcaneovalgus deformity.

Next, examine the foot and look particularly for deformities. These include pes planovalgus (flat foot), pes cavus (claw foot) (Fig. 2.46), congenital talipes equinovarus (**club foot**, or **CTEV**) and **calcaneovalgus** deformities (Fig. 2.47) (p. 352). The commonest deformity is probably the adducted forefoot, or metatarsus adductus, of early childhood (p. 351). The adducted forefoot can be distinguished from a club foot by looking at the hindfoot. Cover up the forefoot; if the hindfoot is normal, the patient does not have a club foot (p. 351).

Palpation

Look for areas of tenderness, particularly over bony prominences and the metatarsal heads.

Movement

The ankle, subtalar and midtarsal joints function as a unit and must be distinguished from each other (Fig. 2.48). The ankle is a hinge joint allowing up and down movement (dorsiflexion and plantar flexion), measured in degrees.

The subtalar joint between the talus and calcaneum is complex and consists of two separate articulations with an oblique axis that allows **inversion** and **eversion**, which are measured as a fraction or percentage of normal.

The midtarsal joint is a collection of small plane joints between the tarsal bones and allows pronation and supination about the long axis of the foot, also measured as a fraction or percentage of normal.

Stressing

Stressing the ankle ligaments may reveal instability, and stressing the ankle, subtalar and tarsometatarsal joints in turn will often determine the site of pain. Longitudinal pressure on the toes (as for the fingers) produces pain if there is a fracture.

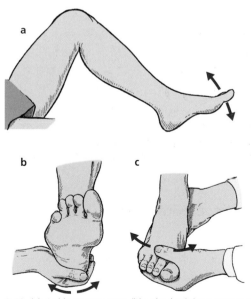

Fig. 2.48 (a) Ankle movement; (b) subtalar joint movement, assessed by moving the calcaneum relative to the leg; (c) tarsal joint movement, assessed by moving the forefoot while holding the calcaneum steady.

Chapter | 3 |

Orthopaedic anatomy

By the end of this chapter you should:
- Be able to identify different types of joint in the body.
- Understand collagen and its function and how this relates to motion/wear.
- Understand the effect of muscles on fractures and the displacement caused.
- Be aware of neurovascular injuries and know which nerves are commonly injured and where.

Joints

Types of joint

First, remember that synovial joints are just one type of joint and that the fibrous and cartilaginous types are just as important.

Synovial joints

The shoulder, elbow, hip, knee and ankle are all synovial joints lined by synovium, which secretes synovial fluid. The articular surfaces are covered with smooth hyaline articular cartilage and movement is determined by the shape of the bones, ligaments, surrounding soft tissues and the joint capsule, which contains the proprioceptors which form the afferent segment of postural reflexes.

Synovial joints can be classified according to shape and the movement that occurs between the bones. Ball and socket joints such as the hip (Fig. 3.1) and shoulder allow movement in all planes, but a hinge joint such as the knee allows movement in one plane only. Condyloid joints such as the radiocarpal joint are elliptical and allow movement in two planes, whereas pivot, or peg, joints such as the superior radioulnar and atlantoaxial joints allow movement about one axis only (Fig. 3.2).

Some joints, such as the patellofemoral joint, have a very large range of movement (Fig. 3.3), but others have much less. The small bones of the tarsus, for example, are linked by plane joints with so little movement that groups of joints must work together to permit a useful range of motion.

The posterior intervertebral, or facet, joints are also plane joints, as is the sacroiliac joint.

Other joints are more complex and more interesting mechanically. The first carpometacarpal joint is saddle-shaped and similar to a universal joint in design (Fig. 3.4). Other joints work in pairs, including the superior and inferior radioulnar joints, which function as a single unit with two bones moving about an axis that passes through the centre of each (Fig. 3.5). The tibiofibular joints are similar; movement of the ankle produces movement at the superior tibiofibular joint (try it on your own leg).

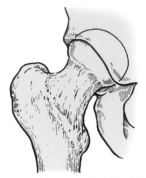

Fig. 3.1 A ball and socket joint. The ball of the femoral head is enclosed by the cup of the acetabulum.

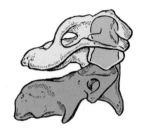

Fig. 3.2 A peg joint. The atlas can pivot on the axis.

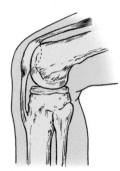

Fig. 3.3 The knee is a hinge joint but the patellofemoral joint is a sliding joint.

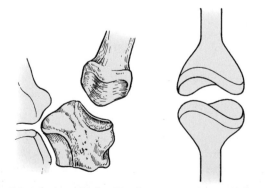

Fig. 3.4 A 'universal' joint. The first carpometacarpal joint has two saddle-shaped joint surfaces.

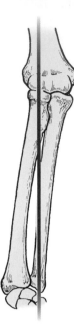

Fig. 3.5 Paired joints. The axis of pronation and supination of the forearm runs through the proximal and distal radioulnar joints.

The subtalar joint also consists of two separate articulations between the same two bones, one convex upwards and the other convex downwards, but movement occurs about an oblique axis which does not pass through the articular surface of either.

Cartilage joints

There are two types of cartilage joints: primary, or synchondroses, and secondary, or **symphyses** (Fig. 3.6). Synchondroses link immature growing bone at the epiphyses in children and have no movement. Symphyses, which are only found in the midline of the body, have a mass of fibrocartilage linking the bones instead of a synovial cavity. The pubic symphysis is the best known but the intervertebral joints with their intervertebral discs and the manubriosternal joint are also symphyses.

Fibrous joints

The flat bones of the skull are linked at the suture lines by fibrous tissue, which prevents any appreciable movement. These linkages are, strictly speaking, joints, but their function is to limit movement rather than encourage it. The inferior tibiofibular joint is the largest syndesmosis in the body and is important for the stability of the ankle (Fig. 3.7).

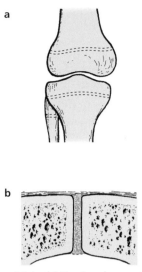

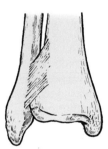

Fig. 3.6 Cartilage joints. (a) Synchondroses at the growing ends of long bones; (b) a symphysis between the two halves of the pubis.

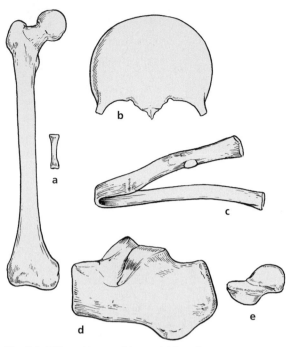

Fig. 3.8 Different types of bone: (a) long bones; (b), (c) flat bones; (d), (e) short bones.

Fig. 3.7 The tibiofibular syndesmosis allows a very slight, but important, degree of movement between the two bones.

Bones

Types of bone (Fig. 3.8)

Long bones

The epiphysis in a growing long bone is separated from the hollow shaft, or diaphysis, by the epiphyseal plate, or physis. The part of the diaphysis next to the physis is the metaphysis. Any bone arranged like this is called a long bone, even if it is quite short – the phalanges of the fingers and toes are 'long' bones in structure. Damage to a growing epiphysis causes deformity.

Flat bones

Flat bones, such as the skull, pelvis and ribs, form in condensations of fibrous tissue and are often called membrane bones. Their function is the protection of soft viscera such as the brain and lungs.

Short bones

Short square bones like those of the tarsus and carpus form in blocks of cartilage and ossify from the centre. They do not have epiphyses.

Accessory ossicles

In addition to the normal bones, accessory ossicles occur as variants of normal. These are entirely innocent structures but can be mistaken for fractures and treated as such. The os trigonum behind the talus (Fig. 3.9a) and the accessory navicular (Fig. 3.9b) are among the most common.

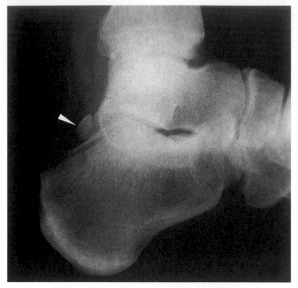

a

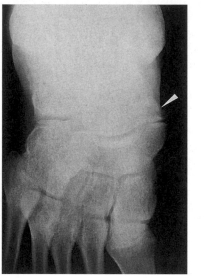

b

Fig. 3.9 Accessory ossicles: (a) the os trigonum: (b) accessory navicular bone.

Epiphyses

Growth of bones

Long bones grow from a physis (epiphyseal plate or growth plate) at each end. Although both ends grow, one will generally grow faster than the other and different epiphyses contribute different amounts to the length of a bone.

The lower femoral and upper tibial epiphyses contribute roughly 60% of limb length, but the proximal humeral epiphysis is responsible for 80% of the length of the humerus. The exact proportions need only be remembered by orthopaedic surgeons.

If all growth is stopped at an epiphyseal plate, the limb will be straight but shorter than normal. If only one side of the plate is stopped, which can happen after a fracture through the growth plate, an unpleasant angular deformity may follow (pp. 102, 218). These problems do not occur in membrane or cartilage bones, which grow by getting gradually bigger in all directions.

Generalized illness in childhood can retard bone growth and leave a dense line on the radiograph that remains throughout life (growth arrest). These lines are called Harris' lines and are of no clinical importance (Fig. 3.10).

Apophyses

A scale of growing bone, or apophysis, is present on some bones. Unlike epiphyseal plates, apophyses do not contribute to the length of the bone. There are many apophyses but the most important are at the acromion, the olecranon, the tibial tubercle and the calcaneum. To the unwary, apophyses look like fractures and can lead to a patient being put in plaster for a fracture that does not exist.

Periosteum

The outer half of the periosteum is fibrous but the inner half contains mesenchymal cells which can differentiate into osteoblasts or osteoclasts. Periosteum, like all living tissue, must be treated gently at operation if its growth potential is to be preserved.

Blood supply

The nutrient artery supplies the bone marrow and some cortex in adult long bones but the periosteal vessels can take over if the nutrient artery is damaged by, for example, a fracture or intramedullary nailing (p. 135) (Fig. 3.11). The circulus vasculosus, the ring of vessels which surrounds most joints, contributes to the supply of the large ends of long bones.

It is easy to forget the blood supply of bone when operating upon a limb with a tourniquet applied but the nutrient artery and periosteum must be respected or the bone may become avascular and die.

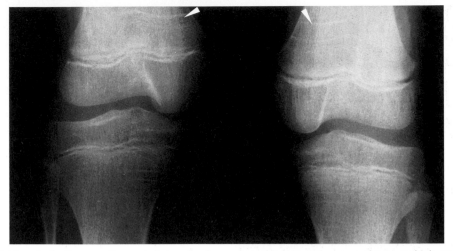

Fig. 3.10 Harris' lines indicating growth arrest during development. In this patient they were due to multiple operations for a congenital anomaly.

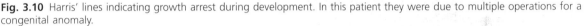

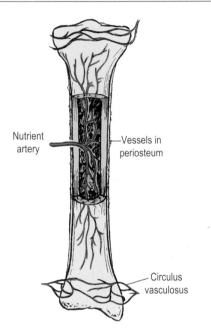

Nutrient artery

Vessels in periosteum

Circulus vasculosus

Fig. 3.11 Blood supply of a long bone.

Cartilage

Types of cartilage

Hyaline cartilage

Hyaline, or articular, cartilage is highly organized tissue consisting of loops of type II collagen within a ground substance of proteoglycans produced by chondrocytes. The proteoglycans are hydrophilic and the tissue tension within the deep layers of hyaline cartilage is considerable. The structure can be compared with an inflatable building or a 'blister' over a tennis court: one is inflated by water drawn in by proteoglycans, and the other by air pumped in by an electric fan. In one, the pressure is contained by collagen loops, in the other by a plastic canopy (Fig. 3.12).

Fibrocartilage

Fibrocartilage varies from place to place according to its elasticity, which depends on the relative amounts of elastin and collagen within it. The fibrocartilage of the ear and nasal cartilages, for example, is different from that of the intervertebral discs.

Collagen

There are many types of collagen, each with different properties. Type I collagen is found in bone and type II is found in hyaline cartilage. Hyaline cartilage heals with fibrocartilage, which contains type III collagen and is less durable than true hyaline cartilage. Type IV collagen is found in flexible structures such as the ear and nose, and other types are found elsewhere.

Muscles

The 'traditional' anatomical teaching was that a muscle arises from bone 'a', is inserted on bone 'b'

37

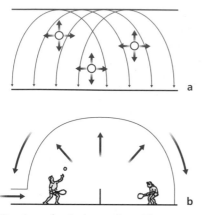

Fig. 3.12 Structure of articular cartilage. The pressure generated by the chondrocytes and ground substance is contained by arches of collagen, just as the air pressure in a tennis 'blister' is contained by its canopy.

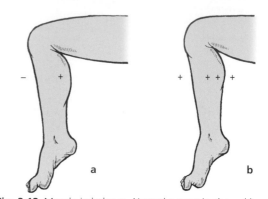

Fig. 3.13 Muscle imbalance. Normal power in the ankle flexors but diminished power in the ankle extensors (a) produces an equinus deformity. Normal power in the extensors and increased power in the flexors (b) also produces a flexion deformity.

and acts on joint 'c'. This is excellent for understanding the workings of the cadaver, but of very limited value in the management of patients. Muscles are only one part of the total motor system and the correct balancing of these muscles, both in direction and in power, is essential if a damaged limb is to work normally.

Agonists and antagonists

Muscles work as balanced groups which oppose each other. If the flexor muscles work more strongly than the extensors, as they do in cerebral palsy, a flexion deformity develops. If the flexors are completely denervated, an extension deformity develops, but only if the extensors are still working (Fig. 3.13).

The agonists and antagonists work in such close harmony that no muscle can be regarded simply as an anatomical structure running between its origin and insertion. Moving an extensor to reinforce a weak flexor is no guarantee of success because the extensor has 'learned' to contract while the flexor is relaxing. Extensive physiotherapy is needed to re-educate the muscle to work in the opposite manner to which it is accustomed. To add to this difficulty, a transferred muscle never works quite as effectively as it did before transfer and loses at least one MRC grade of power (p. 14) when it is moved.

Fractures separating muscle groups

The importance of the relationship between muscles is illustrated by certain fractures. A fracture of the

femur at the junction of its upper and middle thirds leaves the hip abductors and most of the flexors on the upper fragment, and all the adductors and most of the extensors on the lower. The upper fragment therefore swings up into unopposed abduction and flexion while the lower fragment stays on the bed and swings into adduction (Fig. 3.14). Similarly, a fracture of the forearm separates the supinators (biceps and supinator) in the upper fragment from the pronators (pronator teres and pronator quadratus). What happens? The upper fragment supinates as far as it can and the lower fragment pronates to produce a nasty rotational deformity that prevents supination. This means that the patient cannot collect change when shopping.

A variation on the same theme is seen in fractures of the upper end of the femur. With the femur intact, the iliopsoas internally rotates the hip because it lies lateral to the axis of rotation of the joint. If the femoral neck is broken, the iliopsoas cannot act on the hip, but spins the femur about its long axis to produce the characteristic external rotation deformity of a fracture at the upper end of the femur.

Fractures which separate the mechanical linkage between muscle groups are difficult to hold without internal fixation devices.

Compartments

Muscles are contained within fascial compartments (Fig. 3.15). The fascia prevents the damaged tissue swelling and the pressure within the compartment can rise so much that its contents become ischaemic

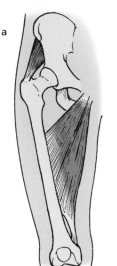
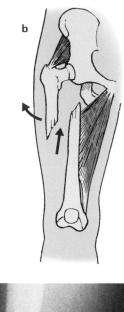

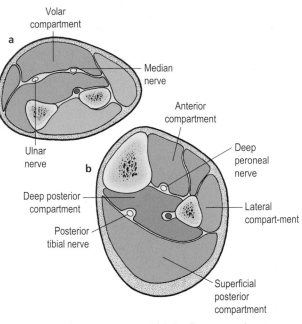

Fig. 3.15 Fascial compartments in (a) the forearm and (b) the calf.

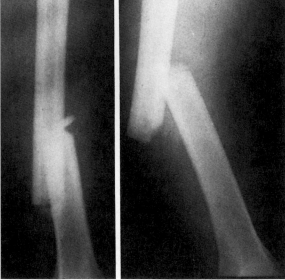

c
Fig. 3.14 Fractures separating muscle groups. When a fractured femur separates the hip abductors from the hip adductors, the bones are pulled apart. (a) Normal. (b) Transverse fracture of the femur showing displacement of the fragments. (c) Radiograph of fractured femur.

and die. Ischaemic muscle is replaced by fibrous tissue, which contracts. Nerves also perish and a serious disability ensues.

Forearm

There are two compartments in the forearm, **ventral** (flexor) and **dorsal** (extensor).

Ventral compartment. The ventral compartment includes the median and ulnar nerves, and the radial and ulnar arteries. Compression of these structures within the fascial sheath can have disastrous consequences.

Dorsal compartment. The extensor compartment is less often damaged than the ventral and includes the posterior interosseous nerve but no major vessels. The consequences of a dorsal compartment syndrome are less serious than ventral compartment compression, partly because it contains fewer important structures and partly because its fascia is less dense.

Lower limb

In the leg there are four compartments and all can cause serious problems (Fig. 3.16).

Anterior tibial compartment. The anterior tibial compartment contains the anterior tibial artery and deep peroneal nerve after it has left the peroneal compartment.

Superficial posterior compartment. There are no important vessels or nerves in the superficial posterior compartment, which includes gastrocnemius and soleus only.

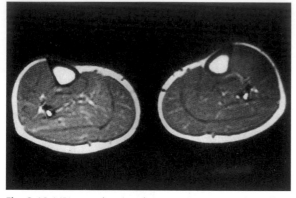

Fig. 3.16 MRI scan showing the compartments in the calf. By kind permission of the MRIS Unit, Addenbrooke's Hospital, Cambridge.

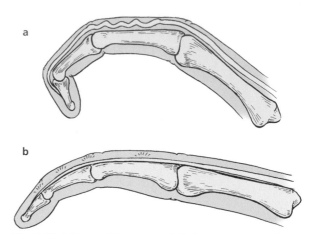

Fig. 3.17 A finger with an excessively long extensor tendon (a) cannot be fully extended. (b) A finger with an excessively short extensor tendon cannot be fully flexed.

Deep posterior compartment. The deep posterior compartment contains the posterior tibial vessels and nerves and the peroneal artery. The consequences of damaging these are serious.

Lateral (peroneal) compartment. The lateral compartment contains the superficial peroneal nerve but it is seldom affected by compression.

Muscle length

Muscles only work correctly over a very small range of movement. If a bone is fractured and unites a centimetre shorter than it was before, the first centimetre of muscle contraction has no effect on the position of the limb and power is reduced (Fig. 3.17). The correct relationship between the length of the muscle and tendon and the length of bone should be maintained whenever possible, but if this cannot be achieved the muscle will eventually adapt to its new length.

Tendons

The direction in which a muscle acts depends upon the direction of its tendon, which can change as it runs through loops, as at the wrist, or around corners, as in the fingers. Tendons do not tolerate friction well and are protected at such points by bursae, synovial sheaths, or the **sesamoid bones**, such as the patella and the fabella in the gastrocnemius tendon at the back of the knee.

Nerves

The orthopaedic surgeon sees many neurological lesions: root lesions caused by prolapsed discs or spinal injury, peripheral nerve lesions caused by trauma, ulnar neuritis, median nerve compression, brachial plexus injuries, spinal stenosis, peroneal muscle atrophy and many others. A few patients are seen with other neurological disorders, particularly if they cause muscle weakness or mimic a disc lesion. These must be recognized and referred to the neurologists.

Orthopaedic surgeons are therefore particularly interested in dermatomes and the root value of peripheral nerves. A knowledge of the root innervation of muscles is also needed to interpret the MRC grading of muscle power. If a muscle is innervated by several nerve roots, one root can be completely divided with only a partial loss of power, but dividing one root will cause a complete loss of power if the muscle is supplied by a single root only.

Dermatomes and root values

The dermatomes in the upper and lower limbs determine the distribution of sensory symptoms arising from pressure on the nerve roots, and must be known in detail (Fig. 3.18).

The distribution of the L4, L5 and S1 roots is specially important because they are involved in 90% of lumbar disc prolapses (Fig. 3.19).

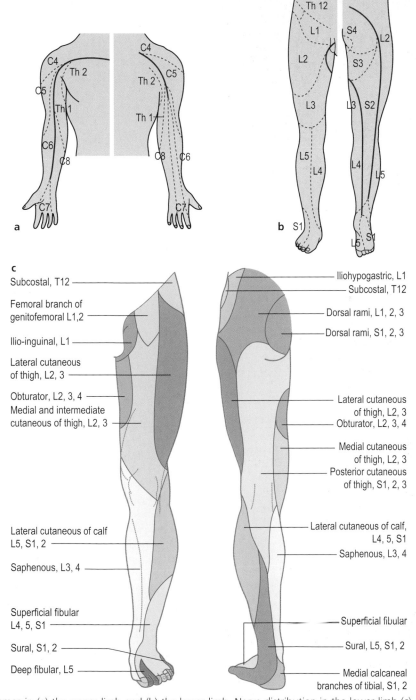

Fig. 3.18 Dermatomes in (a) the upper limb and (b) the lower limb. Nerve distribution in the lower limb (c).

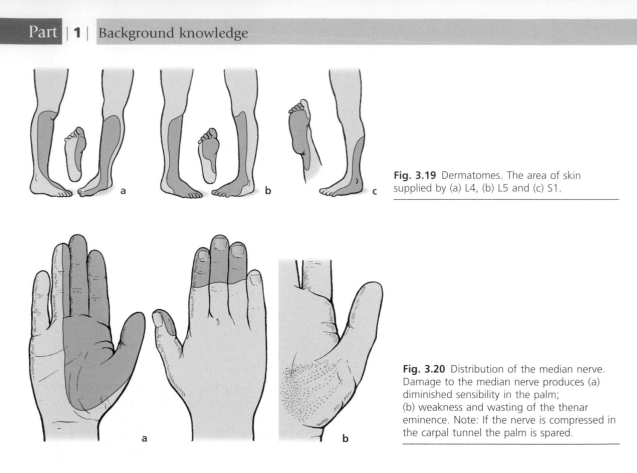

Fig. 3.19 Dermatomes. The area of skin supplied by (a) L4, (b) L5 and (c) S1.

Fig. 3.20 Distribution of the median nerve. Damage to the median nerve produces (a) diminished sensibility in the palm; (b) weakness and wasting of the thenar eminence. Note: If the nerve is compressed in the carpal tunnel the palm is spared.

Peripheral nerves

Damage to the median nerve at the wrist and the ulnar nerve at the elbow (pp. 203, 221) are common problems and provide a good example of the importance of clinical anatomy.

Median nerve

Patients with persistent paraesthesia in the distribution of the median nerve are likely to have compression of the median nerve at the wrist (Fig. 3.20) (p. 387). The fluid retention of pregnancy is one cause but repetitive movements of the flexor tendons of the hand and wrist also lead to a localized flexor tenosynovitis, which in turn causes soft tissue swelling and compression of the median nerve as it enters the hand through the carpal tunnel.

As the median nerve is compressed, sensory symptoms are felt in thumb, index and middle fingers, half the ring finger on the palmar surface and on the back of the fingers. The palm itself is spared because the palmar branch arises before the nerve enters the carpal tunnel.

Variations in the distribution of the median nerve are common.

Ulnar nerve

The ulnar nerve may be irritated at the elbow as it runs behind the medial epicondyle. The nerve can be damaged by trauma, osteoarthrosis, deformity from malunion (tardy ulnar palsy, p. 387), or even pressure on the medial side of the elbow as the arm rests on an operating table. The patient will experience paraesthesiae or numbness in the little finger and the ulnar half of the ring finger, weakness of the hand, or sometimes clumsiness due to weakness of the intrinsic muscles supplied by the ulnar nerve (Fig. 3.21).

Radial nerve

The radial nerve is safe in the forearm but vulnerable in the upper arm. Pressure on the radial nerve from old-fashioned axillary crutches can lead to a troublesome drop wrist but few sensory symptoms (Fig. 3.22). Other causes, now almost historical, are the 'Saturday night palsy' of inebriated patients who fall asleep with their arms over the back of a chair and, in more recent and healthier days, pressure on the medial side of the upper arm from prolonged pressure on the back of a cinema seat.

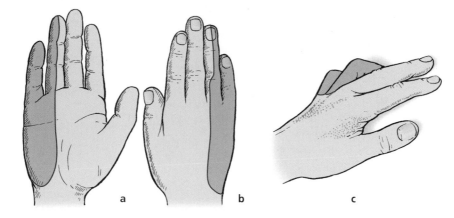

Fig. 3.21 Distribution of the ulnar nerve. Damage to the nerve produces diminished sensibility in: (a) the palm; (b) the dorsum of the hand; and (c) a claw deformity in the little and ring fingers because of damage to their interossei and lumbrical muscles.

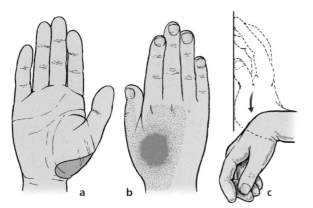

Fig. 3.22 Distribution of the radial nerve. Damage to the radial nerve produces no loss of sensibility in the palm (a) but there may be a small area of diminished sensibility on the dorsum (b) and there will be paralysis of the wrist extensors (wrist drop) (c).

Sciatic nerve

In the lower limb, the commonest peripheral nerve lesion is damage to the lateral half of the sciatic nerve from posterior dislocation of the hip (Fig. 3.23) (p. 182).

Common peroneal nerve

A similar but not identical clinical picture is produced by a lesion of the common peroneal nerve as it passes around the fibular neck.

Vulnerable peripheral nerves (Fig. 3.24)

Upper limb
- Median nerve – hand through glass window.
- Ulnar nerve at elbow – pressure during operation, trauma from fracture.
- Radial nerve – cuts around the elbow, pressure from crutches, etc.
- Digital nerves – cuts around the fingers.
- Brachial plexus – upper cord, downward pressure on the shoulder as when falling off a motorcycle; lower cord, dragging of the arm upwards during road trauma and catching onto things while falling, e.g. scaffolding.
- Cervical nerve roots – prolapsed intervertebral disc.

Lower limb
- Common peroneal nerve – damage at the neck of the fibula through trauma.
- Lumbar nerve roots – prolapsed intervertebral disc.
- Sciatic nerve – damage from dislocation of the hip.

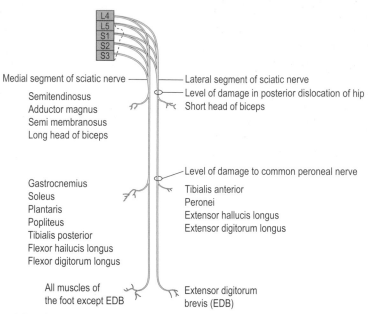

Fig. 3.23 Roots of the medial and lateral components of the sciatic nerve, which become the popliteal and common peroneal nerves behind the knee.

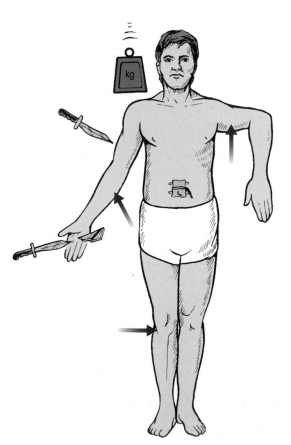

Fig. 3.24 Common sites of peripheral nerve injury include abduction injuries of the brachial plexus, lacerations of the radial nerve, compression of the ulnar nerve, lacerations of the median nerve at the wrist and digital nerves in the fingers, pressure on the radial nerve in the upper arm, root entrapment in the lumbar spine and pressure on the common peroneal nerve at the knee.

Chapter 4

Basic science in orthopaedics

By the end of this chapter you should be able to:

- Understand the general principles of joint lubrication and biomechanics.
- Understand the different types of implant used to fix fractures and orthopaedic conditions and their complications.
- Understand the different types of metals used.
- Have a clear understanding of how fractures heal.

Biomechanics

An understanding of the way the body works as a machine is essential to an orthopaedic surgeon but mechanical considerations must always come second to the clinical assessment of the individual patient. The temptation to regard the patient as a machine must be resisted; people are not machines, even if the body is.

Joint loading

The loads imposed on the joints and the direction of the forces in which they act are not always obvious from gross anatomy (Fig. 4.1a). The load across the hip, for example, is the resultant of the patient's weight acting downwards and muscles pulling the femur medially and upwards at an angle of about 16° from the vertical. This should not be a surprise because the bone trabeculae in the femoral neck and ilium are oriented in the same direction (Fig. 4.1b). According to Wolff's law, which states that the posi-

tion of the trabeculae is dictated by the forces acting on the bone, the trabeculae are the 'materialized trajectory of the force'.

When standing on one leg, the abductors act at a mechanical disadvantage because they are nearer the centre of the hip joint than the patient's centre of gravity (L1). In consequence, they have to lift about three times body weight and the load across the hip joint is correspondingly increased. Because loading a diseased hip is painful, it is useful to reduce the load across the hip by allowing the abductor muscles to work at a greater advantage. Patients need no biomechanical knowledge to walk with an antalgic (pain-relieving) gait and quickly find that leaning the body to the side of the affected hip is less painful than walking upright because it brings the centre of gravity closer to the fulcrum and reduces the load across the joint (Fig. 4.2).

Muscles act at a mechanical disadvantage in other joints as well. The elbow and knee both have flexors and extensors so close to the axis of rotation that they must contract with a force several times greater than the weight they are lifting.

Joint lubrication

Calculations of the shear stresses on a joint surface show, among other things, that the patella has a greater shear stress imposed upon it than any other bone – seven times body weight.

Joint lubrication is complex and depends on three mechanisms (Fig. 4.3).

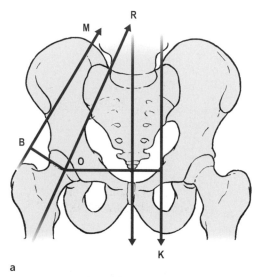

a

Fig. 4.1a Vectors acting at the hip joint.

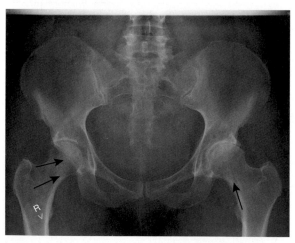

b

Fig. 4.1b Radiograph of the pelvis to show that the trabeculae are arranged according to the line of weight transmission and follow Wolff's law.

Boundary lubrication

Boundary lubrication depends on molecules sliding over each other and is best for heavy loads and slow movements. Graphite is a boundary lubricant. The large hyaluronic acid-based proteoglycan molecules in synovial fluid function in the same way.

Surface lubrication

Compounds which flow between surfaces, such as oils, are the best known lubricants. Synovial fluid acts as a surface lubricant and its efficiency is increased by the 'wedge effect'. The joint surfaces are not a perfect fit and the irregularities create a wedge of fluid at the point of contact, a little like a car 'hydroplaning' on a wet road.

'Boosted' lubrication

To improve lubrication still further, fluid from the articular cartilage is squeezed out when it is compressed. This is 'boosted' lubrication.

Implants

It is often necessary to insert plates, screws, prostheses and other devices in the body and much effort goes into implant materials and design. It was not always so; in the early days of internal fixation, ordinary wood screws were used to fix fractures but these were specifically designed for timber and proved unsuitable for bone. Not only did the screws rust but a wood screw, which is tapered and ideal for a fibrous material like wood, cannot be used on a dense material like cortical bone. Different types of screws, threads and bone are dealt with on page 133.

Stress risers

Bones are more flexible than metal plates. Screwing a metal plate to bone stiffens it and produces a 'stress riser' at each end, which can cause a fracture at the end of the plate (Fig. 4.4).

Similar problems arise around joint prostheses. Not only do fractures occur immediately below the tip of the femoral component of a total hip replacement (THR), but the different stiffnesses of the bone and implant mean that the interface between the two is under strain. Attempts have been made to overcome this problem by developing 'isoelastic' implants with the same elasticity as bone.

Holes

Drilling a hole through bone also produces a stress riser by weakening the bone, but a hole filled with

a screw weakens it much less. These considerations only concern orthopaedic surgeons but it is important to appreciate that there is more to reconstructive surgery than the layman supposes.

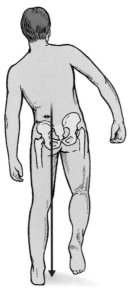

Fig. 4.2 Antalgic gait tilting the pelvis reduces the load on the joint and thus the pain (see also Fig. 2.35).

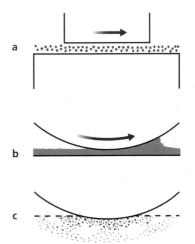

Fig. 4.3 Different types of lubrication: (a) boundary lubrication; (b) surface lubrication; (c) boosted lubrication.

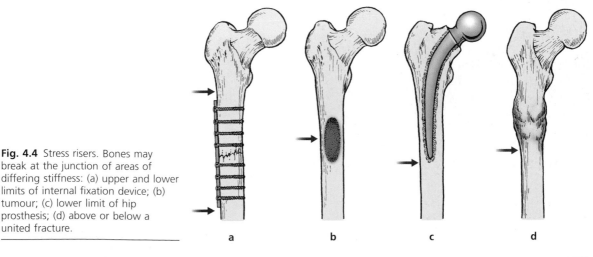

Fig. 4.4 Stress risers. Bones may break at the junction of areas of differing stiffness: (a) upper and lower limits of internal fixation device; (b) tumour; (c) lower limit of hip prosthesis; (d) above or below a united fracture.

a   b   c   d

Materials

Many materials have been used for implants, and most have proved unsatisfactory (Fig. 4.5). The salts of the constituent metals are slowly leached out of the implant over the years and some are toxic or allergenic. The ideal material must be insoluble, strong, non-toxic, non-carcinogenic, and also non-irritant in particulate form.

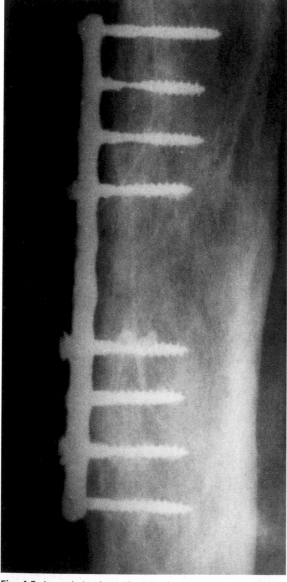

Fig. 4.5 An early implant. The metal was not truly inert and the screws have corroded.

Metals

Stainless steel, perhaps the simplest implant material, contains a cocktail of different elements and is generally satisfactory, although not as strong as chrome, cobalt and molybdenum alloys of which many implants are made (Table 4.1). Prostheses are also made of almost pure titanium. Precious metals such as silver and gold are satisfactory implant materials but lack the strength required of a prosthesis, quite apart from their cost.

Plastic

Most artificial joints consist of a metal and plastic articulation. The plastic usually used is high density polyethylene (HDP), but some early prostheses were made of polytetrafluoroethylene (PTFE, Teflon), which was satisfactory until its wear particles provoked a vigorous foreign body reaction that eroded bone. Particles of HDP also produce an inflammatory response, but it is much milder than that caused by PTFE.

Ceramics (aluminium oxide)

Ceramics are also used in prostheses but they are brittle and their wear particles are irritant.

Fixation

Many patients – and some doctors – believe that once an implant is in position it will stay fixed to

Table 4.1 Composition of some alloys used in orthopaedic implants

	Stainless steel (%)	Chrome/ cobalt (%)	Titanium alloy (%)
Iron	62.2		
Chromium	21.5	28	
Nickel	9		
Manganese	4		
Molybdenum	2.6	5	
Niobium	0.3		
Nitrogen	0.4		
Silicon		0.75	
Cobalt		65	
Titanium			90
Vanadium			4
Aluminium			6

Chapter 4

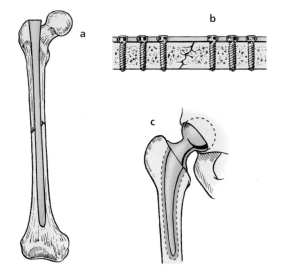

Fig. 4.6 Methods of attaching implants to bone: (a) tight interference fit; (b) screws; (c) bone cement.

bone for ever. This is not so; bone implants do not behave like dental fillings. Teeth have no 'turnover' and do not change throughout life. Bones do not have this advantage and turn over regularly so that after about a year an implant is attached to a different bone from the one in which it was placed. Although the body reproduces itself fairly accurately it does not do so precisely and this leads to loosening, wear particles, a foreign body reaction, more loosening, etc. This is a particular problem in cancellous bone because the trabeculae change shape in response to load.

Implants are fixed to the skeleton in four ways (Fig. 4.6):

1. By being a 'tight fit'.
2. Mechanically with screws.
3. With bone cement.
4. By bone ingrowth.

Interference fit

An interference fit is nothing more than a tight fit like a cork in a bottle or a nail in wood. Some implants have fins and flanges to make them fit more firmly at operation, but sound immediate fixation does not prevent the implant loosening with time.

Screws

Screws produce sound fixation of a plate to bone but are themselves only held by an interference fit and can loosen.

Bone cements

Bone cements are not adhesives; they do not 'stick' to bone but fill up spaces to produce a better mechanical fit. In builders' language, bone cement is a grout, like the material used to fill the cracks between tiles.

The most commonly used is acrylic cement, which is polymethylmethacrylate and chemically the same as Perspex. The cement is prepared during operation by mixing a liquid which contains the monomer (monomethylmethacrylate) and a stabilizer to prevent it polymerizing, with a powder that includes a catalyst to initiate polymerization, a filler consisting of polymethylmethacrylate powder, a radiopaque material such as barium sulphate, and sometimes an antibiotic. The mixture forms a dough-like material which can be forced into the medullary cavity around the implant, where it sets solid. Low viscosity cement with the consistency of thick cream is also available. Although more difficult to handle, low viscosity cement can be forced into cancellous bone, hopefully to achieve more secure fixation.

Acrylic cement is the best available at present but has many disadvantages. While strong in compression, it is weak in tension and breaks when twisted. Once fractured, the two surfaces rub together and produce wear particles which are irritant to bone. A brisk foreign body reaction results, more bone is resorbed, more acrylic cement loosens, more particles are formed and a vicious circle is established, leading to irreversible loosening of the implant and bone destruction.

Bone ingrowth

One way of overcoming the problem of bone fixation is to coat the prosthesis with a porous surface of sintered metal granules, so that bone may grow into the minute passages that cover the prosthesis and thus fix it to the bone. However, even if the bone does grow into the prosthesis, loosening and fracture may still occur unless the prosthesis has the same elastic properties as the bone. A coating of hydroxyapatite to the component can also be used.

This again allows the bone to grow up to the edge of the component and integrate with the coating. Ligament prostheses can be fixed to bone by making a bone/prosthesis/bone sandwich so that the cancellous bone grows through the weave of the prosthetic material. Fixation of fabric prostheses occurs readily in soft tissues, both in arterial grafts and hernia repairs.

Tissue healing

Bone

When a bone is fractured, it normally heals with bone. Bone is the only solid tissue in the body that can replace itself in this way. The rest heal with fibrous tissue that leaves a scar.

Bone healing is simple when it occurs smoothly, complicated when it does not. In ideal circumstances the haematoma that forms around the bone ends coagulates, the clot is invaded by cells which form a hard mass, or callus, that resembles cartilage, and the callus is gradually converted to bone (Fig. 4.7). Fortunately, haematomas in other situations do not normally become converted to bone, the process being initiated by stimuli from the bone itself. These stimuli are to be found in the bone marrow, surrounding osteoblasts and the periosteum, but their exact nature is not known.

Sound bone healing does not always occur, and the bone ends are then joined by either a mat of fibrous tissue or a false joint (**pseudarthrosis**),

neither of which is mechanically satisfactory. Fractures through cancellous bone, with a good blood supply, surrounded by muscle and without associated soft tissue trauma, have an excellent chance of healing whatever is done to them, but fractures at the middle of the shaft of long bones, particularly with extensive soft tissue damage, have a high incidence of non-union (p. 106).

Bone gradually gains in strength and the bone is 'united' when it is strong enough for normal use. This is a variable criterion because a weight-bearing lower limb bone carries more load than a non-weight-bearing upper limb bone and therefore takes longer to 'unite', even though the rate of healing and the strength of the bone may be the same.

Stages of bone healing

1. For the first 2 weeks, bone healing follows the same pattern as the healing of skin or any other wound. The site of the wound is filled with blood and the broken ends of the bone become necrotic.

2. The blood clot is invaded by macrophages and osteoclasts, which remove dead bone, and osteoblasts, which produce bone, instead of the fibroblasts which form fibrous tissue in soft tissue injuries.

3. Between 2 and 6 weeks after injury osteoid tissue develops and forms a firm mass, or callus, around the fracture and ossification of the osteoid begins. Callus forms both outside the bone as subperios-

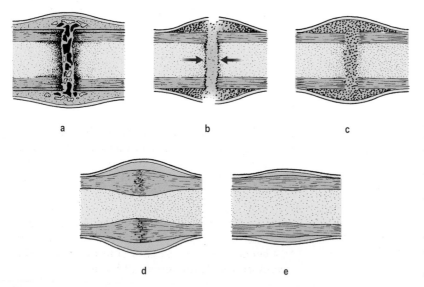

Fig. 4.7 Bone healing: (a) first 2 weeks, blood clot and macrophages form around the fracture; (b) 2–6 weeks, sharp edges are removed by osteoclasts and callus forms within the haematoma and medullary cavity; (c) 6–12 weeks, bone forms within the callus and bridges the gap between the fragments; (d) 6–12 months, the cortical gap is bridged with bone; (e) 1–2 years, remodelling occurs and normal architecture returns.

a   b   c

d   e

teal callus, and inside as endosteal callus. The pH of the tissues increases at this stage and calcium is deposited.

4. Between 6 and 12 weeks, ossification occurs, a solid bony bridge crosses the gap and the bone regains some mechanical strength.
5. Between 12 and 26 weeks, the callus matures.
6. Between 6 and 12 months, the gaps between the cortical ends are bridged.
7. Between 1 and 2 years, remodelling occurs, bony prominences become smooth and normal bone architecture is restored.

The timing is very variable and is much faster in children, in whom callus can be seen at 2 weeks.

Remodelling

In children, remodelling will correct some, but not all, bone deformities. Up to 30° of malalignment in the plane of movement of the joint can be expected to correct itself by remodelling in the young child. Rotational deformities and malalignments in other planes do not do so well (Figs 4.8, 4.9). A further

blessing is that, in children, a broken limb will grow faster than normal and a loss of length of 1–1.5 cm can be accepted under the age of 12 years.

The electrical activity of bone

Bone has piezoelectric properties and produces a small electric current when it is bent, like a crystal in an old-fashioned record player pick-up head. The convex side of the bent bone, which is under tension, has a positive charge relative to the concave side, which is under compression (Fig. 4.10). Bone is formed on the negative concave side and, if a potential difference is applied to the two sides of a bone, bone will form around the negative cathode and be eroded around the positive anode. This suggests that electricity is responsible for bone formation and resorption, an idea supported by the observation that, if screws and plates are made of dissimilar metals, bone resorption occurs between them as a result of the small current that flows between the two different metals.

Against this must be weighed the fact that almost anything has some piezoelectric activity, even a dead twig, and despite many efforts to apply a potential difference to broken bones there is still little convincing evidence that it induces more rapid healing or makes an non-united fracture unite with bone.

Articular cartilage

Hyaline cartilage does not regenerate in the adult. Although superficial damage can heal in the very young, for all practical purposes injuries to hyaline cartilage heal with fibrocartilage and fibrous tissue with inferior weight-bearing properties (Fig. 4.11).

Skin

Unlike bone, skin cannot reproduce itself and heals with a fibrous scar. This can be a special problem to the orthopaedic surgeon because any scar, even a surgical scar, that crosses a joint can contract and restrict movement (Fig. 4.12).

To operate upon a joint and create a scar which limits joint movement is not helpful and the site of incisions around joints must be carefully selected. As a general rule, incisions should never cross skin creases on the flexor surface of joints.

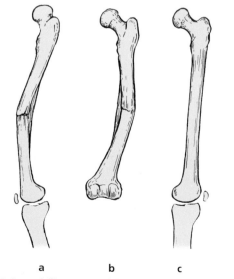

a   b   c

Fig. 4.8 Remodelling occurs: (a) well in the plane of flexion and extension; (b) partly in a plane at right-angles to flexion and extension; (c) not at all in rotation.

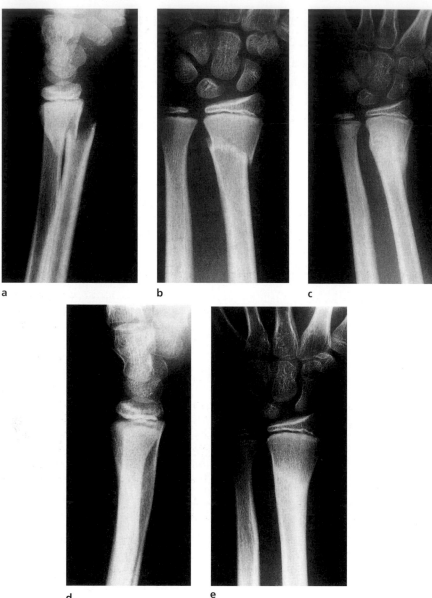

Fig. 4.9 Fracture remodelling in a child: (a), (b) a fracture of the lower end of the radius; (c) remodelling has begun 6 weeks later; (d), (e) the final position 6 months later. The radial epiphysis on the lateral view has regained its normal forward angulation, but the anteroposterior position has not altered.

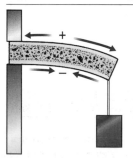

Fig. 4.10 Piezoelectric effect in bone. When a bone is bent, the tension side has a positive charge relative to the compression side.

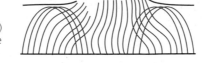

Fig. 4.11 Healing of articular cartilage: (a) the collagen arcades are disrupted; (b) the defect is filled with fibrocartilage but the collagen arcades do not regenerate.

a   b

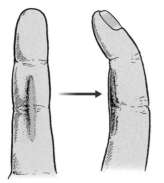

Fig. 4.12 Scars that cross flexion creases may contract to pull the joint into flexion.

Stages of skin healing

1. The wound edges bleed, the space fills with clot and the surrounding vessels dilate. White blood cells invade the clot.

2. During the first 2–3 days, the wound margins fill with macrophages, which remove dead tissue. Fibroblasts and capillary buds appear and the clot is replaced with granulation tissue.

3. Between 3 and 14 days, the fibroblasts form fibrous tissue, vascularity diminishes and the scar contracts to 80% of its original size. After 14 days the wound is healed soundly enough to withstand normal stresses but does not regain its full strength until 3 months.

4. Between 2 weeks and 2 years, the fibrous tissue contracts further. The wound, a dull purplish colour at first, gradually becomes pale. Scars on the flexor aspects of joints tend to produce tight contractures but those on the extensor aspect stretch and leave ugly wide scars.

Nerves

Nerves are often severed in limb trauma and small cutaneous nerves may be divided during operation. When a nerve is cut, changes are seen in the cell body and the axon cylinder distal to the cut degenerates.

Fine fibrils from the proximal end enter the distal sheath and grow down it at the rate of 1 mm per day. Healing of the nerves depends upon the two cut ends of the nerve being so close that the axon can cross from the proximal end of the nerve to the distal and grow down its own axonal tube to the end plate. Although individual nerve fibres may heal well and nerves can be approximated surgically using a microscope so that they appear anatomically normal, there is no guarantee that each individual neurone will find its correct destination. A telephone cable provides a useful analogy: to cut across a large telephone cable and hold the two ends together with tape is unlikely to make all the right connections (Fig. 4.13).

Because the nerve ends cannot be accurately apposed even with the help of a microscope, nerves do sometimes grow down the wrong axonal tube and reach the wrong end organ. The result of this can be that heat or light touch are experienced as pain and the incorrectly innervated skin is hypersensitive. If the cut ends are not approximated, a neuroma will form at the end of the nerve and this also leads to altered sensibility, which can be distressing.

Muscle

Muscle, like skin, heals with fibrous tissue and a cut muscle never regains its full bulk or power, even if it does all that is asked of it in normal use. A few multinucleate muscle cells may be seen. These contribute little to the function of the injured muscle. Areas of ischaemic muscle following arterial damage, compartment syndromes or crushing injuries are replaced with a mass of fibrous tissue that contracts and limits joint movement (Fig. 4.14). In severe cases, the contracture will pull the limb down into a position of extreme flexion, as in Volkmann's ischaemic contracture of the forearm.

Immunology

Bone, like other tissues, evokes an immune response but it is weaker than in other tissues. Some hospitals

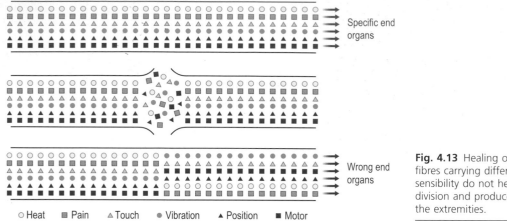

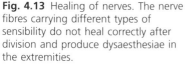
Specific end
organs

Wrong end
organs

Fig. 4.13 Healing of nerves. The nerve fibres carrying different types of sensibility do not heal correctly after division and produce dysaesthesiae in the extremities.

○ Heat ■ Pain △ Touch ● Vibration ▲ Position ■ Motor

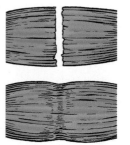

Fig. 4.14 Healing of muscle. Muscle heals with fibrous tissue, which produces a contracture within the muscle belly.

maintain banks of cadaveric bone to fill large bone defects but the bone is never as good as an autograft, which has excellent osteogenic properties, no antigenic potential and will not transmit AIDS or other diseases.

Exposing bone to very low temperatures, in the region of −20°C, diminishes, but does not eliminate, the antigenicity of the transplanted bone. Because of this, deep-frozen allograft 'bank bone' is better than refrigerated bone and will act as a scaffold for gradual replacement with the patient's own bone by creeping substitution, although it is affected by a cell-mediated immune response just like other tissue.

Freeze-dried tissues can also be used and there is some evidence that the HIV does not survive freeze-drying.

Articular cartilage can also be moved from one patient to another with a limited immune reaction, but muscle, nerve and other musculoskeletal tissues evoke too great an immune response to permit useful transplantation.

Chapter | 5 |

Investigations

By the end of this chapter you should:

- Know the different radiographic investigations used and the reasons for ordering different tests.
- Know the risks and benefits associated with each of these individual examinations.
- Have a clear understanding of what type of laboratory investigations can be used and for what reason and when.

Although laboratory and radiological investigation of orthopaedic patients is helpful, the single most important step in establishing a diagnosis and determining the management of a patient is a properly taken history. The clinical history yields information that no laboratory or computer can provide.

The second most useful step in determining management is clinical examination. Only when a proper history has been taken and a clinical examination performed should investigations be requested. When these results are available they should be interpreted in the context of the patient's symptoms, job and home circumstances. To rely on investigations alone, without relating them to the patient's symptoms and individual circumstances, is wrong.

Radiology

Radiographs are essential in orthopaedics, not only to recognize fractures and other bone lesions but also to determine the best way to treat a fracture, the accuracy of reduction and the state of union. Radiographs are so important that it is sometimes forgotten that the bones they show belong to people and it is all too common an error for treatment to be decided on the basis of radiographs alone. Pain and motivation do not show on a radiograph!

Physics of radiology

The visibility of a structure on a radiograph depends upon the atomic weights of its constituent elements. Calcium, with an atomic weight of 40, is easily visible, and so are barium (137) and iodine (127). Fat, water and carbohydrate, which consist of carbon (12), hydrogen (1) and oxygen (16), are hardly visible but the iron (56) of haemoglobin and fascia, which contains sulphur (32) within the collagen molecule, can be seen more clearly. Careful examination of a radiograph will therefore show far more than just bone. The individual muscles and the fascial sheaths around them can be seen, and a fluid level of fat in a joint is a sure indication of an **intra-articular** fracture (Fig. 5.1). Although it is fair to say

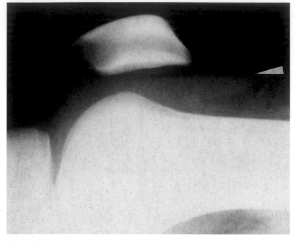

Fig. 5.1 Haemarthrosis of the knee. Note the fluid level, with fat floating on blood, indicating a fracture within the knee.

that many of the abnormalities visible radiologically can be detected more easily by clinical examination, it is still helpful to recognize a joint effusion on a radiograph and know that it consists of blood rather than synovial fluid.

Looking at a radiograph

Orthopaedic radiographs must always be taken in at least two planes because lesions can be missed if one shadow is superimposed upon another, particularly with fractures, where one view may show gross displacement while the other is anatomical. When one view is good and one is bad, the worse position is always correct because displacement can never be an artefact (Fig. 5.2).

All radiographs are eventually examined by a radiologist, but the orthopaedic surgeon has to make a decision on management before the report is available and must therefore examine the films correctly. This is especially true in the accident department, a place rich in pitfalls for the unwary (Fig. 5.3). Undisplaced fractures which are missed always slip when the patient reaches home and impacted fractures never disimpact until the patient has been reassured that he has no broken bones.

If treacherous fractures are not to be missed, every cortex of every bone must be examined systematically on every view. It helps to trace around the cortices with a pencil (without marking the film) when doing this. Meticulous examination of each bony detail can, however, lead to something very

obvious being missed and it is just as important to stand back and view the radiograph as a whole picture, particularly when a structure such as the spine is being examined.

Although bones are easily seen, soft tissues also cast shadows, but the brightness of the viewing box makes them difficult to see. Because the area of viewing box not covered by the radiograph is very bright, the examiner's iris constricts and obscures detail in the darker areas. It is surprising how much more of the soft tissues can be seen if the exposed area of the viewing box is masked; try looking down a tube of rolled up radiograph to confirm this.

Special techniques

Tomograms

The X-ray source and plate are moved to produce a blurred radiograph that leaves only one plane or slice of tissue in focus. Tomograms are useful in the investigation of defects deep within a bone, but they have their limitations (Fig. 5.4). To make tomographic cuts less than 1 cm apart is difficult and lesions less than 1 cm in diameter are easily missed. These shortcomings have made the technique almost obsolete but it is important to understand the principles because it is the forerunner of computed tomography (CT), which has largely superseded plain tomography.

Contrast studies

Structures that are not normally seen on a radiograph can be made visible by coating them with a radiopaque material such as iodine or barium, by filling cavities with gas, or both. The use of two materials, gas and a solution opaque to X-rays, is double-contrast radiography and is particularly useful in the investigation of joints, when it becomes double-contrast arthrography.

Radiculography and myelography. Iodine solutions can be injected into the spinal theca to outline the spinal canal and nerve roots stretched over a prolapsed intervertebral disc.

Arthrography. Double-contrast **arthrography** can outline the menisci and other intra-articular structures with great clarity (Fig. 5.5). A radiopaque medium is injected first, left in the joint long enough to spread over the intra-articular structures, and the joint inflated gently with gas, usually carbon dioxide,

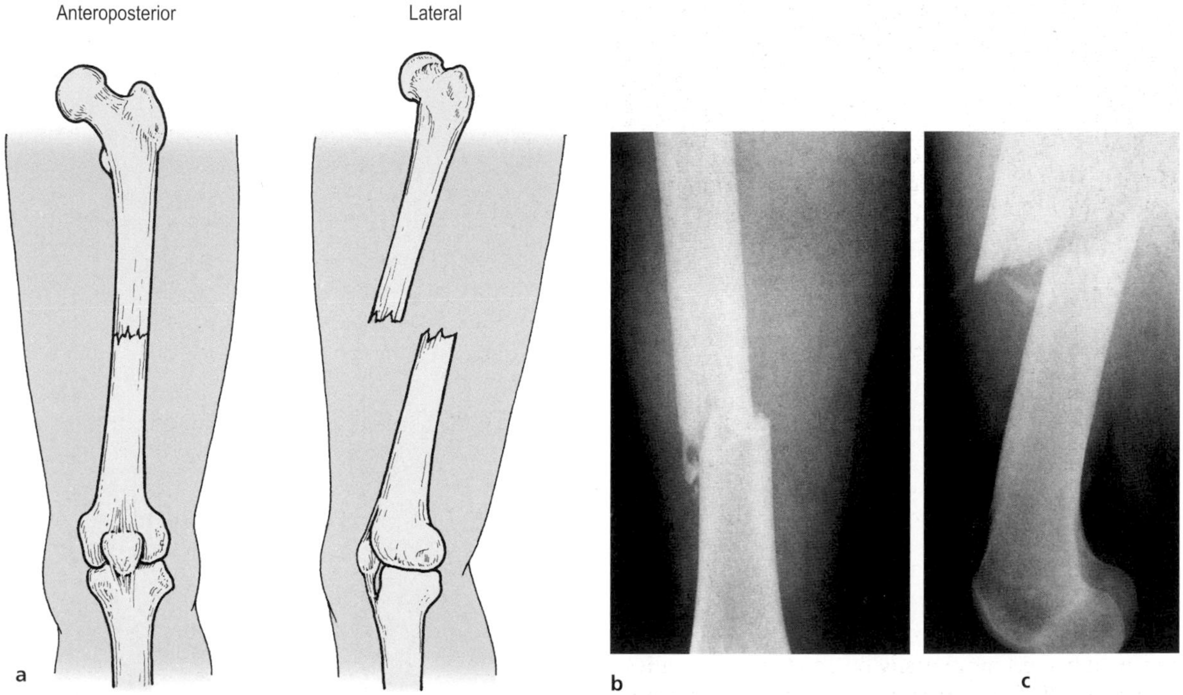

Anteroposterior   Lateral

a   b   c

Fig. 5.2 The worst views are always the most accurate: (a) good alignment may be an artefact but bad alignment can never be; (b), (c) radiographs of the same fracture.

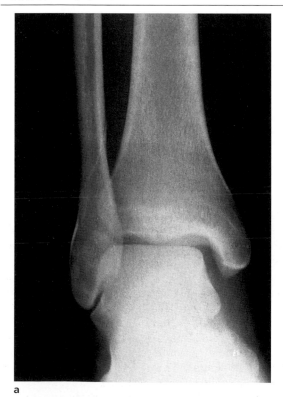

a

Fig. 5.3a The importance of two projections. Can you see the fracture on this X-ray? See (b).

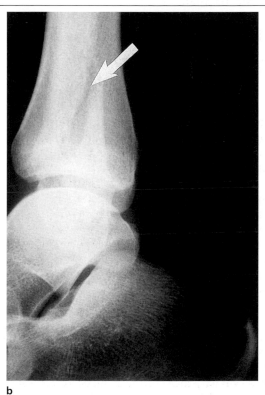

b

Fig. 5.3b The fracture is in the fibula.

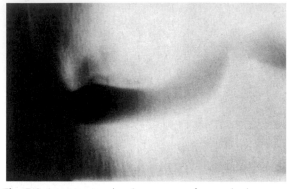

Fig. 5.4 A tomogram showing an area of avascular bone and depressed cortex in a joint.

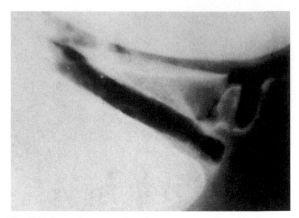

Fig. 5.5 An arthrogram showing a torn meniscus, a deep meniscosynovial sulcus, articular cartilage and bone.

to outline the intra-articular surfaces more clearly. Carbon dioxide is used because it is more rapidly absorbed; if air or nitrogen is used the joint can make an unpleasant squelching noise for as long as a week.

Although double-contrast arthrography is helpful in outlining solid structures, it is less useful in showing irregularities of joint surfaces or inflammation of soft tissue. Particular applications of double-contrast arthrography are in the investigation of internal derangements of the knee or shoulder and in congenital dislocation of the hip in children.

Discography. Radiopaque medium can be injected into the intervertebral discs to demonstrate lesions in the body of the disc. Apart from making the disc lesions visible, the increase of intradiscal pressure caused by an injection may reproduce the patient's symptoms and confirm the diagnosis.

Stress radiographs

Joints with doubtful stability can be examined under load to detect abnormal joint laxity and are particularly useful at the ankle and knee if plain films are unhelpful (Fig. 5.6).

Computed tomography

Slight differences between the radiodensities of various elements can be enhanced by computer. If radiographs are made at different angles and in different planes, the computer can integrate the information to produce pictorial 'slices' of the body and demonstrate structures not recognizable on a standard radiograph or tomogram. New develop-

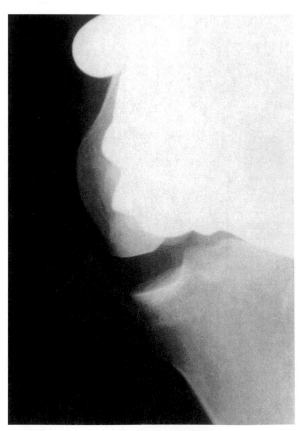

Fig. 5.6 Stress radiographs. Stress is applied to a knee with a ligament rupture. The shadow is the surgeon's hand in a lead glove.

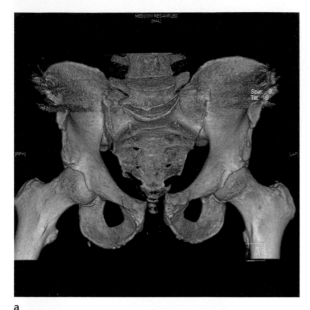

a

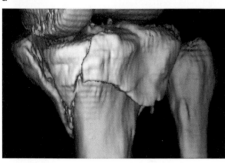

b

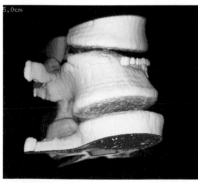

c

Fig. 5.7 (a) CT 3D reconstruction of pubic diastasis and damage to sacroiliac joint; (b) reconstruction tibial plateau fracture; (c) reconstruction vertebral crush fracture.

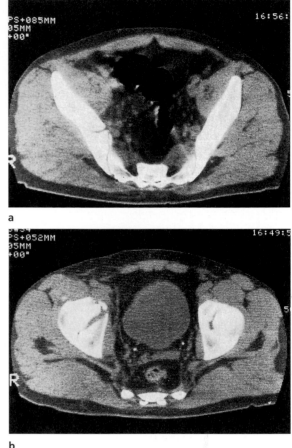

Fig. 5.8 CT scans showing (a) fracture through the ilium; (b) fracture of the right acetabulum.

ments include a 'three-dimensional' presentation of the image which displays an entire bone as if it were a shaded drawing (Fig. 5.7). A disadvantage, doubtless soon to be overcome, is an inability to show metal without distorting the rest of the image.

CT has made an enormous impact on the management of soft tissue lesions in the abdomen and central nervous system, including prolapsed intervertebral discs, and is now essential to determine the exact anatomy of complicated spinal and pelvic fractures (Fig. 5.8). CT scans give precise information and reveal spicules of bone that might damage nerve roots or the spinal cord. A practical problem is that CT equipment is so large and cumbersome that severely injured patients and those with multiple fractures cannot easily be examined, and this limits its usefulness.

59

Magnetic resonance imaging

Magnetic resonance imaging (MRI), sometimes known as nuclear magnetic resonance (NMR), depends on the behaviour of protons in a magnetic field rather than radiodensity. The protons, or hydrogen nuclei, are first made to line up by exposing the body to a powerful magnetic field. Once they are aligned, the body is exposed to a radiofrequency stimulus which reorientates the nuclei. When the radiofrequency stimulus is withdrawn, the nuclei swing back to their previous position and this movement can be displayed visually (Fig. 5.9).

Different elements behave differently and the technique can be used to display, for example, the distribution of phosphate. Hydrogen is generally used because it provides the best images of soft tissues, which are shown more clearly than with CT and without the need to expose the patient to radiation.

MRI is invaluable in the investigation of intracranial lesions but is less useful in bone, which contains less water and thus fewer hydrogen nuclei. It can also show changes in the vascularity of bone following trauma and degenerative change in the intervertebral discs and ligaments. It is now widely used in soft tissue injuries around a joint, assessing the chondral surfaces, menisci and ligamentous structures. It is also very useful in the assessment of benign and malignant bone tumours, their characteristics, spread and involvement of other tissues. MRI is now a routine investigation.

Radioisotope scanning

Radioactive isotopes (radioisotopes) can be used to 'tag' radicals, such as phosphate, which are metabolically active in bone and other skeletal structures. Compounds made radioactive in this way can be injected intravenously and will find their way to the target tissue, where they can be demonstrated by scanning the body for radioactivity.

Available radioisotopes

The choice of radioisotope depends on the specificity of the radioisotope for individual tissues, its half-life, and its availability.

The preparation of the radioisotopes poses practical problems. Most must be prepared in an atomic pile and used promptly before the radioactivity decays. A short half-life minimizes the dose of radiation to the patient but, if too short, it can be impossible to get the isotope into the patient before it decays. Technetium-99m is widely used because it has a half-life of only 6 hours but can be prepared daily in the hospital by eluting with saline an ion-exchange column containing molybdenum-99.

Patients are often concerned, and rightly so, about the dosage of radiation from a 'whole body nuclear isotope scan'. Comparison of radiation doses from different investigations is not as simple as it might appear because the amount of radiation received by the skin, bone marrow and the deep structures is not strictly comparable. In simple terms, a skeletal scan involves a higher dose of radiation than a chest or pelvis radiograph, but not as much as a barium meal or intravenous urogram.

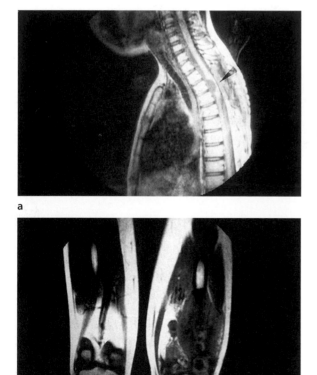

a

b

Fig. 5.9 MRI scans showing: (a) a space-occupying lesion in the spinal canal of a child; (b) a tumour in the tissues in the back of the right thigh in a child. By kind permission of the MRIS Unit, Addenbrooke's Hospital, Cambridge.

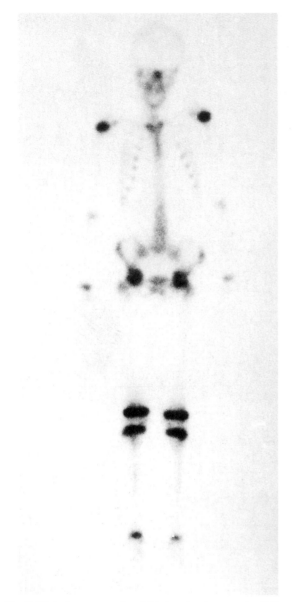

Fig. 5.10 Isotope scan of a child showing increased activity at the most active epiphyses. Note that there is more activity at the knees than at the hips or ankles, and at the shoulders than at the elbows or wrists.

Technetium-99m

Technetium-99m combined with a phosphate compound is deposited in areas of osteoblastic activity, and is commonly used to outline bone lesions. The compound is only taken up by bone that is being laid down or resorbed – 'coming and going bone'. Areas of dead or sclerotic bone appear as 'cold' areas (Figs 5.10, 5.11). Although this limits its value,

there is no other way to demonstrate the metabolic state of individual areas of the skeleton and the technique is complementary to conventional radiography (Fig. 5.12). In children with acute osteomyelitis (p. 311), the technetium scan is usually positive long before radiographs show the lesion.

Gallium-67

Gallium-67 has less affinity for bone but is taken up by proteins found in healing bone and many tumours. Gallium-67 gives a fair indication of the presence of infection, although it is far less specific for pus than technetium-99m is for bone lesions.

Indium-111

Indium-111 can be used to label leucocytes, which are found at sites of infection. It is better than gallium-67 for soft tissue infections but gallium is more reliable for infections in bone.

'Blood pool' image

To learn as much as possible from the investigation, the body is scanned twice, once shortly after injection of the radioisotope and the second time a little later. The first 'blood pool' image shows how quickly the radioisotope reaches the lesion and is an indication of its vascularity. The delayed image, obtained several hours later, shows how long it remains in the lesion and demonstrates its osteoblastic activity.

Indications

Isotope scans are particularly useful in the investigation of persistent pain for which no clinical or radiological cause can be found. A fatigue fracture of the tibia, for example, may not be visible radiologically but shows up clearly on a radioisotope scan as a hot spot, as do small vascular lesions such as osteoid osteomas (Fig. 5.13). Conversely, a normal radioisotope scan can confirm that there is no abnormal bone activity, and that if pathology is present it probably lies elsewhere.

A specific use of bone scanning is in the assessment of prosthetic joints that are painful after joint replacement. If the prosthesis has loosened and there is a foreign body reaction around the prosthesis, the affected area will be seen on the bone scan as a hot area. A technetium scan

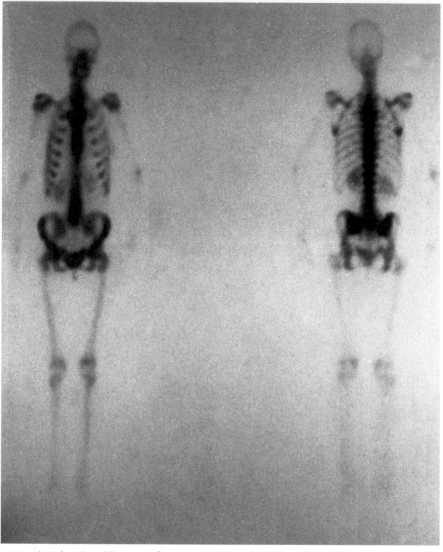

Fig. 5.11 Isotope scan. A technetium-99m scan of a normal adult skeleton from front (*left*) and back (*right*).

will not show if there is infection as well as loosening, but a gallium scan may give some indication of this.

Thermography

Thermography creates a pictorial representation of the warm areas around a joint, which gives an indication of blood supply and thus areas of inflammation or vascular disease.

Because the instruments are very sensitive, great care must be taken to avoid artefacts. The ambient temperature must be carefully controlled and the affected area must be allowed to reach a steady temperature before the investigation is performed, particularly if the patient has been wearing a bandage or dressing. The limb must also be positioned correctly and consistently.

Thermograms can be used to assess the progress of chronic joint disease, particularly rheumatoid arthritis and its response to treatment, but it is a non-specific investigation in that it will determine only where the areas of inflammation are and not the pathology that is responsible for them. Like a radioisotope scan, the thermogram provides an

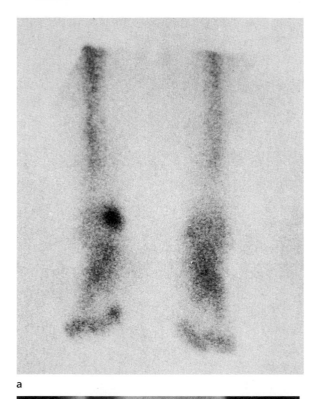

a

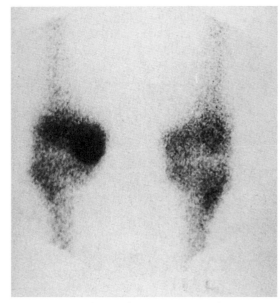

Fig. 5.13 Isotopic hot spots. An isotope scan showing an area of increased activity in the medial femoral condyle of a knee.

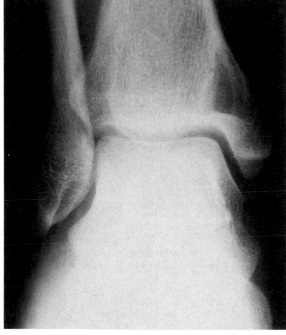

b

Fig. 5.12 (a) An isotope scan to show a destructive lesion of the bone; also visible radiologically (b).

indication of tissue activity unobtainable in any other way.

Arthroscopy

An arthroscope is nothing more than a telescope used to look inside joints and inspect nooks and crannies not accessible even through a full arthrotomy. Fine detail, including the synovial capillaries, can be seen. Arthroscopy involves more than just the visual inspection of the interior of a joint. The individual structures can be manipulated with a probe or hook, and the movement of one structure on another observed as the joint is moved (Fig. 5.14).

The principal use for arthroscopy is in the management of internal derangements of various joints, most commonly the knee. It is possible to operate inside the knee and other joints while looking through the arthroscope and perform extensive surgery through two small puncture wounds instead of the long incision of an arthrotomy. The technique is now developed to the point that open procedures upon these joints are seldom required. Even major reconstructive work can be done with relative ease.

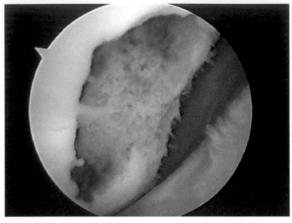

Fig. 5.14 Arthroscopic view of an osteochondral defect in the medial femoral condyle of a knee.

The main disadvantage of arthroscopy is that it is an invasive procedure usually done under general anaesthetic and, like all endoscopic operations, it is technically difficult.

Examination under anaesthetic

It is difficult to examine a painful joint thoroughly with the patient awake, particularly if ligamentous instability is suspected. Examination with the patient asleep and fully relaxed allows the integrity of the ligaments to be assessed and the range of movement measured accurately. In practice, examination under anaesthetic (EUA) is usually combined with arthroscopy and is seldom performed as an isolated procedure.

Laboratory investigations

Orthopaedic surgeons make few routine demands upon the laboratory.

Uric acid or urate estimation is needed if gout is included in the differential diagnosis but is not a routine investigation. Remember that the levels are variable and that a single normal level does not exclude the diagnosis of gout.

Tests for rheumatoid arthritis vary from hospital to hospital and it is sensible to use the same tests as the local rheumatologists. The Rose–Waaler, or sheep cell agglutination test (SCAT) and the latex test are both used but, like the uric acid estimation, need not be performed as routine.

Biochemical investigations, including serum calcium, phosphorus and alkaline phosphatase, are essential in the investigation of metabolic bone disease, as described on p. 317.

Synovial fluid may be examined for crystals, cells and blood. Viscosity and biochemical investigations on synovial fluid are also possible.

Preoperative assessment

Routine investigations for patients having operations are the same as those for other surgical patients.

Haemoglobin estimation

Haemoglobin estimation and white cell count should be done in every patient if blood loss is likely or anaemia is a possibility, but can be omitted before very minor elective procedures.

Cross-match

The appropriate quantity of blood should be cross-matched after giving the laboratory adequate notice.

MRSA

Swabs should be taken from elective surgery patients to screen for MRSA.

Urea and electrolytes

These should be estimated in patients over 60 and those who have been taking diuretics or non-steroidal anti-inflammatory drugs (NSAIDs) for long periods, or have a history of renal disease.

Erythrocyte sedimentation rate

An erythrocyte sedimentation rate (ESR) is useful if a total joint replacement is to be performed because patients with a loose or infected prosthesis usually have a raised ESR and a preoperative figure is useful as a baseline for comparison. The test is also valuable in investigating acute infections and tumours. Although a normal ESR cannot exclude a condition completely, a normal reading makes it most unlikely that the patient has a bone infection, tumour or rheumatoid arthritis.

Blood gases

PCO_2, PO_2 and pH should be measured in patients who have suffered major trauma.

Electrocardiogram

An electrocardiogram (ECG) is advisable for men over 55, women over 65, and anybody with cardiovascular disease.

Chest radiograph

A chest radiograph is needed for the following:

- Patients over 65.
- Patients with symptoms or signs in the respiratory or cardiovascular systems.
- Patients with a history of chest disease.
- Patients with malignant disease.
- Recent immigrants.

Radiographs

A recent radiograph of the part to be operated on is needed unless it is soft tissue only.

Electrical studies

Nerve conduction studies

Nerve conduction studies are tedious to perform, uncomfortable for the patient, and may be difficult to interpret. They should not be requested without a very good reason.

The conduction velocity in the myelinated fibres of a peripheral nerve can be measured by stimulating the nerve with a square wave pulse of 50–250 V lasting 0.05–0.2 ms using surface electrodes and recording its arrival either further along the nerve or at the muscle it supplies.

Pressure on a peripheral nerve may cause local demyelination or axonal degeneration, which slows conduction through the damaged segment and reduces the amplitude of the recorded response, yielding information about the performance of the nerve.

Demyelination slows nerve conduction or blocks it completely and this reduces the amplitude of the recorded response.

Abnormalities may be localized, as in traumatic lesions, or generalized, as in a peripheral neuropathy, but lesions of the central nervous system, such as multiple sclerosis, show no abnormality in the peripheral nerves.

Motor nerves

The normal conduction velocity in a peripheral motor nerve is about 50 m/s in the arm and 45 m/s in the leg, but the velocity varies with temperature and the age of the patient. Conduction is slower in neonates and the elderly, and the velocity falls 2 m/s for every 1°C drop in temperature. The values may vary according to the technique and equipment used and most laboratories have their own set of 'normal' values.

Sensory nerves

The conduction velocities in peripheral sensory nerves are similar to those in motor nerves, but a little faster, and subject to the same variables.

Sensory conduction can be measured orthodromically; i.e. as the impulse travels towards the central nervous system, or antidromically, in the opposite direction. Antidromic stimulation, e.g. by stimulating the median nerve at the wrist and recording the arrival of the impulse in the index, is easier to perform and gives greater amplitudes.

Electromyogram (EMG)

The electrical activity of muscles can be detected with a needle electrode in the muscle belly and demonstrated visually on an oscilloscope or audibly through a loudspeaker. At rest, a normal muscle is silent but if its nerve supply has undergone axonal degeneration the individual muscle fibre will contract spontaneously and rhythmically. This activity can be recorded easily in relaxed muscle as 'positive sharp waves' or 'fibrillation potentials'; these indicate serious damage to the nerve but may take as long as 3 weeks after injury to appear (Fig. 5.15).

Different lesions cause different appearances. The individual wave formations are called 'units'. Large units can indicate anterior horn disease, while small polyphasic units are seen in inflammatory muscle disease and peripheral neuropathies. The duration and stability of a unit can also give useful information but careful interpretation is needed.

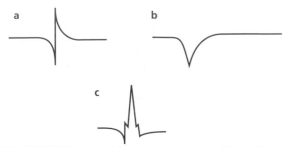

Fig. 5.15 EMG traces: (a) normal appearance; (b) positive sharp wave of denervation; (c) polyphasic wave seen in myotonia.

Bacteriology

Culture and sensitivity

Obscure infections with fungi or exotic bacteria are seen occasionally and need the closest possible cooperation with the bacteriology department. Because many bacteria are very difficult to culture in the laboratory, it is essential that the right specimen reaches the laboratory, in the best condition possible, and in the correct transport medium. In many instances, there is only one chance to obtain a good specimen and a brief telephone call to the laboratory before it is sent can avoid the catastrophe of finding that the specimen reached the laboratory in an unusable condition. Polymerase chain reactions may improve the sensitivity of the normal culture methods.

Smear

Do not forget that a simple smear and Gram stain may sometimes yield valuable information in less than 10 minutes.

Serology

Serological tests for infection, such as the antistreptolysin and antistaphylolysin titres, may also be needed, but the cases in which they are relevant are so rare that it is wise to discuss the problem with the laboratory beforehand to ensure that the investigations are appropriate. New investigations and new antibiotics are constantly being introduced and it is impossible for the clinician to keep absolutely up to date with all of them.

Case report

The following is an example of the way in which an orthopaedic patient might be investigated.

History

A 68-year-old retired farmer, who lives with his wife in a two-storey cottage, attends hospital with pain in the groin following total hip replacement 2 years earlier. The pain is worse when he bears weight on the leg and the hip is painful at the extremes of movement. The patient is otherwise well.

Examination

On clinical examination, the patient appears fit and the hip movements are as follows:

- Flexion: 80°.
- Extension: 30° (i.e. a fixed flexion deformity of 30°).
- Internal rotation: 20°.
- External rotation: 30°.
- Abduction: 20°.
- Adduction: 20°.

Inspection, palpation and stressing the joint reveal nothing.

Investigations

Radiographs

Plain radiographs show the prosthesis in good position but there is a narrow transradiant line between cement and bone near the tip of the femoral component.

Laboratory investigations

Haemoglobin and white cell count are normal, but the ESR is raised at 45 mm/h, compared with 15 mm/h before operation, which is consistent with either loosening or infection around the prosthesis. Urea and electrolytes, requested because the patient is over 60, are normal.

Isotope scan

A technetium bone scan is performed and reveals a hot spot around the lower end of the prosthesis. A gallium scan is also hot in this area, suggesting that there may be an infection.

Operation

The patient's symptoms become worse and it is decided to explore the hip prosthesis and, if possible, replace it. An ECG is normal; 4 units of blood are cross-matched; 500 mg flucloxacillin is given intramuscularly with the premedication and the bacteriologist told that this has been given.

Bacteriology

The bacteriologist requests specimens of cement from the area of the hot spot, swabs from the cavity in the femoral shaft, and tissue from the same area.

No frank infection is found at operation, the cavity is curetted thoroughly and fresh specimens are sent to the laboratory. Aerobic, anaerobic and micro-aerophilic cultures are set up within 30 min of collection and a new hip prosthesis is secured with antibiotic-loaded cement.

The laboratory cultures *Staphylococcus albus* from the specimens. *S. albus* is normally found on the skin and is not usually considered to be a pathogen, although it can give rise to a low grade infection in the presence of a foreign body such as a prosthesis. It is sensitive to flucloxacillin.

Progress

The patient made a satisfactory recovery and 2 years later still had a pain-free hip.

Chapter | 6 |

Methods of treatment

By the end of this chapter you should:

- Appreciate the value of physiotherapy and occupational therapies.
- Understand the different types of walking aid available and when these are used.
- Appreciate the value of community services in the management of orthopaedic patients.
- Be aware of different drug treatments for arthropathies.
- Have a clear understanding of the different types of operative management of bones and joints.

When asked to describe the treatment of any condition, it is a good principle and a safe answer to reply that treatment may be conservative or operative. This is particularly true in orthopaedic surgery, where there are more things to offer the patient than operation. Before selecting the right treatment for the individual patient, the physical requirements of work, home circumstances and motivation, as well as the patient's likely cooperation with treatment and rehabilitation, all have to be considered.

It must also be remembered that many conditions get better on their own and there is a great temptation for doctors to 'ascribe to their own skill the kindly work of time' (John of Salisbury 1180).

Physical therapy

Physiotherapy

An injured limb can be made to work again by a programme of graded exercises to increase the range of joint movement and muscle power using weights, springs and other devices in the ward or gymnasium. Rehabilitation and the supervision of day-to-day progress are essential parts of orthopaedic treatment, but only part of the physiotherapist's role; a good physiotherapist will also build up the patient's morale to achieve goals previously thought impossible.

Physiotherapists can also reduce inflammation and swelling in injured areas by ultrasound, electrotherapy and the cautious application of ice and heat. Electrotherapy includes pulsed electromagnetic fields (PEMF) and interferential treatment, which depends on two slightly different electrical waveforms crossing within the area to be treated and raising the temperature at their point of intersection. Short wave diathermy was once in general use but is now becoming less popular.

Muscles can be made to contract by applying an intermittent current (faradic stimulation or 'faradism') if the patient is unable to contract the muscle voluntarily. Faradism will not work if muscle is denervated, although interrupted direct current and other types of electrotherapy are effective.

Physiotherapists also manipulate the spine and other joints when necessary.

Remedial gymnastics, which once required a separate qualification from physiotherapy, takes the physical rehabilitation of the patient further than routine physiotherapy and is helpful to the young patient with physical or sporting ambitions.

Occupational therapy

The popular concept of occupational therapy is centred on handicrafts such as raffia and wickerwork, but this has little in common with modern occupational therapy, which concentrates on rehabilitating the patient through tasks relevant to work and everyday activities.

Occupational therapy departments include a small kitchen, a bath and a lavatory so that problems can be overcome before the patient leaves hospital, rather than after discharge when there is no help available. The department may also include a small printing press, so that patients can regain fine finger movement while they set type, and a treadle-operated woodworking machine to improve the coordination and strength of the legs, as well as the manual skills of carpentry. Apart from encouraging physical coordination, to produce something useful is tangible evidence of recovery and excellent for morale.

Occupational therapists also provide special cutlery for patients with hand deformities, 'pickups' for those who cannot bend and simple gadgets to help with dressing and other activities of daily living (Fig. 6.1).

Chiropractors and osteopaths

Chiropractors and osteopaths practise manipulation with great skill but do very little else, and generally work outside the hospital system. 'Manipulative medicine' is only one component of physiotherapy and is best conducted where there is access to other forms of treatment.

Walking aids

Frames

Frames provide a firm base to lean on and are particularly helpful for the elderly, but they are cumber-

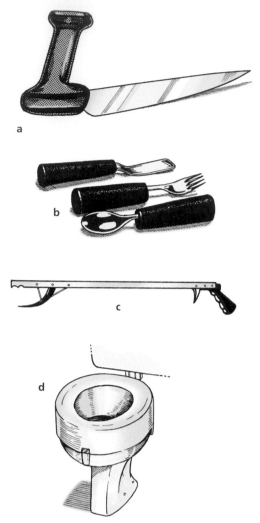

Fig. 6.1 (a) Knife for patients with rheumatoid arthritis of the hand. (b) Thick handled cutlery for patients with poor grip. (c) 'Pick-up'. (d) 'Doughnut' to increase the height of the lavatory seat for patients with poor hip movement.

some, and most patients want to progress rapidly from the frame to crutches. Wheeled frames ('Rollators') are useful in hospital but only work on smooth floors (Fig. 6.2).

Crutches

Crutches reduce the load on the lower limbs in patients with fractures or painful joints and help with balance. Three types are in common use (Fig. 6.3).

Axillary crutches. The traditional axillary crutch has the great disadvantage that leaning on the upper end presses the radial nerve against the humerus and

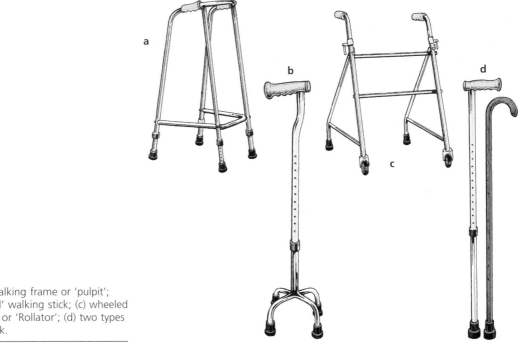

Fig. 6.2 (a) Walking frame or 'pulpit'; (b) 'quadrupod' walking stick; (c) wheeled walking frame or 'Rollator'; (d) two types of walking stick.

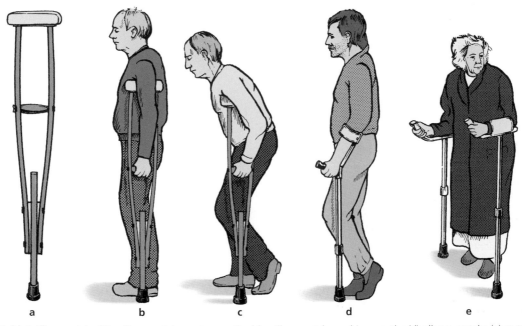

Fig. 6.3 (a) Axillary crutch; (b) axillary crutch used correctly; (c) axillary crutch used incorrectly; (d) elbow crutch; (e) gutter crutch.

causes a 'crutch palsy'. When axillary crutches are used, the elbows should be locked straight; the upper end is not for weight-bearing.

Elbow crutches. To avoid this problem, elbow crutches may be used and are preferable to axillary crutches, but have the disadvantage of being easily broken, particularly by heavy patients.

Gutter crutches. Patients with deformed hands cannot use either axillary or elbow crutches effectively and prefer gutter crutches so they can use their forearms for weight-bearing.

Walking stick

A walking stick reduces the load on an injured limb if it is pushed against the ground when the injured limb is taking weight. Stand on a bathroom scale and press a stick against the floor to see how this happens (Fig. 6.4). Used correctly, a third of the body's weight can be taken through the stick, but only if the stick is put to the ground at the same time as the injured leg. This usually means holding the stick in the hand opposite the injured limb, but right-handed patients with injuries of the right leg find this difficult.

Appliances

Surgical appliances include splints and braces to support limbs, **prostheses** to replace absent parts of the body, surgical shoes and spinal supports. Appli-

ances are expensive, although economical by comparison with hospital admission.

Orthoses

Orthoses, or braces, are used to support limbs (Fig. 6.5). A leg with no active dorsiflexors of the ankle is helped by a device to lift the foot, and an unstable knee is helped by a simple exoskeleton or caliper. The design and development of orthoses has advanced enormously in recent times and many heavy and unsightly devices of the past (Fig. 6.6) can be replaced with lightweight cosmetic orthoses. Close cooperation with the fitter, or orthotist, is essential if the patient is to receive the best appliance for his or her own requirements.

For patients with paraplegia, complex braces can also be made that support the lower limbs well enough to stand, and in some cases walk, unaided (Fig. 6.7).

Weight reduction

In the past, it was considered important to relieve the weight taken by an injured or diseased limb and many devices existed to achieve this (Fig. 6.8). Protection from full load-bearing is still important for some conditions, particularly healing fractures.

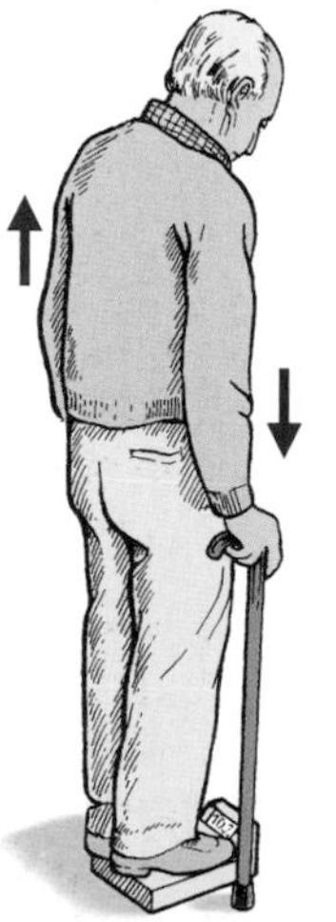

Fig. 6.4 Mechanism of action of a walking stick. When the stick is pushed against the floor, the patient's weight on the limb is reduced, relieving pressure on joints.

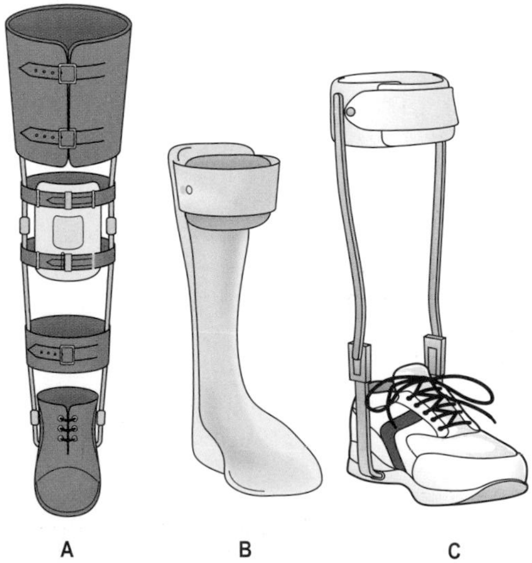

| A | B | C |

Fig. 6.5 Modern types of orthosis: (a) weight-relieving caliper; (b) below-knee caliper with T strap; (c) cosmetic drop foot splint.

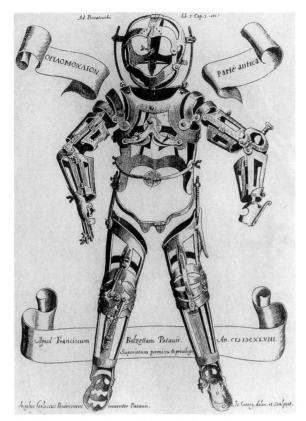

Fig. 6.6 An early orthosis. From Fabricius ab Aquapendente, *Opera Chirurgica* (1647), Padua. By kind permission of the Wellcome Institute Library, London.

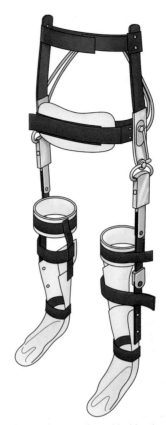

Fig. 6.7 A modern orthosis with padded leather waistband and steel limb supports.

Prostheses

Artificial limbs, or 'exoprostheses', have also improved in recent years (Figs. 6.9, 6.10), and fitting limbs is now a specialty in its own right. This service is provided at Artificial Limb and Appliance Centres (ALACs), which are established regionally and are not available in every city.

Everyday problems of maintaining artificial limbs, including repair and replacement of the limb, and practical problems such as pressure sores on the stump are best managed by these centres and it is always worth discussing difficulties with the appropriate specialist at the limb centre. The limb centre can also help by explaining the practical problems of amputation with the patient before operation, which not only helps the patient adjust to the inevitable problems but also helps the surgeon choose the right prosthesis for the individual and ensure that the stump is as good as can be achieved.

Prostheses for the upper limb present a number of different problems. A working prosthesis to replace the hand usually includes a hook of some type if it is to be of practical use; these can be unsightly. Cosmetic substitutes for the hand are seldom functional. Many patients have two prostheses, one for the working day and another for social occasions where appearance is more important than function.

The design and selection of prostheses is a subject in itself.

Spinal supports

Spinal supports were once used extensively for tuberculosis and other infections. These diseases are now uncommon and have been replaced by low back pain as the commonest indication for a lumbosacral support (Fig. 6.11). Spinal supports restrict movement of the lumbar spine and should be prescribed sparingly, especially in obese patients, who

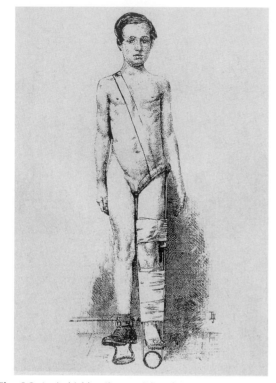

Fig. 6.8 An ischial-bearing, weight-relieving, patten-ended caliper. From Thomas H O (1876) *Diseases of the Hip, Knee, and Ankle Joints*. By kind permission of the Wellcome Institute Library, London.

can expect little support from a lumbosacral corset that cannot get near the pelvis because of fat.

Collars

Collars to support the neck are used after trauma and for patients with acutely painful necks. Do not use the term 'cervical collar': a collar cannot be worn anywhere else.

Footwear

Surgical shoes or boots are prescribed for patients with foot deformities. Normal shoes are designed for normal feet and patients with abnormal feet are sometimes disabled only because they cannot find shoes that fit. Many patients with quite severe deformities can cope in soft shoes such as trainers, but specially made shoes will be needed if these are unsatisfactory. There are several types of appliance (Fig. 6.12):

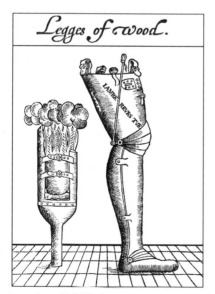

Fig. 6.9 An early artificial limb. From *A Discourse of the Whole Art of Chirurgerie* (1612). By kind permission of the Wellcome Institute Library, London.

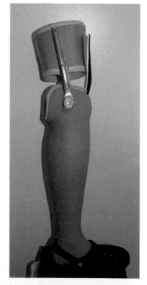

Fig. 6.10 A modern socket (without waistband).

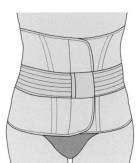

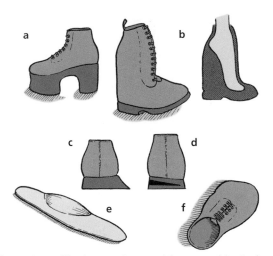

Fig. 6.12 Modifications to shoes and footwear: (a) raised sole and heel; (b) boot to accommodate fixed equinus deformity; (c) float to heels; (d) wedge to heel; (e) an insole; (f) surgical shoe for foot deformity.

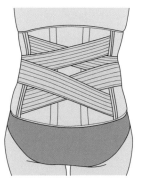

Fig. 6.11 A lumbosacral support.

- Special shoes made by taking a cast of the foot and building the shoe around it.
- Boots with a firm ankle support for patients with unstable ankles.
- Floats to the sole and heel for feet that tend to roll over.
- Insoles: soft insoles are helpful for patients with prominent metatarsal heads; firm moulded insoles support flat feet.
- Raises to the sole or heel to compensate for limb inequality.

These simple devices may be enough to make operation unnecessary.

Community services

Social services

Many patients have been helped more by social services or modifications to their home than by hospital treatment. Elderly patients unable to fend for themselves may need a home help to assist with housework and shopping rather than a total hip replacement, and the insuperable problem of climb-ing stairs can sometimes be solved by fitting a stout handrail.

These aspects of patient care cannot be ignored just because they happen outside hospital.

Warden-controlled accommodation is suitable for many elderly or infirm patients and allows them to live an independent existence in a home of their own. As the age of the population increases, small developments of single-storey accommodation designed specifically for the elderly are seen more often.

Those who cannot cope with warden-controlled accommodation need long-term residential care. Such accommodation may be provided either by local authorities or by private individuals but is under great pressure and the level of care offered is very variable.

If a patient is to be cared for by the family it is important to consider before discharge the impact such arrangements will have upon the rest of the family. Home visits from social workers, occupational therapists and the local health visitor are very helpful.

Resettlement

Patients who cannot be restored to their former work need to be resettled or retrained. A man engaged in heavy manual work and unable to lift after a back injury must find another job; a builder's labourer with a stiff foot needs work that does not involve walking over rough ground. These problems

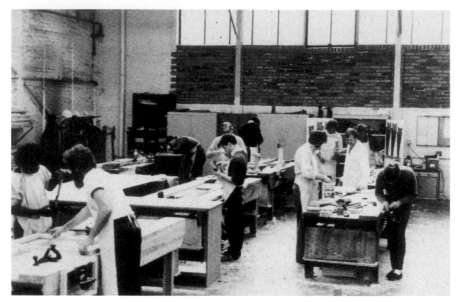

Fig. 6.13 A skill centre for retraining injured patients. By kind permission of Skills Training Agency, Sheffield.

commonly occur in patients with little academic aptitude and the selection of a new job can be difficult.

Advising a patient to give up his or her work and undergo retraining involves a great deal of thought and sympathetic assessment to determine the patient's own particular skills (Fig. 6.13). This is best done in a resettlement or retraining centre, contacted through the local Disablement Resettlement Officer. It is not uncommon to find that a resettled patient can earn more in the new job and enjoys it better. On the other hand, 'outdoor people' are always unhappy at the prospect of working indoors, seated at a bench doing repetitive manual tasks, and need much encouragement.

Rehabilitation centres

Rehabilitation of the severely injured patient requires a coordinated approach and a sense of direction, which is missing when the patient is an outpatient receiving a little physiotherapy here and some occupational therapy there while they wait their turn for industrial retraining. Combining all these facilities under one roof, where patients receive more concentrated and continuous treatment than an ordinary hospital can offer, makes the task of rehabilitation a full-time occupation. This can achieve results not possible if patients are at home dwelling on their problems.

Drugs

Non-steroidal anti-inflammatory drugs (NSAIDs)

Non-steroidal anti-inflammatory drugs are used for the conservative management of joint disease. Many such drugs are available and there is little to choose between them, but patients often do not react predictably. One patient may be completely relieved by a drug that has no effect on a patient with the same condition, and several may have to be tried before finding one that 'suits' the individual.

NSAIDs are the first line of treatment for most joint pains but they are not a panacea. They may not be effective and they have complications, of which the commonest is gastrointestinal irritation. Newer types (COX-2 inhibitors) may reduce this risk, but they can have their own complications, e.g. sudden cardiac death. They may also impair renal function if given for long periods. Urea and electrolytes should be measured before operation in patients who have been taking NSAIDs.

Steroids

Steroids, gold, hydroxychloroquine, sulfasalazine, methotrexate and penicillamine are all used in the management of rheumatoid arthritis. Patients requiring such treatment are better treated by rheumatologists than by orthopaedic surgeons. Great care should be taken when using methotrexate because of potential fatal blood dyscrasias.

Colchicine

Colchicine is effective in acute attacks of gout but a larger dose of a non-steroidal anti-inflammatory is also effective and causes fewer side-effects.

Antibiotics

Antibiotics are used prophylactically before implant procedures, such as joint replacement, and in the treatment of joint infections. They are also used to treat both acute and chronic infections, including osteomyelitis.

Prophylactic antibiotics

An appropriate prophylactic regimen for joint replacement is flucloxacillin 500–1000 mg, given intravenously in the anaesthetic room and continued for three doses thereafter. It is also acceptable to give 1 g 6-hourly for 24 h. It is important that the antibiotic is given before the incision is made so that there is a high blood level at the wound site.

If the patient is sensitive to penicillin, cephalosporins may be adequate but 10% of patients with penicillin sensitivity are also sensitive to cephalosporins. In those patients over the age of 60 there is high incidence of *Clostridium difficile* infection with the use of cephalosporins. A single intravenous dose of vancomycin is an alternative but the levels of this should be monitored.

Therapeutic antibiotics

In acute infections, the correct choice of antibiotics varies from place to place. Flucloxacillin 500 mg four times daily with ampicillin 500 mg four times daily, intravenously or orally, is a good 'best guess' for treatment in children before the laboratory results are known. The dose can be increased to 1 g of each drug in adults.

Anticoagulants and deep vein thrombosis

Deep vein thrombosis of some degree occurs in up to 60% of patients over the age of 40 after ortho-paedic operations. The majority are 'silent'; i.e. they are not apparent clinically.

Death from pulmonary embolus occurs in about 0.5% of patients following hip or knee replacement and is a constant anxiety. The risks following orthopaedic operations are far greater than those after other procedures, partly because of the trauma to the tissues surrounding the deep veins and partly because of difficulties in moving injured limbs in order to maintain venous flow.

Prophylactic anticoagulation

There is no agreement on prophylactic measures for anticoagulants after orthopaedic procedures. There are several reasons for this:

1. Prophylactic anticoagulants may reduce the incidence of deep vein thrombosis after operation but this is not the same as reducing the incidence of fatal pulmonary embolus.

2. Anticoagulants can cause their own complications. These include increased blood loss both before and after operation. Wound haematomas predispose to infection and delayed wound healing, and the complications of the additional blood replacement following increased blood loss may outweigh its benefits.

3. The incidence of pulmonary embolus is so low that huge numbers of patients must be studied before a statistically valid conclusion can be drawn.

Various methods of prophylaxis have been used, including elastic support stockings, faradic stimulation of the opposite limb during surgery, intermittent compression of the calf during operation, low dose warfarin and subcutaneous heparin. None has been shown to be completely effective. Low molecular weight heparin may decrease the risk of complications associated with anticoagulation.

If a deep vein thrombosis is suspected, an ultrasound of the superficial and deep veins is done initially. A venogram may be used when in doubt but this is invasive and often painful for the patient. The d-dimer blood test is also sensitive in predicting a thrombosis. Patients with large thrombi in proximal veins require full anticoagulation as there is a great risk of these clots breaking off and ending in the lung.

Established deep vein thrombosis

Anticoagulants are required in patients with established deep vein thrombosis. Full therapeutic anticoagulation is best conducted by the haematologist and should be continued after discharge for at least 6 months.

Intra-articular steroids

Intra-articular steroids should only be given when a diagnosis has been confirmed. They should not be given without careful thought and are more generally used by rheumatologists than by orthopaedic surgeons. They are most effective in patients whose disease is well controlled by drugs.

Hydrocortisone acetate 25 mg is a useful preparation for injection into painful areas, particularly at the bone–muscle or ligament–bone interface. Other preparations, e.g. triamcinolone, are used for intra-articular injection, but when injected subcutaneously they can cause fat necrosis and therefore skin atrophy. They should not be used for subcutaneous injection.

Operative management

There are more different operations in orthopaedic surgery than in any other surgical specialty.

Operations on tendons

Tendons can be (Fig. 6.14):

- Cut – tenotomy.
- Made longer – tendon lengthening.
- Moved – tendon transposition (transfer).
- Released – tenolysis.
- Fixed to bone to stabilize joints – tenodesis.
- Repaired.

Tenotomy

Dividing a tendon is a simple way to stop a muscle working and can be done either percutaneously, through a short stab incision, or by open operation.

Example: the adductor spasm of cerebral palsy can be relieved by subcutaneous adductor tenotomy.

Tendon lengthening

Tendons can be lengthened either by making a Z-shaped cut and joining the two ends together or by cutting the two halves of the tendon and allowing them to slide over each other inside the tendon sheath. Tendon lengthening relieves a fixed deformity without defunctioning the muscle altogether, as a tenotomy does.

Example: the Achilles tendon can be lengthened to reduce the equinus deformity of talipes.

Tendon transposition

A tendon can be transposed from its normal insertion to another so that the line of action of the muscle is altered, or power restored to a denervated muscle group.

Example: drop foot from common peroneal palsy can be relieved by transposing the tibialis posterior from the back of the leg to the front so that it acts as a dorsiflexor.

Tendon release (tenolysis)

Tendons which run through fibrous sheaths may become inflamed where they enter the fibrous tunnel or adherent to the sheath after trauma.

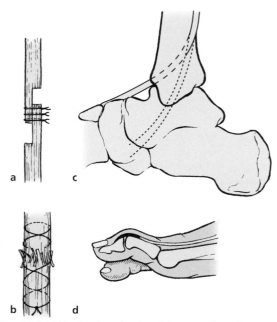

Fig. 6.14 (a) Tendon lengthening; (b) repair of tendon injuries; (c) tendon transfer; (d) tenodesis.

Example: thickened nodules within the digital flexor tendons as they enter the flexor tunnel in the palm cause 'locking' of the finger in flexion, relieved by dividing the sheath (p. 380).

Tenodesis

Tendons can be converted to ligaments and used to stabilize unstable joints by attaching the tendon to bone immediately above the joint upon which it acts.

Example: a fixed flexion deformity of the big toe caused by unopposed action of the flexor hallucis longus can be controlled by fixing the tendon of extensor hallucis to the neck of the first metatarsal to create a 'dorsal ligament'.

Tendon repair

Tendons can be repaired if they are torn or divided.

Example: repair of a ruptured Achilles tendon.

Operations on bones

Bones can be (Fig. 6.15):

- Cut – osteotomy.
- Joined – osteosynthesis.
- Grafted.
- Lengthened.
- Smoothed – exostectomy.
- Drained.

Osteotomy

An **osteotomy** is done either to correct deformity or to alter the stresses on a joint. An osteotomy is a surgical fracture and must unite like a fracture, but the site of the 'fracture' is carefully selected and the operation done so that the bone has the best chance of uniting uneventfully.

Example: tibial osteotomy to relieve the pain of osteoarthritis at the knee by correcting the varus deformity that follows wear of the medial compartment (p. 407).

Osteosynthesis

Fractured or osteotomized bones can be joined together using plates, screws or nails (Figs 6.16,

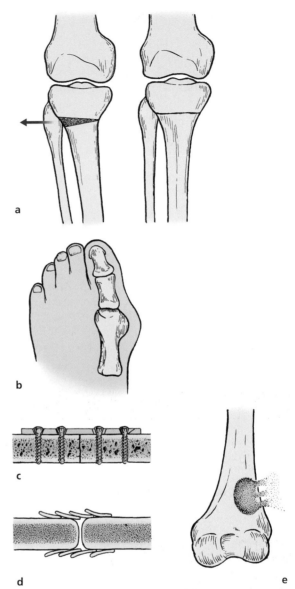

Fig. 6.15 (a) Osteotomy to correct malalignment; (b) exostectomy to remove bony prominences; (c) osteosynthesis with plate and screws; (d) bone grafting; (e) decompression of bone abscess.

6.17) (p. 132). Fixation devices do not make bones unite; they only hold the bones together in the correct position while natural bony union occurs. If this does not happen, even the strongest metal plates and screws will eventually break or pull out of the bone (Figs 6.18, 6.19).

Example: internal fixation of unstable fractures (p. 81).

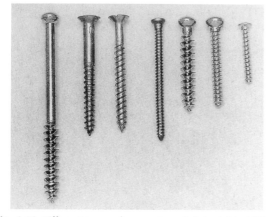

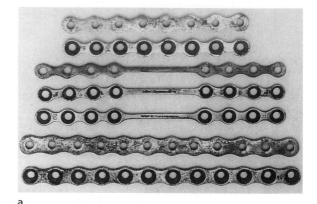

a

Fig. 6.16 Different types of screw. From left to right: ASIF cancellous lag screw; ordinary wood screw with tapered shank; chipboard screw with parallel-sided shank; self-tapping bone screw with fluted self-tapping tip; ASIF cancellous screw; ASIF cortical screw; ASIF small fragment screw (compare with Fig. 9.22).

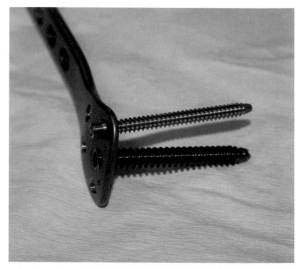

Bone grafting

> **There are three types of grafted tissue:**
>
> 1. Autograft – from elsewhere in the patient.
> 2. Allograft – from another human.
> 3. Xenograft – from another species.

b

Fig. 6.17 Different types of plate. (a) Very old plates. Note the pitting and corrosion and the very flimsy design. These plates were not strong enough for rigid fixation. (b) Modern locking plate with screws.

Autografts. Autografts are used to encourage bone union or replace lost bone. In the past, a strip of cortical bone was taken from a site such as the tibia and screwed across a fracture site as a 'cortical inlay graft' to hold the ends together. Although a neat surgical exercise, the bone was being used as an internal fixation device and not as living tissue. Modern metal plates are far stronger than devitalized cortical bone and have largely replaced the cortical bone graft.

Instead, slivers or chips of cancellous bone, which contain osteoblasts and bone marrow, are taken from a site such as the iliac crest and laid around the bone, without disturbing the fracture site, to induce ossification. This technique uses bone as a biological agent and does not have an analogy in other branches of surgery.

Example: cancellous bone from the iliac crest is placed between the transverse processes and the sacrum in an intertransverse lumbosacral fusion.

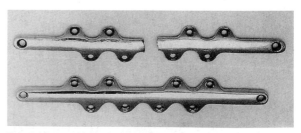

Fig. 6.18 An old tibial plate which has broken.

80

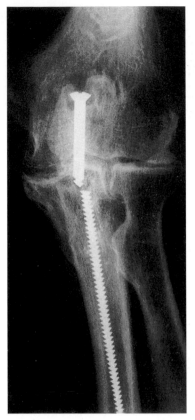

a

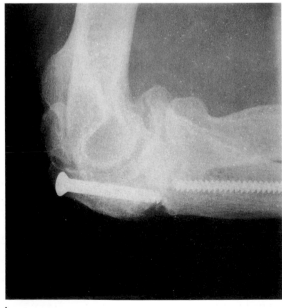

b

Fig. 6.19 (a), (b) Fractured internal fixation. The screw used to fix a fractured olecranon has itself fractured because the fragments did not unite.

Allografts. Allograft bone is used to replace lost bone when insufficient autograft is available or when whole segments of structural bone are required. The revision of joint replacements in which there has been extensive bone loss is a common use for allografts.

Allograft bone is likely to be used more frequently as practical problems are overcome. The allograft must be stored sterile and has a limited shelf life that varies according to the method of preservation. When whole bone segments are used, a large range of sizes for both left and right sides must be kept.

Achilles tendon, patellar tendon and tibialis posterior tendon can be used to replace the anterior cruciate ligament and other ruptured ligaments.

A particular anxiety, common to all donor materials, is the possible transmission of infections, e.g. the hepatitis virus and HIV. This is a justifiable fear because patients have contracted AIDS in this way. Freeze-drying and irradiation have been claimed to reduce the risk of disease transmission but this may be at the expense of the mechanical properties of the graft.

Xenografts. Xenografts (tissue from another species) are treated to remove protein and fat, leaving only the mineralized structure intact. These grafts are essentially foreign bodies which act as a skeleton for creeping substitution rather than a true osteogenic bone graft. They have little, if any, osteogenic potential but are useful to fill spaces and hold osteotomies open.

More recently, bone morphogenic proteins (BMP) have been used with encouraging results. These stimulate the natural healing mechanism.

Other materials. Inert sponges of many materials containing calcium have been used as scaffolds for creeping substitution. Among the most recent to be offered for general use is coral, which has been machined to exact sizes, sterilized and packed ready for insertion. ('Full fathom five thy father lies; Of his bones are coral made;' William Shakespeare, *The Tempest*, Act I, Scene 2.)

Lengthening bones

Bones can be lengthened in a number of ways. A variety of techniques have been used in the past, including periosteal stripping, implantation of a foreign substance, alteration in the blood supply, sympathectomy, bioelectrical stimulation, hormone therapy and surgery. Unfortunately many of these

81

techniques were unreliable. The use of growth hormone in particular led to tragedy as some of the hormone was obtained from human pituitary glands and was contaminated with the Creutzfeldt–Jakob disease (CJD) agent; a few of the patients treated in this way have contracted this disease.

Operations are more reliable. Simple division of the bone in a step cut fashion with subsequent distraction of the two bone ends and refixation at the desired length is possible, but only small segments can be lengthened at a time. The lengthened segment of bone is also weaker than normal and recovery may be prolonged.

In the immature skeleton a bone can be lengthened by stretching the growth plate (physeal distraction). This is achieved by the application of an external fixator across the growth plate and slowly distracting the physis. The degree of lengthening achieved is variable and the technique is limited to those patients with an open physis and potential for growth. Complications are frequent and the results are often unpredictable.

An easier and more reliable method is by callotasis. In essence this consists of cutting the bone (corticotomy) and progressive stretching of the healing callus that forms. After approximately 7–10 days following the corticotomy, the callus is stretched at a rate of approximately 1 mm per day. Distraction is achieved using either a monolateral external fixator or a ring fixator (see Fig. 9.20b). Once the desired length has been achieved the fixator is clamped and the bone is allowed to consolidate (Fig. 6.20). Patients can walk on the limb with the fixator in situ until the bone has remodelled and strengthened. There is always concern for the soft tissues, nerves and blood vessels while the distraction of the bone is in progress. Meticulous care of the pin sites is needed and patients should be prepared for a prolonged period of treatment. Patients should also be advised not to smoke while treatment is in progress because smoking interferes with ossification.

Exostectomy

Exostoses and other lumps can be levelled, preferably making a slight depression at the site of the original bump so that the fibrous tissue which forms at the site of operation lies in the depression.

Example: levelling an exostosis on the dorsum of the foot.

Draining infection

In days gone by, bone infection was a common problem and orthopaedic surgeons spent much of their time letting pus out of abscesses and removing sequestra. These operations are, thankfully, seldom required now but it is still occasionally necessary to perform a sequestrectomy and unroof infected bone cavities (p. 312).

Example: drilling acute osteomyelitis (p. 312).

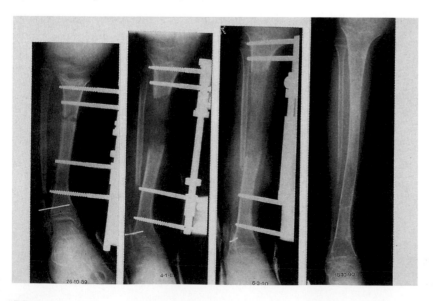

Fig. 6.20 X-rays of limb lengthening using callotasis.

Operations on joints

Joints can be

- Stiffened – arthrodesis.
- Opened – arthrotomy.
- Refashioned – arthroplasty.
- Subjected to excision of the synovium – synovectomy.
- Mobilized – arthrolysis.
- Looked into – arthroscopy.
- Aspirated.
- Manipulated.

Arthrodesis

Stiffening a joint, or **arthrodesis**, is achieved by removing the articular surfaces of the joint and holding the bone ends together so that they unite like a fracture. The operation is indicated for irreparable damage or instability of a joint and will produce a sound and painless limb that lasts a lifetime, but the loss of movement is a serious disadvantage in large joints such as the hip and knee (Figs 6.21a, 6.22, 6.23).

The effect of arthrodesis is usually irreversible but can be predicted by immobilizing the joint in plaster, after which the patient may decide that a painful joint that moves a little is preferable to a painless limb that will not move at all.

Arthrodesis should not be performed if there is a chance of other joints becoming stiff. A patient can manage with one arthrodesed hip but to manage with two is extremely difficult. If both hip and knee are arthrodesed in the same limb, problems are inevitable: hold your own hip and knee stiff and try to imagine the difficulties yourself.

Example: arthrodesis of the proximal interphalangeal joint of the second toe for hammer toe (p. 440).

Arthrotomy

Any operation that opens a joint is an **arthrotomy** but the term is usually applied to an exploratory arthrotomy. With arthroscopy and other modern investigative techniques, exploratory arthrotomy is seldom performed alone and is largely obsolete.

Arthroplasty

Any operation that creates or reshapes a joint is an **arthroplasty**. There are several types (Fig. 6.24).

Excision arthroplasty. **Excision arthroplasty**, in which the bone surfaces are removed and the space between them is allowed to fill with fibrous tissues, is the simplest and sometimes the most satisfactory arthroplasty, but leaves an unstable joint.

Example: excision arthroplasty of the hip (Girlestone's procedure) as a salvage procedure for failed total hip replacement (p. 403).

Interposition arthroplasty. Rather than leave the two bone surfaces of an excision arthroplasty exposed, a prosthetic or organic material can be laid between the two. A stainless steel cup or mould was inserted in the hip joint before the advent of total hip replacement and a similar operation was performed at the knee.

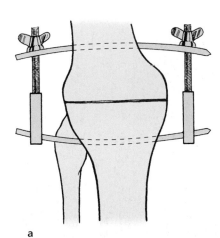
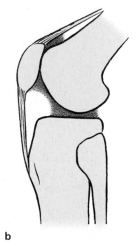

Fig. 6.21 (a) Compression arthrodesis; (b) adhesions within joints can be released by arthrolysis.

a

b

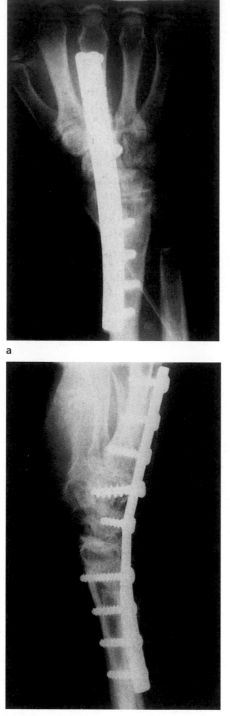

a

b

Fig. 6.22 Anteroposterior (a) and lateral (b) views of an arthrodesis of the wrist using ASIF internal fixation. The radiograph was taken immediately after operation and the drain is still in position.

Example: silastic spacers inserted in the metacarpophalangeal joints in rheumatoid arthritis.

Replacement hemiarthroplasty. If one surface of a joint is replaced with an artificial material such as metal, the operation becomes a replacement hemiarthroplasty, or simply a hemiarthroplasty.

Example: fractures of the femoral neck may be treated by replacing the femoral head with a metal prosthesis. This is satisfactory but the hard metal of the prosthesis may erode the acetabulum.

Total joint replacement. A metal prosthesis will erode bone affected by osteoarthritis or other disease. Because of this, it is usual to replace both joint surfaces in osteoarthritis and perform a total joint replacement, one of the most successful operations in orthopaedic surgery (Fig. 6.25).

Problems arise if the hip becomes infected or the components loosen, when it may be necessary to remove the artificial material and convert the total hip replacement to an excision arthroplasty.

Example: total hip replacement for osteoarthritis (p. 395).

Synovectomy

Synovium affected by rheumatoid arthritis or any other chronic inflammation may need to be removed. Without synovium, the joint develops a new lining which differs slightly from the original.

Example: synovectomy of the elbow for rheumatoid arthritis.

Arthrolysis

For a joint to function normally the bone surfaces must be free to slide over each other and the synovial cavity must be free of adhesions. If there has been bleeding or infection in the knee, fibrous adhesions will form between the two synovial surfaces and between articular cartilage and synovium, restricting movement severely. Division of the adhesions restores joint movement but they can reform (see Fig. 6.21b).

Example: mobilization of the knee following trauma.

Arthroscopy

Joints can be looked into with a telescope, an invasive procedure usually done under general anaesthetic (Fig. 6.26).

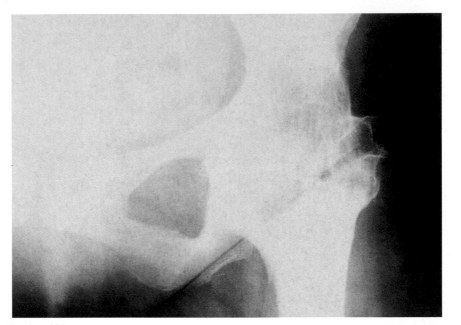

Fig. 6.23 An arthrodesed hip.

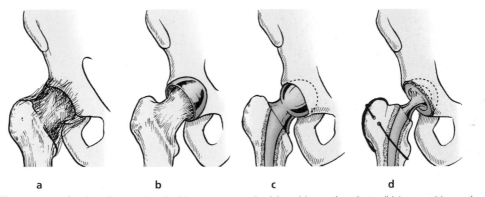

a   b   c   d

Fig. 6.24 Different types of arthroplasty using the hip as an example: (a) excision arthroplasty; (b) interposition arthroplasty; (c) hemiarthroplasty; (d) total hip replacement.

Aspiration

Joints can be aspirated; i.e. fluid can be drawn out of them: (1) to relieve the tension of a haemarthrosis; (2) to remove fluid for culture; (3) to remove synovial fluid for examination.

Aspiration requires little more skill than any ordinary injection but full sterile precautions must be taken to prevent infection. The aspiration can be done under local anaesthetic, provided that joint capsule, synovium and skin are infiltrated.

Example: diagnostic aspiration of a painless joint effusion.

Manipulation under anaesthetic

Joints can be manipulated under anaesthetic to break down adhesions or assess movement. Manipulation is helpful in restoring movement after haemarthrosis or joint replacement; however, over-enthusiastic manipulation of a joint can tear ligaments or break the bone.

Example: manipulation of a stiff joint after a fracture.

85

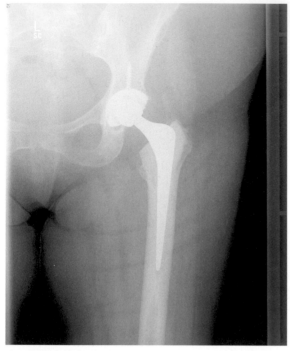

Fig. 6.25 Postoperative hip X-ray.

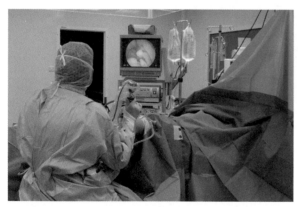

Fig. 6.26 Arthroscopy of the knee.

Operations on ligaments

Ligaments can be (Fig. 6.27):

- Repaired when torn.
- Replaced or reconstructed.
- Shortened – plication or capsulorrhaphy.

Repair

Ligaments are strong and complex structures. If a ligament is even a millimetre too long, the joint that it controls may be unstable; if it is a millimetre too short, joint movement will be restricted. Even if the ligament can be accurately resutured so that it is a perfect length and in perfect position, the chances that the repaired ligament will have the same 'stretchiness' as the original are slight. Because of this, repairing ruptured ligaments is not generally successful.

Example: repair of the ulnar collateral ligament of the first metacarpophalangeal joint (p. 232).

Replacement or reconstruction

Because of the difficulty of repair, ligaments are sometimes replaced with a length of tendon (p. 421) or prosthetic material, but none of these procedures is entirely satisfactory.

Example: reconstruction of the anterior cruciate ligament of the knee for instability.

Plication and capsulorrhaphy

Ligaments can be tightened by advancing the attachment to bone or plicating the joint capsule to restrict movement.

Examples: distal advancement of the medial ligament of the knee for instability (p. 422); the Putti–Platt operation for recurrent dislocation of the shoulder (p. 365); inferior capsular shift for multidirectional glenohumeral instability.

Operations on nerves

Nerves can be (Fig. 6.28):

- Decompressed.
- Repaired.
- Freed – neurolysis.
- Grafted.

Decompression

The most commonly performed operation on nerves is decompression for dysfunction caused by outside pressure.

Example: decompression of the median nerve at the wrist for carpal tunnel syndrome (p. 387).

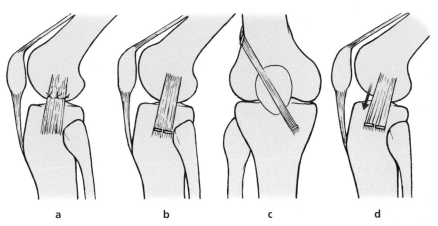

Fig. 6.27 Operations on ligaments: (a) repair; (b) reattachment; (c) replacement with tendon or prosthesis; (d) advancement of ligament attachment.

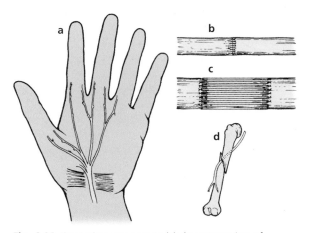

Fig. 6.28 Operations on nerves: (a) decompression of compressed nerve; (b) repair by suture of the perineurium; (c) cable grafting of large defects; (d) neurolysis. Tethering of the nerve to bone or other tissues can be released by operation.

Grafting

Large gaps in a nerve can be replaced with a cable graft made from cutaneous nerves. These operations are unreliable but are sometimes an attractive alternative to accepting a serious disability.

Example: replacement of the upper cord of the brachial plexus with a graft made from the sural nerve.

Operations on skin

Skin can be:

- Repaired.
- Grafted.
- Changed in shape – plastic surgery.

Repair and grafting are dealt with in Chapter 9.

Repair

Nerves divided by injury can be repaired (p. 141).

Example: repair of the median nerve at the wrist following a laceration.

Neurolysis

Nerves can become involved in dense scar tissue, which interferes with function.

Example: mobilization of the median or ulnar nerve following a laceration of the wrist.

Plastic operations

Small areas of skin can be changed in shape to release tension, but complex plastic procedures are better done by plastic surgeons. If you find these procedures difficult to understand, try cutting out the patterns in Figure 6.29 on a separate piece of paper and move the flaps to see the effect.

Example: Z-plasty for Dupuytren's contracture (p. 88).

87

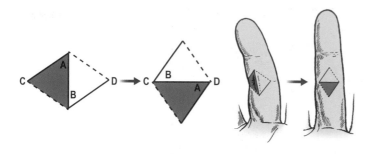

Fig. 6.29 Z-plasty. A Z-plasty can change the shape of a piece of skin and the direction of the contracture.

Case reports

The way in which the different services are necessary for the management of orthopaedic patients is illustrated by comparing the fate of three imaginary 78-year-old women of identical size and weight who had identical fractures treated by identical operations on the same day.

Patient A (Fig. 6.30a)

This patient is a bright and active woman without relatives who fended well for herself before operation and lived alone in a bungalow (1). Her operation was uneventful and the next day, rather against her will, she sat out of bed. The following day, again under protest, she began to walk with a walking frame (3) and within 2 weeks had discarded the frame and was using elbow crutches. While in hospital, the occupational therapist made certain that the patient was able to wash and dress herself, use the lavatory, and prepare a meal while still using crutches (4). A few simple aids were necessary to help her dress but with practice she was well able to cope.

The social worker visited the patient in hospital and arranged that after discharge a home help would assist with housework, and that 'meals on wheels' would call so that she would have at least one hot meal every few days even if she could not cook her own. The community nurse visited her and arranged for the health visitor to call after discharge. The patient's family doctor was notified of the time and date of her discharge and a telephone call to the patient's neighbours ensured that the house was heated and that fresh food was available when she arrived home (5). She was visited at home by the health visitor later on the day of discharge and by her family doctor the following day.

The patient discarded her crutches 6 weeks after operation (6) and a few weeks later was again looking after herself without assistance.

Patient B (Fig. 6.30b)

Also a bright 78-year-old woman living in a bungalow (1). The postoperative X-ray of this patient was so good that the surgeon decided she really did not need much physiotherapy or occupational therapy. The patient felt tired after operation and her kind surgeon felt so sorry for her that he let her stay in bed for a full week (2). Thereafter she spent longer and longer every day sitting out of bed (3) until about 3 weeks after operation, when she was given a pair of crutches and taken home by ambulance late one afternoon (4). Her home was unheated and the only food in the house, which was bought before her operation, had gone bad. The family doctor and health visitor did not know she was going home and none of the neighbours saw the ambulance arrive. The patient was unable to feed herself and could neither attract attention nor get herself to bed. The following day, neighbours noticed that a light was on and found the patient unconscious in an armchair (5). She was readmitted to hospital (6) with hypothermia and after intensive rehabilitation in the geriatric department made an excellent recovery, but she might not have been so fortunate.

Patient C (Fig. 6.30c)

This elderly woman lived in her old family home, a large rambling building which she could not

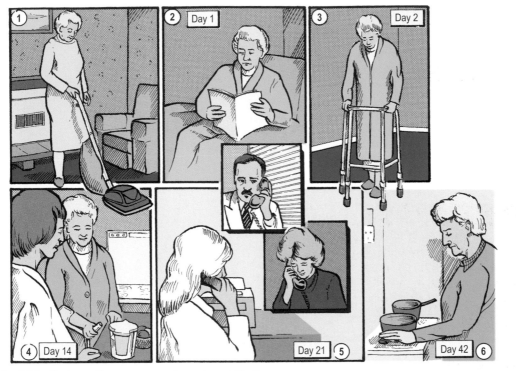

Fig. 6.30a Postoperative management – early mobilization.

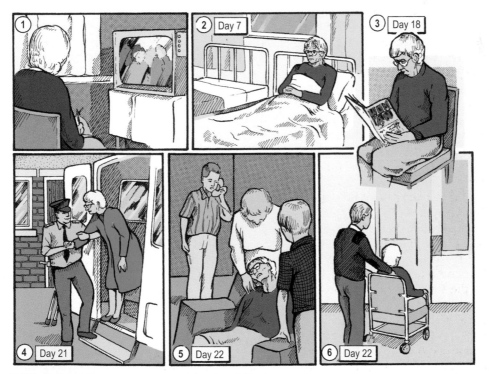

Fig. 6.30b Postoperative management – delayed mobilization.

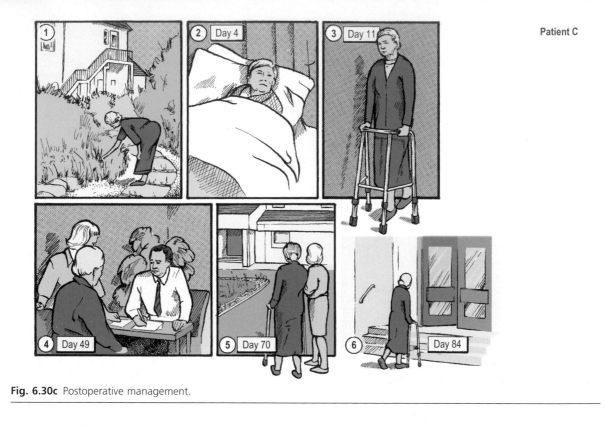

Fig. 6.30c Postoperative management.

manage even before she broke her hip (1). She had not been feeding herself properly and was not as fit or alert as the other two patients. Perhaps because of this, she did not recover as quickly from the effects of operation (2). Despite excellent physiotherapy and occupational therapy, she could not be made as fit as she was before the accident and could only walk with a frame (3). The occupational therapist and social worker visited the patient's home and discussed the problem with her family doctor (4). All agreed that she would be unable to return to her home and the decision was made to find warden-controlled accommodation, which the social worker arranged. The patient visited the home, liked the accommodation and the warden agreed that she would be a suitable resident (5). The social worker helped the patient dispose of her house and the patient, using a walking frame, was discharged to her warden-controlled home (6).

Moral

The only straightforward part in the management of these three patients' injuries was the operation. The doctor who believes that his or her responsibilities stop when the patient leaves the operating theatre should not take up orthopaedic surgery.

Part | 2 |

Trauma

Chapter | 7 |

The principles of managing trauma

By the end of this chapter you should be able to:
- Make a simple diagnosis of a fracture and be able to classify common injuries.
- Appreciate the common complications.
- Diagnose different joint injuries and the damage to soft tissue supporting structures.

Fractures

Trauma and fractures are not the same thing. When a limb is broken, every tissue in it is damaged. The fact that the bony injury is the only one visible on the radiograph does not make it the most serious. Radiographs do not show severed nerves, crushed muscles, ruptured blood vessels or torn ligaments, any more than they tell whether a wound is contaminated, how the injury occurred or how it should be treated.

The severity of an injury is greatly influenced by the violence of the impact. A leg broken by a car travelling at 95 km/h (60 m.p.h.) will be more seriously injured than one broken by tripping over the cat (Fig. 7.1). In the high speed injury there will be damage to all the soft tissues as well as bone, and possibly damage to the blood vessels. The bone ends will be crushed and devitalized, nerves stretched or severed, and muscles crushed. Although the bone may unite soundly and in good position, so that it is even stronger than before the injury, damaged

muscles cannot be restored, and severed nerves will never be the same, however meticulously they are repaired.

To understand the damage to the soft tissues, imagine the position of the limb at the moment of impact when the bone ends were widely separated (Fig. 7.2). By the time the patient reaches hospital, the soft tissues will have bounced back almost to their normal position and the radiographs give no indication of the extent to which the soft tissues were stretched. This is not a difficult concept, yet inexperienced casualty officers frequently decide how to treat a patient just by examining the radiograph and this can lead to disaster.

Even if the fracture is treated correctly in the accident department, soft tissue injuries can still spoil the result of the finest fracture management. This is easily forgotten when the patient is sitting in the fracture clinic with an injured limb hidden inside a cast. If the radiographs look normal it might be imagined that all that needs to be done for the limb to work normally again is to remove the cast. This is not so.

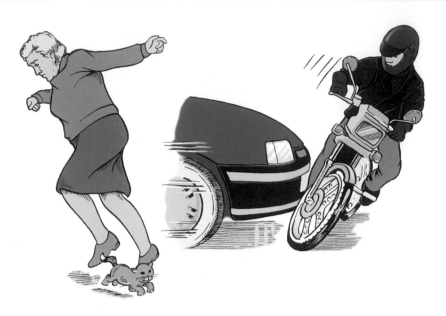

Fig. 7.1 Violence of impact. Cats cause less damage than cars.

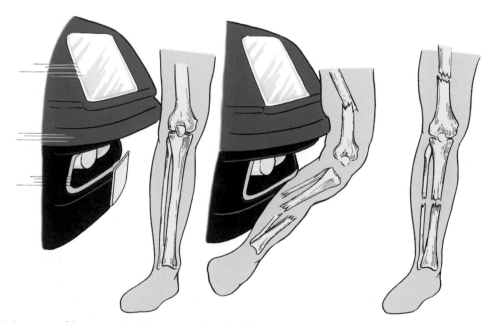

Fig. 7.2 Displacement of fragments. Soft tissues recoil and pull bone fragments back together after an impact. Try to imagine how the fragments and soft tissues must have been at the time of greatest displacement.

Three stages of fracture management

1. Deal with any open wounds.
2. Attend to the fracture until it is united.
3. Mobilize the joints and rehabilitate the limb.

Fracture management can therefore be divided into three phases. Early management is directed to converting contaminated wounds to clean wounds, and the second stage to joining together those things that have broken, notably bone. The third stage consists of separating those things that have stuck together but should be separate, particularly muscles and joint surfaces.

There is no point in achieving a perfect radiograph with solid bone if the muscles cannot operate the joints. On the other hand, it is equally bad to start early rehabilitation and produce excellent muscles around a malunion. A balance must be struck between these two conflicting aims. The correct approach is to start mobilization and vigorous physiotherapy as soon as it is safe to do so, but to choose the right moment takes experience.

Recognizing a fracture

The physical signs of a fracture

- Abnormal movement in a limb due to movement at the fracture site.
- Crepitus or grating between the bone ends.
- A deformity that can be seen or felt.
- Bruising around the fracture.
- Tenderness over the fracture site.
- Pain on stressing the limb by bending or longitudinal compression.
- Impaired function.
- Swelling at the fracture site.

Although it is usually easy to know when a bone is broken, it is surprisingly easy to miss a fracture and some are notorious for the number of times they escape recognition.

If either of the first two signs on the list above are present, there is a fracture, but these signs are absent if the ends are impacted. Undisplaced fractures cause no deformity, bruising can take hours to appear and unconscious patients cannot report pain or tenderness.

The following fractures are often missed (Fig. 7.3):

1. Impacted fractures of the femoral neck.
2. Fractures of the ribs.
3. Fractures of the skull, particularly the base of the skull.
4. Facial fractures, particularly the zygoma.
5. Fractures of the radial head.
6. Fatigue fractures before the callus has appeared.
7. Fractures of the scaphoid.

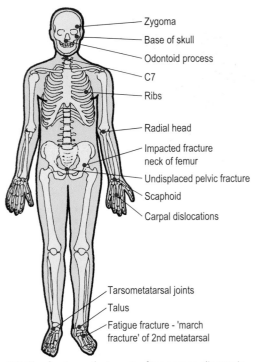

Fig. 7.3 The fractures that most often escape diagnosis.

8. Fracture dislocations of the carpus, particularly the lunate.
9. The seventh cervical vertebra.
10. Undisplaced fractures of the pelvis.
11. Fractures of the odontoid.
12. Fracture dislocations of the tarsometatarsal joint.
13. Fracture of the talus.

Natural history of fractures

Grass grows without gardeners and bones unite without orthopaedic surgeons. Like a gardener, the orthopaedic surgeon tries to make nature's task easier, but nothing will 'make' a bone unite if the circumstances are not right.

Untreated, fractures can do one of several things. At best, they unite soundly in good position to give a perfect result, but they may be slow to unite (**delayed union**), fail to unite at all (**non-union**) or unite in the wrong position (**malunion**) (Fig. 7.4).

There is no hard and fast rule to say how any one fracture will behave without treatment but, in general, fractures in cancellous bone unite soundly and non-union is seldom a problem, although there

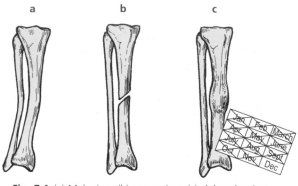

Fig. 7.4 (a) Malunion; (b) non-union; (c) delayed union.

may be malunion. In contrast, the long bones are susceptible to non-union, particularly if there is poor blood supply to the bone ends as a result of extensive soft tissue damage.

Patients are, understandably, very eager to know how long their bone will take to join, but fractures unite gradually and the question 'Has the fracture joined yet?' is impossible to answer. A bone is only united when it is strong enough to take its normal load; this varies from bone to bone, but a good rule of thumb is to say that most bones join in 8 weeks, lower limb bones take twice as long and fractures in children take half as long.

A very rough guide to fracture healing

Bones join in 8 weeks, but double this in the lower limb and halve it for children.

Fracture healing

The healing of bone explains the clinical behaviour of a uniting fracture. Immediately after the fracture the bone ends rub together and cause crepitus, which is distressing to the patient. After about 14 days, fibrous tissue has replaced the blood clot between the bone ends and the crepitus ceases but the fracture remains mobile.

At about 4 weeks the fracture becomes 'sticky' and movement is less obvious. During the next 2 months the bone becomes solid but not always strong enough to do all that is asked of it, particularly if it is a weight-bearing bone in the lower limb.

As healing proceeds, the mass of tissue around the fracture becomes hard and produces a fusiform callus. Patients are often alarmed by the swelling and think they have cancer. They must be reassured

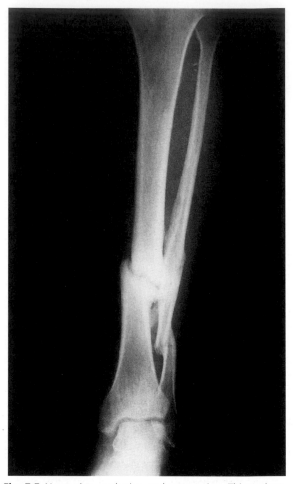

Fig. 7.5 Non-union, malunion and cross-union. This patient had non-union of the tibia, malunion of the fibula and cross-union between the two.

that it is a sign of good fracture union. The callus never disappears completely but becomes smaller with time as the soft tissue swelling around it diminishes and remodelling occurs.

Malunion

The term malunion is applied to a bone that has united soundly but in the wrong position (Fig. 7.5). This sounds alarming but does not always matter greatly. Fractures of the clavicle almost always unite with a little shortening and overlap, which is quite acceptable and does not affect the functional result, but in fractures where the fragments are pulled apart by the unopposed action of different muscle groups, the functional result of malunion is poor.

If the morbidity of the operation to fix the fracture and prevent malunion is less than the morbidity of the malunion, then the operation is worthwhile. If this is not so, it is better to leave the malunion rather than submit the patient to an operation with a doubtful outcome.

Cross-union. Cross-union, in which two adjacent bones become linked by new bone, is a variety of malunion. Cross-union in the forearm blocks pronation and supination.

Non-union

If the healing process fails, the bone ends do not unite and remain separate. This is a serious problem in a weight-bearing bone but may cause less disability in other situations, such as a fractured metacarpal. Two types of non-union are seen: (1) hypertrophic, and (2) atrophic.

Hypertrophic non-union is characterized by a massive cuff of bone around the ends of the fractures that looks a little like an elephant's foot (Fig. 7.6a). These fractures are trying desperately to heal and can be helped to do so by realigning the limb and preventing movement between the bone ends. Prevention of movement can be done by rigid internal fixation, or intramedullary or extramedullary stabilization.

Atrophic non-union shows rounding of the bone ends (Fig. 7.6b), sometimes so marked that the tips of the bone ends resemble pencils, and the medullary cavity may be closed. This is indicative of a poor blood supply to the bone ends.

A pseudarthrosis forms in some patients (Fig. 7.7). If there is no sign of osteogenesis, treatment must aim to 'kick start' this by bone grafting with fresh cancellous bone or marrow.

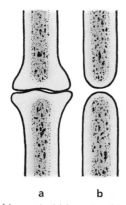

a   b

Fig. 7.6 Shape of bones in (a) hypertrophic non-union and (b) atrophic non-union.

Delayed union

A fracture with delayed union takes longer to unite than normal but eventually does so. It is important to distinguish delayed union from non-union, as delayed unions will unite with time and attention to correct immobilization of the fracture fragments. Non-unions, however, may need operative intervention in order to allow the bone ends to unite. Separation of the two types can be difficult. Unless there are positive signs of non-union, such as closing of the medullary cavity of the fragments, which makes the diagnosis easy, or an improvement between one radiograph and the next, diagnosis rests on comparing the rate of bone union with the normal rate of healing of a fracture in the same situation.

Classification of fractures

Simple and compound

Fractures can be classified in many ways but the simplest and most practical was the ancient classification of the old military surgeons who regarded all fractures as simple or compound.

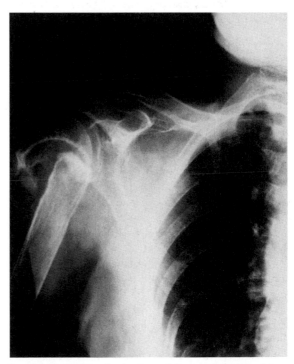

Fig. 7.7 Non-union of a fracture of the surgical neck of the humerus. A pseudarthrosis has formed at the site of the fracture.

Compound fractures, in which there was soft tissue damage and an open wound, were treated by immediate amputation, whereas **simple fractures**, which had intact skin, were not. The reason for this heroic approach was the scourge of infection, particularly tetanus. Without antibiotics or a proper understanding of the management of infection, patients with contaminated wounds often died and amputation was an attractive alternative.

Potentially infected fractures can now be treated and immediate amputation is a thing of the past, but anaerobic bacteria are just as lethal as ever. Any fracture beneath a contaminated wound should be regarded as 'compound' in the ancient sense and treated energetically (pp. 132, 312).

Open and closed

Modern treatment of 'compound' fractures is so effective that the term is no longer applicable. Apart from this, fractures with intact skin can be far from 'simple' to treat and 'compound' may be confused with complicated, comminuted or multiple. 'Simple' and 'compound' have been replaced by '**closed**' and '**open**' but 'compound' is sometimes used to describe how the skin has been damaged (Fig. 7.8). A fracture in which the skin has been penetrated by a bone fragment from inside the leg is sometimes referred to as 'compound from within' to distinguish it from a true open fracture and to emphasize the potential danger.

Shape

Fractures can also be classified according to the shape of the fragments and this is helpful in deciding management (Fig. 7.9).

Transverse fractures are the result of a direct blow or a pure angular force applied to the bone. The shape of the bone ends helps transverse fractures to stay aligned more easily than fractures which do not fit together so neatly.

Oblique or spiral fractures. Most long bone fractures are caused by a violent twisting movement about the long axis of the bone rather than the sideways bending which causes a transverse fracture. A sharp twist to the leg while the foot is stuck in a rabbit hole produces a spiral fracture of the tibia, even if radiographs suggest that the fracture line is oblique. In fact, oblique fractures are rare and are almost always a radiological artefact.

The fragments of a spiral fracture are more difficult to balance against each other than the square end of a transverse fracture and are very unstable. The bone spikes damage blood vessels, nerves or skin and the tips of the spikes can themselves break off to produce a triangular fragment known as a 'butterfly' fragment.

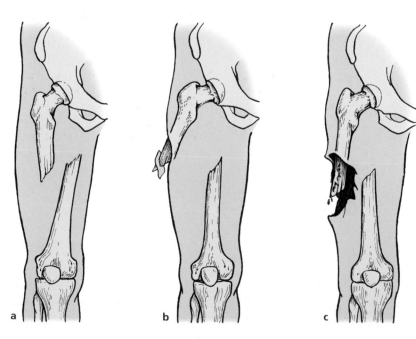

Fig. 7.8 Open and closed fractures: (a) closed fracture; (b) 'compound from within'; (c) an open fracture with contamination.

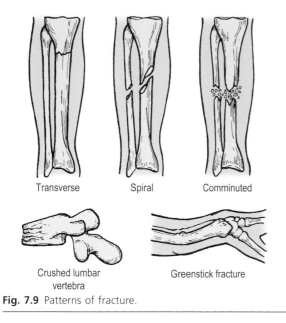

Transverse   Spiral   Comminuted

Crushed lumbar vertebra   Greenstick fracture

Fig. 7.9 Patterns of fracture.

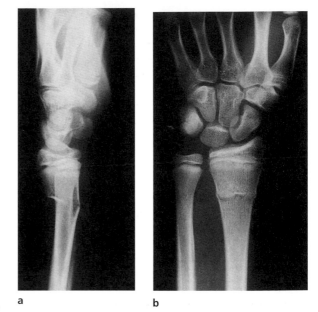

a   b

Fig. 7.10 A greenstick fracture of the radius with buckling of the dorsal cortex and a crack in the anterior cortex.

Comminuted. Applied to a fracture where the bone is splintered into more than two fragments, **comminuted** implies that exact anatomical reconstitution is difficult or impossible. Comminuted fractures occur most often in bone damaged by direct trauma.

Crush fractures. A fracture in which cancellous bone is squashed or crushed presents a difficult problem because there are no fragments left to manipulate back into position. If the fracture site is opened up and the cortex of the bone replaced in its normal position, a large cavity remains and the bone can only be restored to its normal shape by packing the space with bone graft or holding the sides of the cavity apart by external fixation.

Crush fractures are typically seen in the lumbar vertebrae, tibial plateaux and calcaneum.

Greenstick fractures. When a green stick breaks, it does not snap cleanly but bends so that one 'cortex' buckles while the other remains intact. If the force is very great, one side may snap while the other remains intact – try it. If a green stick fractured in this way is straightened it bounces back slightly but will not hold its correct position.

Fractures of long bones in children behave in the same way. The compressed cortex first buckles to produce a 'buckle' fracture. If the force continues, the cortex under tension will fracture (Fig. 7.10). Because of the resilience of the bone, reduction is only possible if the fracture is made complete or if

three-point pressure (p. 127) is applied. Fortunately, fractures in children remodel well enough to restore the normal anatomy and the deformity of most greenstick fractures can be accepted.

Mechanism of injury

Fractures can be caused in several ways (Fig. 7.11).

Direct violence

Bones can be broken by a direct blow and many patterns are seen. A sharp blow on the front of the knee may shatter the patella into many small fragments held together by soft tissue, like a boiled sweet broken in its wrapper (p. 254), but the fragments of a tibia fractured in a road traffic accident will be widely separated.

Indirect violence

More fractures are caused by indirect violence than direct violence. In this type of trauma, usually a twisting injury, no violence is applied to the site of the fracture itself. Open fractures are therefore uncommon, although the bone fragments can penetrate the skin from inside, making the fracture 'compound from within'.

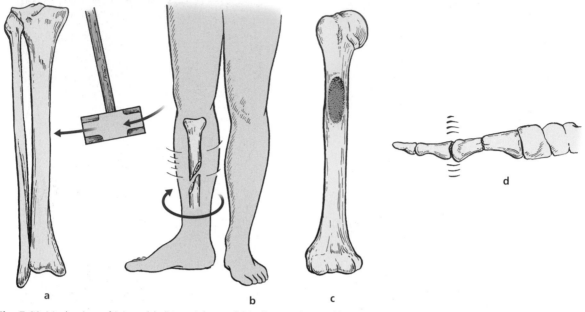

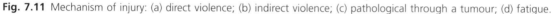

Fig. 7.11 Mechanism of injury: (a) direct violence; (b) indirect violence; (c) pathological through a tumour; (d) fatigue.

Pathological fractures

Pathological fractures occur through abnormally weak bone. Tumours, cysts and osteoporotic bone are common sites of pathological fractures (Fig. 7.12).

Fatigue fractures

Repeated small bending stresses will break any material (Fig. 7.13), including bone. The commonest example is a fracture of the second metatarsal in young adults who walk excessive distances. Classically, military recruits suffered this injury after route marches and the fracture is still known in English as a 'march fracture' and in French as '*pied du jeune soldat*'. **Fatigue fractures** are also seen in the tibiae of long-distance runners and hurdlers, and in the pars interarticularis of fast bowlers and javelin throwers.

Other terms (Fig. 7.14)

Undisplaced fractures

The fragments in an undisplaced fracture are in almost anatomical position and manipulative reduction is not required.

Impacted fractures

If cancellous bone is compressed in its long axis the two bone ends are so firmly thrust together that the fracture is stable unless the fragments are pulled apart. On a radiograph, the impacted bone is seen as an area of increased bone density – the opposite of a normal transradiant fracture line, and easily missed. Occasionally, impacted fractures become disimpacted after a few days, producing a troublesome deformity and a difficult clinical problem that requires careful explanation to the patient.

Segmental fractures

Segmental fractures are those in which a long bone is broken in two places, creating a large free segment of bone that is not attached to the rest of the skeleton. The free fragment is difficult to hold without internal fixation.

Stable fractures

A stable fracture is one in which the two bones are lying in a position from which they are unlikely to move. Stable fractures are often undisplaced but some are stable even though the bone is misshapen.

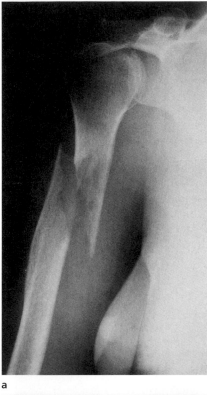

a

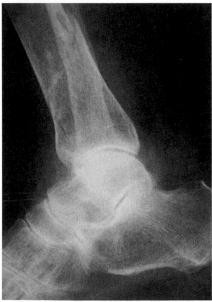

b

Fig. 7.12 Pathological fracture (a) through a metastasis in the humerus; (b) of the tibia through porotic bone.

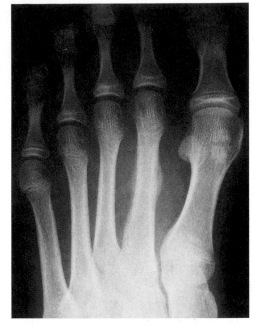

Fig. 7.13 Healed fatigue fracture through the second metatarsal – a 'march fracture'.

Complicated fractures

A **complicated** fracture is one that has a complication, such as infection or vascular damage. The term is seldom used but must be distinguished from compound and comminuted.

Multiple fractures

This term is applied when there are several separate fractures in the same patient. It is not to be confused with a comminuted or compound fracture.

Epiphyseal injury

Injury to the epiphyses of growing bone can cause severe deformity in later life if a bony bridge forms across the fracture site and prevents growth on one side of the bone.

The following five patterns of injury (Fig. 7.15) were described by Harris and Salter:

1. A fracture along the epiphyseal line.

2. Separation of the epiphysis with a triangular fragment of shaft attached to it (Fig. 7.16).

3. Fracture of the epiphysis, part of it remaining attached to the shaft.

101

4. A fracture line passing through both epiphysis and shaft.

5. A crushing injury (Fig. 7.17). This is difficult to recognize at the time of injury, either clinically or radiologically. This type of injury is more commonly associated with later growth arrest or retardation.

Students often have difficulty in accurately describing fractures seen on a radiograph. As already mentioned, there are a number of terms used and these can be confusing. You might find it useful to imagine that you are describing the radiograph to someone on the other end of a telephone line and they obviously do not have the advantage of looking at the film. You cannot, therefore, point at the fracture or the bone and instead you have to have a method of accurate description.

A useful method is to go through the following steps:

1. This is an X-ray of . . . (and describe which bone and which patient).

2. There is a . . . (transverse/oblique/spiral/convoluted/segmental/greenstick, etc. type of fracture).

3. Of the . . . part of bone (e.g. midshaft of the tibia).

You should then describe the degree of displacement or the angulation of the distal segment.

You will not be able to state with certainty from looking at the film whether the fracture is open or closed, but this will be readily apparent when you examine the injury in detail.

Complications

As elsewhere, the complications of fractures and soft tissue injuries can be classified in two ways:

1. Immediate – within a few hours
   Early – within the first few weeks
   Late – months and years later.

2. Local
   General.

Immediate complications

- Haemorrhage.
- Damage to arteries.
- Damage to surrounding soft tissues.

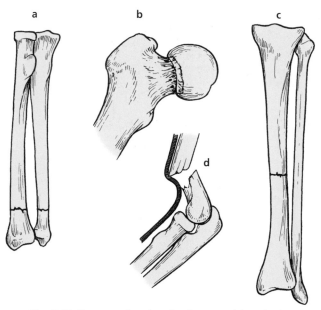

Fig. 7.14 Terms used to describe fractures: (a) undisplaced; (b) impacted; (c) stable; (d) fracture with complications.

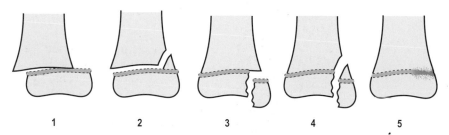

Fig. 7.15 Harris and Salter classification of epiphyseal injuries: (1) epiphyseal slip only; (2) fracture through the epiphyseal plate with a triangular fragment of shaft attached to the epiphysis; (3) fracture through the epiphysis extending to the epiphyseal plate; (4) fracture through the epiphysis and shaft crossing the epiphyseal plate; (5) obliteration of the epiphyseal plate.

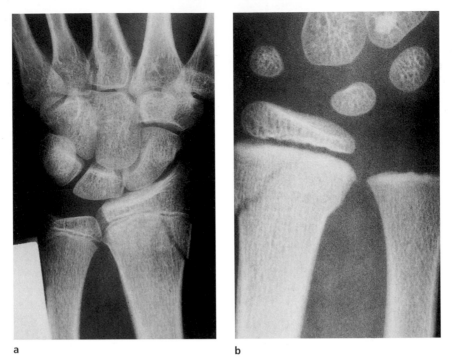

a   b

Fig. 7.16 A type 2 Harris and Salter fracture: (a) of the lower radial epiphysis; (b) with the slight variation of a greenstick buckle on the intact cortex.

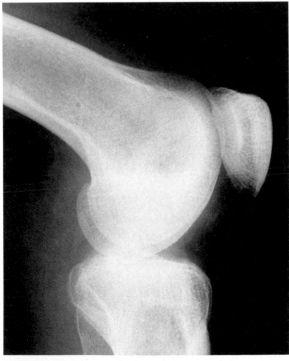

Fig. 7.17 Growth arrest in the anterior part of the upper tibial epiphysis following trauma.

Table 7.1 Blood loss from common fractures

Units (litres) lost		
1–3 (0.5–1.5)	2–4 (1–2.5)	3–5 (1.5–3)
Tibia	Femur	Pelvis
Ankle	Knee	Hip
Elbow	Shoulder	
Forearm	Humerus	

Haemorrhage

Bones are vascular structures and bleed when they are broken. Apart from blood lost from the bone itself, the sharp ends of the bone can damage the surrounding muscle or the blood vessels, and severe blood loss can occur into the soft tissues (Table 7.1).

The normal blood volume is about 5 litres or 8 units, and serious problems occur if more than one-third of the blood volume is lost from the circulation. From this, it follows that patients with two fractured femora or a fractured pelvis can go into

103

hypovolaemic shock or exsanguinate unless prompt action is taken. It is possible for a patient to bleed to death from a fracture without a drop of blood leaving the body.

Damage to arteries

> ### The arteries most commonly damaged at the moment of injury are:
>
> - The middle meningeal artery in temporoparietal skull fractures.
> - The brachial artery in supracondylar fractures of the humerus in children.
> - The popliteal artery in fractures and dislocations at the knee.
> - The aorta in fractures of the 4th and 5th thoracic vertebrae.
> - The femoral artery in fractures of the femur.

Damage to surrounding structures

> ### Serious problems can also arise from damage to neighbouring structures:
>
> - *Broken rib* – perforated lung – pneumothorax.
> - *Fractured sternum* – ruptured aorta – exsanguination.
> - *Broken ribs* – ruptured liver – exsanguination.
> - *Broken neck* – paraplegia with paralysis of phrenic nerve (C3, 4, 5) – asphyxia.
> - *Broken skull* – brain damage.
> - *Fractured face or mandible* – obstructed airway – suffocation.

Viscera. Complications also arise from damage to the surrounding viscera and a complete list would be endless. Only by awareness can potential complications be anticipated and avoided.

Early complications

- Wound infection.
- Fat embolism.
- Shock lung.
- Chest infection.
- Disseminated intravascular coagulation.
- Exacerbation of generalized illness.
- Compartment syndrome.

Wound infection

Wound infection from open fractures can lead to septicaemia and tetanus or gas gangrene from anaerobic infection.

Fat embolism

Fat embolism is an uncommon complication which leads to hypoxia from pulmonary insufficiency. The likelihood of developing fat embolism syndrome is not proportional to the severity of the injury and death can occur from an apparently straightforward transverse fracture of the tibia with little displacement. At postmortem examination, the alveoli are found to be crammed with small fat globules.

Cause. Two mechanisms have been suggested. The most obvious is direct embolization of fat globules from the fracture site, but this is too simple an explanation. The alternative is that circulating triglycerides split into glycerol and fat, generating many small particles of circulating fat. Whatever the cause, the hypoxia of fat embolism syndrome is a serious problem and there is no effective prophylaxis.

Clinical features. These are as follows:

1. The patient shows signs of hypoxia, including a change of mood, drowsiness and eventually loss of consciousness.
2. There is tachypnoea.
3. Petechiae are seen.

Investigations. These reveal that:

1. The arterial PO_2 is low.
2. Chest radiographs show patchy consolidation (Fig. 7.18).
3. The platelet count is low.
4. Serum lipase is raised.
5. Fat globules may be present in the urine.

Treatment. Once established, oxygen is the mainstay of treatment, and assisted ventilation may be required. Systemic and intratracheal steroids may be useful.

Shock lung

Shock lung, also known as wet lung or adult respiratory distress syndrome, can follow slight fluid overload and is made worse if there is any damage to the lungs, aspiration into the lung or overtransfusion. Oedema and electrolyte retention secondary to the trauma also contribute to the adult

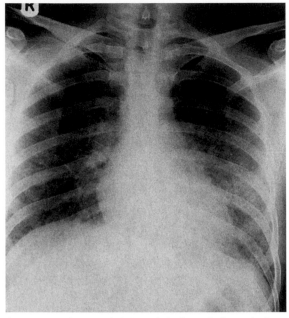

Fig. 7.18 Patchy consolidation of the lungs in fat embolism.

respiratory distress syndrome, described in more detail on page 173.

Treatment is by oxygen and ventilation. Do not over-transfuse with crystalloids!

Chest infection

Chest infection can be fatal in the elderly patient or patients with shock lung. Early mobilization and vigorous chest physiotherapy are the best prophylaxis.

Diffuse intravascular coagulation

Diffuse intravascular coagulation (DIC) can follow any injury and is due to a disturbance of the clotting mechanism. The help of the haematologist is needed in treatment, which may require fresh frozen plasma or platelets, and heparin.

Exacerbation of generalized illness in unfit patients

Diabetes, chest disease, coronary insufficiency and any other pre-existing problem can be exacerbated by a fracture.

Compartment syndrome

See page 112.

Infection

Orthopaedic textbooks of the 19th century describe infections of closed fractures, presumably from a bacteraemia, with the patients dying of septicaemia. This complication is, thankfully, rarely seen in modern times.

Late complications

- Deformity.
- Osteoarthritis of adjacent or distant joints.
- Aseptic necrosis.
- Traumatic chondromalacia.
- Reflex sympathetic dystrophy.

Late complications include malunion, non-union and delayed union, which are dealt with elsewhere (pp. 96–97).

Deformity

Deformity due to malunion may require late correction. Angular deformities greater than 5° can cause degenerative arthritic changes in the joints above and below the fracture. When treating a broken bone it is important, therefore, not to accept an angular deformity unless there is a real possibility that the fracture will remodel. Patients less than 9 years of age with a deformity close to the growth plate and in the axis of joint movement may remodel the fracture over a period of 1–2 years but remodelling in other planes, and in older patients, is much less satisfactory.

Deformities can be corrected by an osteotomy with fixation of the bone or by angular corrections using external fixators and bone lengthening techniques (p. 82). These limb-lengthening techniques can also be used to correct shortening as a result of bone loss, etc.

Where there is a large bony defect or an established non-union, bone can be grown across the defect to unite with the distal bone segment (bone transport). This technique of distraction in healthy bone, transportation of normal bone across the defect and subsequent union to the distal segment has been performed using a ring fixator or a conventional external fixator frame. Slow angular corrections using a circular frame can realign the limb in three planes at the same time. A conventional external fixator applied to the side of the bone alone may only correct the rotational abnormality in two planes at best.

Osteoarthritis of adjacent joints

Joint surfaces broken at the time of the fracture are much more likely to develop osteoarthritis than is an intact joint because of abnormal mechanical wear on the rough joint surfaces.

Osteoarthritis of distant joints

The joint surface does not have to be broken for osteoarthritis to develop (Fig. 7.19). If there is a malunion of the tibia, excessive load will be taken by both the knee and the ankle, and this causes early degenerative change. The same mechanism damages distant joints. If the leg is short after a fracture, the patient will walk with a tilt to one side, compensated for by a curve in the spine. This causes excessive wear on the facet joints on the side opposite the fracture and degenerative osteoarthritis will follow.

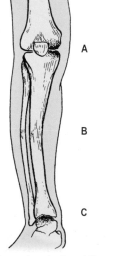

Fig. 7.19 Complications of malunion: (*A*) osteoarthritis of the knee; (*B*) deformity at the fracture site; (*C*) osteoarthritis of the ankle.

Aseptic necrosis (avascular necrosis)

If the fracture interrupts the blood supply to bone the affected bone dies, the bone collapses, the joint is destroyed and the patient develops a stiff and painful joint.

Aseptic necrosis often takes 2 years to develop, and it cannot be excluded until then. This is important if the injury is the subject of litigation. If a patient with an excellent result 12 months after injury is reassured that there has been a perfect recovery and settles the claim on this basis, he or she will be very disappointed if aseptic necrosis develops 12 months later.

Aseptic necrosis is common in bones that derive most of their blood supply from the medullary cavity rather than the surrounding soft tissues or periosteum. Three bones are particularly susceptible (Fig. 7.20):

- *The femoral head* following a femoral neck fracture.
- *The scaphoid* – the proximal pole of the scaphoid, because the blood supply of the scaphoid often enters through the distal pole.
- *The head of the talus*, because the blood supply enters through the sinus tarsi and the neck of the talus. If the neck of the talus is broken, aseptic necrosis of the body will occur.

Radiologically, the affected bone appears denser than the surrounding bone for three reasons:

- *Bone collapse*, which packs the calcified tissue into a smaller area.
- *Disuse osteoporosis* – because there is no blood supply the calcium cannot be removed from the dead bone, but the surrounding bone suffers disuse osteoporosis and is decalcified. This makes the living bone appear denser on the radiograph.
- *Calcium deposition* – calcium salts from the extracellular fluid are deposited on the dead bone, as they are on any dead or foreign material.

Traumatic chondromalacia

Articular cartilage may be damaged by a blow that leaves the bone intact. The articular cartilage softens and eventually disintegrates. The patient is aware of pain and crepitus, which may take as long as 2 years to develop. Once established, traumatic chondro-

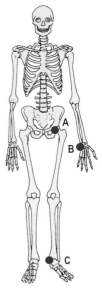

Fig. 7.20 Common sites of aseptic necrosis: (*A*) femoral head; (*B*) scaphoid; (*C*) talus.

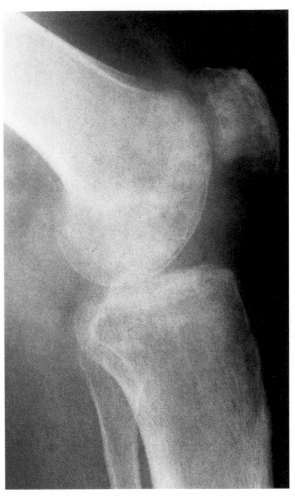

Fig. 7.21 Reflex sympathetic dystrophy around the knee. Note the patchy osteoporosis in the patella and femoral condyles.

malacia is likely to be followed by osteoarthritis. Injuries to the patella are the commonest cause of traumatic chondromalacia.

Reflex sympathetic dystrophy

Reflex sympathetic dystrophy is a curious condition similar to causalgia. It affects bone and can follow any injury, particularly a fracture. The clinical features are that the skin feels cold, goes blue or changes colour, and the limb is excruciatingly tender. The patient cannot move the limb normally and in severe cases the skin is thin and shiny. Radiologically, there is patchy osteoporosis (Fig. 7.21).

The mechanism of reflex sympathetic dystrophy is unclear but it is probably due to a perversion of the sensory fibres which interpret temperature change as a painful stimulus. This over-activity of the sympathetic nerves at the wrist is called Sudeck's atrophy or algodystrophy.

Injuries to joints

Three grades of joint injury occur
(Fig. 7.22):

1. Subluxation (partial dislocation).
2. Dislocation.
3. Fracture dislocation.

Subluxation

Joints that are subluxed, or where there is partial contact between joint surfaces, seldom need active treatment, and normal stability usually returns when the periarticular tissues have healed. If symptoms of instability follow, the joint may need to be stabilized.

Dislocation

Joints that have been completely dislocated (no contact between joint surfaces) must be treated more energetically than those that have subluxed. The joint must be reduced and immobilized until the soft tissues have healed, and some joints, such as the knee, may need open repair.

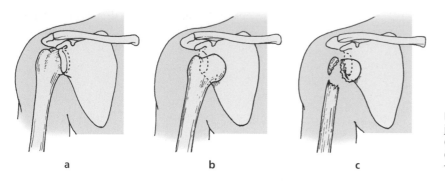

Fig. 7.22 Types of injury to a joint: (a) subluxation; (b) dislocation; (c) fracture dislocation.

Complications. Dislocations may be followed by recurrent dislocation (recurrent dislocation of the shoulder, p. 365, and patella, p. 426), aseptic necrosis, chronic instability or osteoarthrosis if the joint surfaces are damaged.

Fracture dislocation

Dislocations accompanied by a fracture around the joint often heal more soundly than a simple dislocation because bone unites more soundly than ligament, but early management is more difficult. The bony fragment may become jammed in the joint, or the joint may be very unstable because bony congruity is lost.

Treatment often involves fixation of the bony fragment; management is described in the appropriate sections.

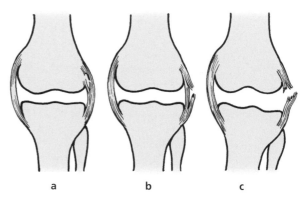

Fig. 7.23 Grades of ligament injury: (a) sprain; (b) partial tear; (c) complete rupture.

Injuries to ligaments

> **Three grades of ligament injury are recognized** (Fig. 7.23):
>
> 1. Sprain, in which stability is maintained.
> 2. Partial rupture, in which there is some loss of stability but some fibres remain intact.
> 3. Complete rupture, with loss of both stability and continuity of the ligament.

Sprains

A sprain, or strain, is a partial tear of a ligament or joint capsule which does not make the joint unstable. The site of the tear is tender, there may be bruising, and the physical signs are similar to those of an undisplaced fracture.

Sprains are treated symptomatically but the joint must be protected from stress until healing is complete.

Partial rupture

Partially ruptured ligaments can be treated conservatively if it is certain that the rupture is incomplete. Cast immobilization for 6 weeks may be required but rest and analgesics are usually adequate. Recurrence is common.

Complete rupture

Ruptured ligaments do not heal soundly even if they are accurately repaired because the scar tissue that forms at the site of repair is never as tough as the original. Surgical repair is often attempted but conservative management may be equally effective.

Injuries to soft tissues

Blood vessels

> **Blood vessels can be damaged in four ways** (Fig. 7.24):
>
> 1. Division.
> 2. Stretching.
> 3. Spasm.
> 4. Crushing.

Complete division

Vessels can be completely divided by penetrating metal objects or the sharp ends of bones. This is a comparatively rare cause of vascular damage.

Stretching

If the deforming force continues after the bone is broken, the blood vessels and other soft tissues will be stretched. This can cause intimal damage, which may be complicated by intravascular clotting, and is common near the elbow and the knee.

Spasm

Spasm of blood vessels can follow intimal damage and is said to be especially common in supracondylar fractures of the humerus in children. Painting the artery with papaverine may relieve the spasm but any intimal damage must also be treated.

Crushing

Direct violence causes intimal damage and sometimes ruptures or severs the vessel completely.

Nerves

Neurapraxia, axonotmesis and neurotmesis are well known. Real-life injuries can seldom be classified so neatly.

> **Injuries to nerves**
>
> - *Neurapraxia* – transient loss of function caused by outside pressure. Early recovery.
> - *Axonotmesis* – loss of function due to more severe compression but without loss of continuity of the neurone. Recovery in weeks or months.
> - *Neurotmesis* – division of the nerve, no neural continuity. No recovery unless repaired.

Like blood vessels, nerves can be damaged by division, stretching or crushing, but most direct injuries to the nerve involve a combination of all three.

Only if the nerve is cleanly divided on a piece of glass or metal is it reasonable to attempt a precise

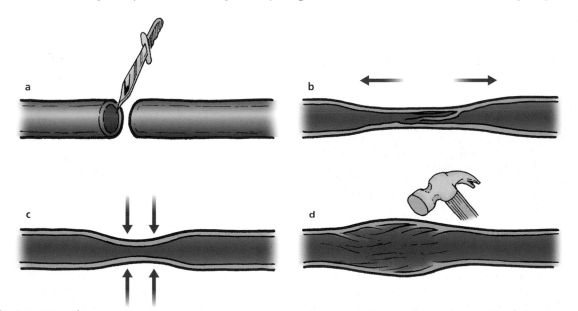

Fig. 7.24 Types of injury to blood vessel: (a) complete division; (b) stretching, with intimal flap; (c) spasm; (d) soft tissue damage to the wall.

surgical repair immediately after injury because of the problems of healing (p. 141). The common sites of damage to peripheral nerves are shown in Figure 3.24.

Ischaemia

Ischaemia also impairs nerve function; gradual loss of sensibility involving a whole limb should suggest the possibility of ischaemia. Compartment syndromes or direct pressure are the commonest causes.

Muscle

Muscle can be damaged in four ways:

1. Crushing.
2. Laceration.
3. Ischaemia.
4. Ectopic ossification.

Crushing

Muscle crushed by direct force heals with fibrous tissue, which shortens the muscle and restricts joint movement.

Laceration

Muscles divided transversely will not hold sutures well enough to stop muscular contraction pulling the edges apart. Fascia surrounding a muscle can be repaired, but the risk of a compartment syndrome (p. 112) makes this unwise.

Ischaemia

Muscle is very vascular and its blood supply is critical. If the blood supply is impaired by arterial damage, a compartment syndrome or a tight plaster, the ischaemic muscle is replaced by fibrous tissue which contracts and pulls the associated joints into an unnatural position. This is a real problem in fracture management.

Ectopic ossification

Ossification in the fracture haematoma is usually confined to the area around the bone, where it is most useful. Sometimes, however, ossification can occur in haematomas within the muscle belly, where it limits joint movement (Fig. 7.25). The quadriceps is a common site. The ectopic bone is sometimes gradually absorbed but, if it is not, severe restriction of the joint movement is likely. The bone can form again and excising it from the muscle belly is seldom helpful.

Bone can also form around joints well away from muscle (Fig. 7.26). A large staghorn of bone may develop at the lower end of the humerus, its spikes wrapped tightly around vessels and nerves. The fragment can be removed and some movement restored but the operation is technically difficult.

Both these types of ectopic ossification must be distinguished from myositis ossificans progressiva, a disease of unknown origin in which many muscles undergo ossification, and from the ossification seen around the joints of paralysed limbs.

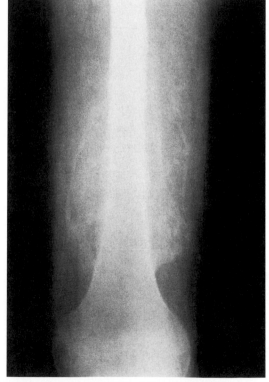

Fig. 7.25 Ectopic ossification within muscle following fracture.

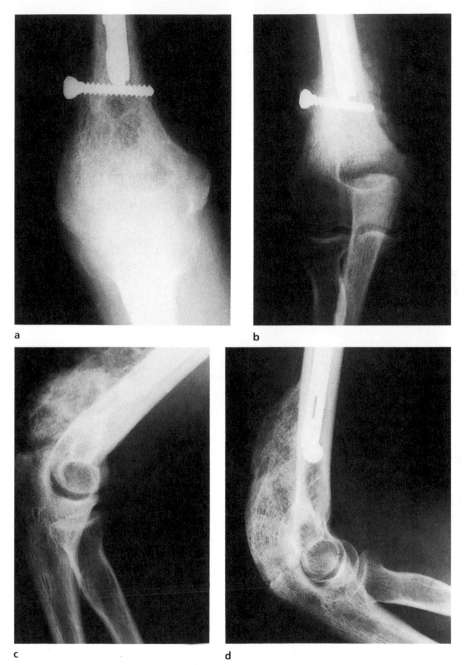

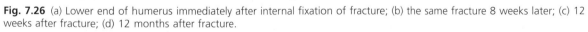

Fig. 7.26 (a) Lower end of humerus immediately after internal fixation of fracture; (b) the same fracture 8 weeks later; (c) 12 weeks after fracture; (d) 12 months after fracture.

Skin

Skin can be damaged by:

- Direct trauma.
- Stretching.
- Degloving.
- Undermining at operation.

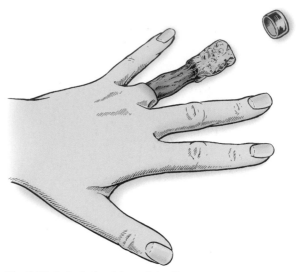

Fig. 7.27 A degloving injury of the finger.

Direct trauma

If a limb is hit hard enough to break bone, the skin at the point of impact is bound to be damaged. Fortunately, areas of skin damaged by direct trauma are small but they are always near the fracture site and make wound closure difficult.

Stretching

Like other soft tissues in a broken limb, skin is stretched at the moment of impact. The damaged skin may die but more often the stretching causes a transient ischaemia that leads to 'fracture blisters'.

Fracture blisters form within 48 h of an injury and complicate internal fixation operations because they are a potential source of infection.

Degloving

If a limb is caught firmly and pulled violently at the moment of impact, the skin may be peeled back over the bones for a considerable distance, perhaps over the whole leg or forearm (Fig. 7.27). These injuries are called 'degloving' injuries but the same problems can arise just by the skin being stripped off the underlying tissues without being rolled back like a glove. This type of degloving is common in fractures of the tibia and fibula.

Treatment. Degloved skin is dead and should be replaced as if it were a free skin graft. If the replaced skin does not survive, the problem of skin cover is best dealt with by a plastic surgeon.

Operation

Skin that has survived the original injury may be damaged at operation, particularly if it is stripped unnecessarily widely from the underlying tissues or stitched too tightly.

If skin does not come together easily, stitch it loosely and close the wound by delayed primary suture (p. 140).

Viscera

Soft organs, such as liver, spleen, heart, lungs and brain, can all be damaged by direct trauma. This possibility must never be forgotten. The ways in which soft viscera can be damaged are too numerous to classify.

Compartment syndromes

Any injured tissue swells and must have room to expand, because if there is no room for expansion the tissue will become ischaemic. The different compartments are described on page 38.

A similar problem arises if limbs or digits are crushed. Fingers caught between rollers, for example, will be crushed and the skin split (Fig. 7.28). If the skin is stitched meticulously together over the soft tissues, the soft tissues will die. It is much better to leave such wounds open and elevate the limb to encourage the swelling to subside more rapidly.

With increase in the pressure in a tight fascial compartment there can be impairment of venous drainage and, ultimately, occlusion of the arterial input. This alteration in the perfusion of the muscles and nerves results in cell death and, in the case of

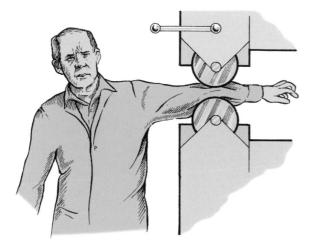

Fig. 7.28 Roller injury. Pressure on the arm between rollers can cause extensive soft tissue damage without fracture.

muscle, fibrosis on healing. This fibrosis causes contractions of the muscle.

Clinical features

The symptoms and signs of an ischaemic limb are:

- Pain, greater than expected.
- Pallor of the limb, usually patchy.
- The limb is cool.
- Pulses are absent.
- Movement, particularly passive extension, is exceedingly painful.

Treatment

The fascial compartments and the skin must be divided so that the muscle can swell. The wound is left open until swelling has subsided, when it may be closed or the defect grafted. The management of the different compartment syndromes is described in the chapters on the areas affected.

Case reports

These three cases represent the management of this potentially limb threatening condition.

Patient A

A 23-year-old motorcyclist was involved in a road traffic accident in which he was hit from the side, sustaining a transverse fracture of the left mid-shaft tibia and fibula. He had no other injuries and was taken by ambulance to the accident and emergency department.

When seen there by the casualty officer he was noted to have a swollen leg and the obvious fracture on both clinical examination and radiographs. Because the fracture was relatively undisplaced his leg was immobilized in an above-knee plaster of Paris backslab and he was admitted to the orthopaedic ward, where he remained overnight. No further observations were made and on review the following morning it was noted by the nursing staff that he had required large quantities of opioid analgesics and was writhing around in great pain and discomfort.

On clinical review it was clear that he had pain on passive extension of the ankle plantarflexors and had started to develop an area of dysaesthesia over the web space between the great and second toe. A clinical diagnosis of an acute compartment syndrome was made; he was taken to theatre immediately and a large anterior lateral fasciotomy was performed. This confirmed necrotic muscle in the anterior lateral compartment, which required excision. The tibia was subsequently stabilized but unfortunately for the motorcyclist he had lost the vast majority of the muscles over the front of the shin, resulting in an inability to dorsiflex his foot thereafter.

Patient B

A 55-year-old man sustained relatively minor trauma to the front of the left shin following a fall. He noted increasing pain and discomfort over the shin and, despite analgesics, this failed to settle.

He was referred to the accident and emergency department, where he was subsequently admitted to the hospital with a painful, swollen leg. It was clear on medical review that he was on warfarin for a cardiac abnormality and, when tested, the INR was significantly elevated.

On clinical examination it was noted that the anterior lateral musculature was very swollen and he had marked pain and discomfort with passive flexion of the ankle. He was monitored reasonably closely with circulatory checks and review of the distal neurology. This confirmed a palpable pulse and normal neurology.

The swelling failed to subside and the warfarin anticoagulation was stopped. This took approximately 3 days to settle and during this period of time the patient continued to have significant pain and dysfunction. The decision was then taken to do a fasciotomy and this confirmed necrosis of the muscles as a result of a large bleed. The vast majority of the muscles were excised, leaving a weakness of ankle dorsiflexion and a large scar, which required subsequent correction with plastic surgery.

Patient C

A 30-year-old rugby player sustained a twisting injury to his right lower leg and was admitted to the orthopaedic ward with a spiral fracture of the mid-third of the tibia.

Because of concerns about compartment pressure, a compartment pressure monitor was inserted as soon as he was admitted and this confirmed a raised pressure. At this stage he had normal distal perfusion and sensibility. The decision was taken to operate immediately and the bone was stabilized using an intramedullary unreamed nail, and a wide fasciotomy was performed.

At the time of the procedure the muscle was slightly 'dusky' in appearance but viable. This patient went on to make a good recovery, although he had to return to theatre to have the fasciotomy scars closed secondarily.

Moral

Compartment syndromes can be devastating for the patient. There should be a high awareness of this by both nursing and medical staff. These syndromes are not always associated with high energy trauma and in those cases where there could be a reason for an increase in the intracompartmental pressure (for example, bleeding) this can easily happen with a relatively trivial trauma.

Early recognition and appropriate treatment with a fasciotomy to relieve the intracompartmental pressure avoids muscle necrosis and therefore long-term dysfunction.

Chapter | 8 |

Immediate care and major incidents

By the end of this chapter you should:
- Appreciate the rationale for a systematic early assessment of the trauma patient in a structured manner.
- Be conversant with major incidents / disasters and how to cope with multiple casualties.

Immediate management of multiple injuries

The management of a patient with multiple injuries depends upon an organized and disciplined approach. The most spectacular injury is seldom the most dangerous while the one that goes unseen can kill the patient. If the 'ABC' routine below is followed, life-threatening conditions will be dealt with first and undiagnosed injuries kept to a minimum.

Immediate action

A – Airway.
B – Bleeding.
C – Circulation.

Check the airway

An obstructed airway causes death most rapidly and must be dealt with first. Complete obstruction of the airway is easily recognized but partial obstruction causes a gradually increasing hypoxia which can go unnoticed until the partial pressure of oxygen (PO_2) falls to critical levels and the patient loses consciousness. *Always check the airway.*

The airway can be obstructed by blood, vomit, broken teeth or dentures, soft tissue swelling around injuries to the neck or larynx, or facial fractures (Fig. 8.1). The first step in resuscitation is to check that the mouth and pharynx are clear (Fig. 8.2).

Respiratory failure can also be caused by chest injuries such as a pneumothorax or flail chest, even if the airway is clear. Pain can also inhibit breathing, and respiratory failure can follow cervical spine fractures above C3 because the phrenic nerve (C3, 4, 5) is damaged, but this complication is so serious that the patients seldom reach hospital. Chest movement and respiratory rate should be checked regularly.

Endotracheal or nasotracheal intubation, or even tracheostomy may be needed to establish an airway.

Stop bleeding

Bleeding is best stopped by external pressure with a thumb or fist over the bleeding point, but a tourniquet may be needed to control bleeding from a limb. Whenever a tourniquet is used, the time of

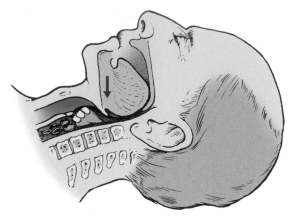

Fig. 8.1 Obstruction of the airway. The tongue, broken dentures, blood, vomit or a fractured mandible can all obstruct the airway.

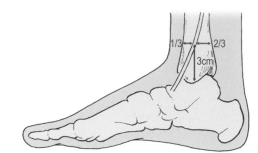

Fig. 8.3 Site for saphenous cut-down. The long saphenous vein lies 3 cm above the medial malleolus, one-third of the way between the anterior and posterior surfaces of the tibia.

Restore blood volume

A large intravenous infusion line should be set up as soon as the airway is established and bleeding controlled. Entering a vein is difficult in the deeply shocked or hypovolaemic patient because the vessels will have collapsed. If the usual veins in the forearm cannot be entered, try the cephalic or external jugular. If these cannot be entered either, cut down onto a vein. The long saphenous vein at the ankle is convenient and is reliably found 3 cm above the tip of the medial malleolus and one-third of the way back from the anterior edge of the tibia (Fig. 8.3).

In a well-organized accident department there will be enough people to do all these things at once while the patient's clothes are removed – it is better to cut clothing off rather than pull it over limbs that may be fractured.

A skilled resuscitation team can establish an airway, arrest bleeding, remove the patient's clothes and set up an intravenous line within minutes of the patient entering the resuscitation unit.

Monitoring and complete examination

When these steps have been taken, the resuscitation team is in control of the situation and less immediate problems can be dealt with.

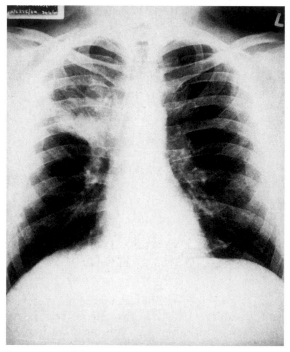

Fig. 8.2 Consolidation of the right upper lobe after inhalation of a foreign body by an unconscious patient.

application must be recorded carefully and the tourniquet released after proper control of the haemorrhage has been achieved, or once every hour, to avoid gangrene.

If there is venous bleeding from a limb, lift the bleeding point above the level of the heart. This will stop the bleeding and improve blood pressure.

When immediate action is complete:
1. Begin charts.
2. Examine the patient completely.
3. Record ECG.
4. Set up central venous pressure (CVP) line.
5. Check the patient again.
6. Notify appropriate specialists.
7. Grade injury.

Charts

Set up a record of the pulse rate, blood pressure, respiratory rate and neurological signs, including level of consciousness and pupil sizes, as soon as possible.

Complete examination

The entire patient should be inspected for wounds, including the back. If there is any possibility of a spinal injury the patient should be 'log rolled', until radiographs are available, to minimize the risk of displacing the fracture. The cervical spine should be protected at all times.

If this thorough inspection is not done very early, injuries will be missed. It is not only embarrassing but reprehensible to save the life of a patient and then find that he cannot work because of a malunited finger that needed only a few turns of adhesive strapping to achieve a perfect result.

Measure the wounds. Bruises and lacerations should be inspected, measured and recorded. Look particularly at the abdominal skin: bruising or imprints of clothing mean that there has been a violent blow to the abdomen and intra-abdominal bleeding should be suspected. Look also for signs of seat-belt bruising.

Examine every bone in the body. This does not take long. The superficial bones, including the skull and clavicle, can be felt with the fingers, the ribs and pelvis 'sprung' (p. 24), and long bones stressed. Fingers and toes can be checked by longitudinal pressure and suspicious areas examined radiologically.

Record ECG

ECG leads should be applied, if not done already, and the ECG displayed on a monitor.

CVP line

If there has been severe blood loss, set up a CVP line. The normal CVP is 4–8 cmH$_2$O and this level should be maintained. In some centres pulmonary capillary wedge pressure is preferred to monitor the restoration of blood volume.

Check the patient again

To be sure that there is no deterioration, check the patient again and again. Pulmonary contusion causing respiratory failure and hypotension from intra-abdominal bleeding may first be apparent at this stage.

Other specialties

If any injuries need specialist attention, the relevant specialists should be informed. Faciomaxillary surgeons, ophthalmic surgeons, neurosurgeons, thoracic surgeons and plastic surgeons may all be needed, as well as 'general' surgeons for the management of abdominal injuries.

Advanced trauma life support (ATLS)

Courses on advanced trauma life support are now mandatory for all surgical trainees and not just for those involved in immediate care. The courses teach internationally agreed techniques to a high standard and are very effective.

These courses advise the primary survey and the secondary survey. The primary survey means attending to the airway, breathing and circulation while ensuring no damage is done to the spinal column, etc. The secondary survey involves a full systematic review of all body parts and systems.

Grading

Several systems are used to grade the severity of injury and give a score that can be used to assess the prognosis. Calculate the scores and record them.

First aid at the scene of an accident

There is a tendency for doctors, but especially medical students, to try to save life at the scene of an accident rather than attend to practical matters. In practice, very few accident victims require urgent medical care, and those that do usually need equipment found only in an ambulance or accident department.

If you are the first person at the scene of an accident, with nobody to help, take the following steps:

Check the airway

Check the patient's airway and clear it if it is obstructed.

117

Feel the pulse

If the radial pulse cannot be felt, feel for the carotid.

Recovery position

If the patient is unconscious, place them in the recovery position but take special care of the spine if there is any possibility of spinal injury. Protect the cervical spine at all times.

Stop oncoming traffic

Stop traffic before it collides with the crashed vehicle(s) or the patient and send for help from police and ambulance services.

Treat the patient

This done, more time can be spent with the patient. Cover exposed bone with the cleanest material available, arrest bleeding and comfort the patient.

Do not be tempted to pull trapped patients out of cars, unless they are on fire, or start definitive treatment such as reducing fractures. Confirm that the emergency services are on the way, wait for the ambulance and give a clear account of events to the crew.

When the patient is in the ambulance, the first aider's task is done and it is neither necessary nor desirable to accompany the patient to hospital. Ambulance teams have great experience in dealing with road accidents and know their own equipment and routines well. They do not need help from a stranger, however gifted.

Trapped patients

If a road accident victim is trapped in a car, leave the individual there until the rescue services arrive. Access to the patient will be difficult because the doors of crashed vehicles are usually jammed and to drag an injured patient with broken limbs or a fractured spine through a broken window is only justified if there is a risk of fire. The rescuers should wear stout gloves to protect their own hands from lacerations on broken glass or torn metal.

If the engine compartment has been pushed backwards the patient may have broken legs and be pinned in the car by the steering wheel. The rescue service has the necessary equipment to cut the

window pillars and remove the roof of the car to give easy access to the patient (Fig. 8.4). The patient can then be secured to a support placed behind the back and lifted directly into the ambulance, if necessary after intubation and setting up an intravenous line (Fig. 8.5).

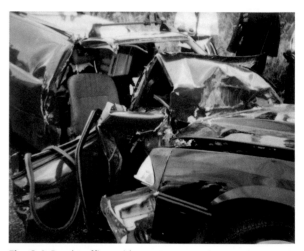

Fig. 8.4 Road traffic accident.

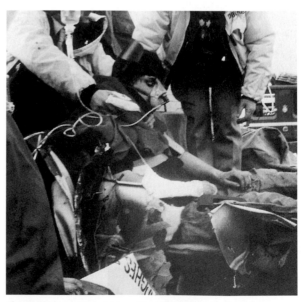

Fig. 8.5 Emergency rescue. An unconscious patient has an intravenous line and is receiving oxygen before being removed from the vehicle. The roof of the vehicle has been removed for access.

Medical rescue team

In many rural areas general practitioners operate accident rescue services to assist the ambulance crew. The general practitioner's car will have equipment to intubate the patient or set up an intravenous line before the ambulance arrives, and narcotics to provide analgesia while the patient is removed from the wreck.

Major disasters and major incidents

A major disaster is an event which requires an extraordinary mobilization of the emergency services (fire, police, ambulance), and a major incident is one which stretches the resources of the accident department and hospital. Not all major disasters are major incidents. Evacuating families after a flood may not generate even one patient, for example.

Major incident procedure

All accident departments have contingency plans for handling a major incident and carry out regular practice drills. As with the management of multiple injuries, success depends upon a well planned and disciplined approach.

The precise details of major incident routines vary from area to area but a typical plan would be as follows.

Designated hospital

The first people to know of a major incident are usually the police. It is they who initiate the major incident procedure routine and select the hospital to which the casualties will be sent, known as the designated hospital. Although criteria vary from area to area, 15 or more patients likely to require hospital treatment are usually enough to trigger the major incident procedure.

The major incident procedure cannot be instituted by concerned members of the public.

Notifying the hospital

The hospital is notified and the switchboard operators initiate the routine at the hospital, which involves almost every department. The medical records staff, portering staff, mortuary technicians,

security staff, administrators and nursing staff all have specific duties, and medical staff are only one part of the team.

Duties of individuals

Any member of staff likely to be involved in a major incident will have an action card which lists their duties and they will refer to this when summoned to take part in a major incident routine (Fig. 8.6).

Some of the duties might be as follows.

Medical Controller. There is always one doctor in charge of coordinating the medical services, usually the consultant in accident and emergency.

The consultant surgeon or consultant physician on call will go to a predetermined ward and create a certain number of beds (perhaps 20) to cope with the anticipated number of victims by discharging or transferring patients well enough to be moved.

The director of the accident service or senior orthopaedic surgeon takes charge of the accident department and allocates staff to other areas, but until then the senior doctor present takes charge. To avoid

ACTION CARD
INSTRUCTIONS IN THE EVENT OF A
MAJOR ACCIDENT ALL *MEDICAL STAFF*

1. When advised of a MAJOR INCIDENT, you are to report to the Accident Service and select an Action Card appropriate to your speciality, or as designated by the Co-ordinating Medical Officer.

2. If all Action Cards have been removed you are to take instruction from the Co-ordinating Medical Officer.

3. If you are not required for duties at that time you are requested to report to the Sisters Lounge adjacent to the hospital staff dining room and await further instructions.

TELEPHONES ARE TO BE KEPT CLEAR FOR INCOMING CALLS.

YOU ARE EXPECTED TO CARRY THIS CARD ON YOU AT ALL TIMES.

Fig. 8.6 Action card. A typical action card for medical staff who may be involved with a major incident. By kind permission of Cambridge Health Authority.

confusion and conflicting orders, the senior doctor wears a brightly coloured tabard, or sometimes a coloured hat for identification.

Theatre staff. All on-call nurses and operating department assistants go to the operating theatre and await instructions.

Medical records department. All casualties are issued with an emergency record number and a set of case notes. Special sets of records are kept available, with identifying bracelets to attach to the injured patients. In some areas, the recording of injured patients is undertaken by the police.

Medical staff. All available medical staff should go directly to the accident service and place themselves under the direction of the senior doctor. They will usually be given an action card appropriate to their grade.

Medical students. There is seldom any shortage of medical staff during a major incident, and a wealth of untrained individuals such as medical students can be a real handicap. By all means ask if there is anything that can be done but be prepared to do something mundane, such as acting as a runner carrying samples for the laboratory or helping to move patients.

Organization at the hospital

When patients arrive, they are assessed by medical staff and placed in one of three categories (Fig. 8.7):

1. Those requiring immediate and energetic treatment.
2. Those with minor injuries, or none at all.
3. Those with serious but non-urgent injuries who do not fit into either of the other categories.

This classification of patients is known as 'triage' and was devised by French military surgeons during the Napoleonic Wars. Although ancient, it is still the best way of handling large numbers of casualties. It is best done by senior surgeons.

Organization at the scene of the incident

Incident Control Officers. Events at the scene of the incident are under the direction of the Incident Control Officer (ICO), usually the senior police officer present, or the senior fire officer if the incident is a fire. Each service – Fire, Police and Ambulance – also has its own ICO at the scene.

Incident Medical Officer. The ICO will request the presence of an Incident Medical Officer (IMO) whenever there are casualties. An accident and emergency consultant from another hospital or a general practitioner from the accident rescue service, if one is available, are common choices for such tasks because they are not needed at the designated hospital. The IMO takes charge of assessing patients, preparing them for transfer to hospital and any treatment that may be required at the scene. The IMO is not responsible for the organization of rescue services, which remains with the ICO.

In some circumstances, the IMO will ask for a mobile surgical team to be sent to the scene of the incident. The mobile surgical team includes nurses and other staff, who take with them equipment kept ready in the accident department for such a request.

First- and second-line hospitals

It is unusual for there to be so many accident victims that the designated hospital cannot cope, but major incident routines include provision for this with a 'second-line' or back-up hospital, nominated if more than a certain number of patients (usually 30) is anticipated. No patients are sent to the second-line hospital until the full quota has gone to the designated hospital. Thereafter, all patients go to the second-line hospital and, if necessary, a third-line hospital when that is full.

Patients sent to the second-line hospital are usually more seriously injured than those sent to the designated hospital, because this receives patients most easily accessible and most easily moved.

Military surgery

Although only a few surgeons are involved in the treatment of battle injuries, the principles are important for all wound management because much of the surgery of warfare concerns the management of contaminated soft tissue injuries in fit young men, without the resources of a modern hospital.

On the conventional battlefield, wounds are usually contaminated with earth, and delay allows time for infection, particularly anaerobic infection, to become established. All such wounds are potentially lethal, which is why the old military surgeons treated open fractures by immediate amputation (see 'Simple and compound' fractures, p. 97).

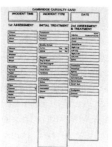

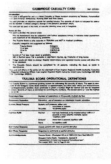

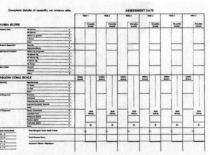

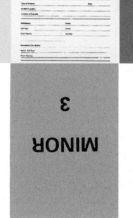

Fig. 8.7 Cambridge casualty card. One side carries a clinical record. The card can be folded so that the other side displays the state of the patient in a distinctive colour. The card is then placed in a plastic envelope and attached to the patient. By kind permission of Carl Wallin Consultancy Services.

Modern transport cuts the delay in treatment to a minimum and avoids some of these problems. A battle injury is usually treated first by the victim's friends, then by medical attendants near the place of injury, and the patient is then transferred to a simple hospital, called a field ambulance, a few miles away. If the injury is particularly serious, the patient will be evacuated to a base hospital, but there is still a considerable delay before the injured patient reaches a specialist surgeon with access to a well-equipped operating theatre.

In urban warfare, the position is different. Patients can be seen by specialist surgeons in ideal circumstances less than an hour from injury. However quickly the patient receives treatment, the mainstay in the management of gunshot wounds is still wide excision and delayed primary suture (p. 141).

Chapter | 9 |

Methods of managing trauma

By the end of this chapter you should:
- Understand and be able to discuss the various methods of management of skeletal trauma.
- Understand the rationale for these different methods of management and the reasons for the difference.
- Be aware of the complications of the various common injuries and their management.

Fractures

The principles of fracture management are:

1. Reduction of the fracture.
2. Immobilization of the fracture fragments long enough to allow union.
3. Rehabilitation of the soft tissues and joints.

Methods of reduction are:

1. Traction.
2. External splints/braces.
3. External fixation.
4. Internal fixation.

Some fractures, when seen, are not displaced and therefore do not require reduction. Others, however, will require reduction in order to keep the bones in the correct position.

Traction

Pulling on a broken limb draws the bones into line, just as a string of beads straightens when it is pulled

at each end. Muscular contraction will shorten any limb unless there is a bone to hold its ends apart and the traction must therefore be strong enough to overcome the muscle power, but not so strong that it holds the ends apart (Fig. 9.1).

Traction can be applied to the limb in a variety of ways.

Skeletal traction

Traction is applied to pins passed through the bone. Although metal pins passing straight through a limb may look unkind, they are more comfortable than skin traction, and allow substantial loads to be applied accurately to the bone itself. The commonest sites for the insertion of skeletal pins are the upper end of the tibia, the calcaneum, the distal femur or the olecranon, but traction can also be applied to the skull, pelvis and many other sites.

Two types of pin are in common use (Fig. 9.2). A *Steinmann pin* has a trocar point and smooth sides. Although easy to insert, it can slip sideways after being in position for a week or more, which is both uncomfortable and unhygienic. *Threaded pins*, such

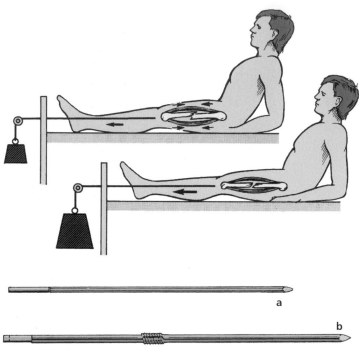

Fig. 9.1 Traction. Traction should be sufficient to pull the bones out to length and overcome local muscle contraction.

Fig. 9.2 Types of pin for traction: (a) Steinmann pin; (b) Denham pin with threads standing proud of the pin shaft.

as a *Denham pin*, have threads which grip the bone and prevent lateral slippage. Although slightly harder to insert, they are better in the long term.

> **Skeletal traction is easy to set up and manage, provided attention is paid to the following points:**
>
> 1. The pins should be drilled through the bone with a hand drill or T handle.
> 2. If the pin is inserted using local anaesthesia, the skin and periosteum must be carefully infiltrated at the points of entry and exit.
> 3. Never try to hammer the pin through the bone – this does not work and breaks the bone.
> 4. Keep the point of entry clean to avoid infection of the pin track but do not wind a bandage round the pin like a cleat: this causes skin necrosis.
> 5. Check whether the pin is threaded or smooth before removing it; smooth pins can be removed with a straight pull but a threaded pin must be unscrewed.
> 6. If the pin area is painful and the bone is tender to percussion, suspect a pin track infection.

Skin traction

Skin traction is applied by means of adhesive strapping stuck directly onto the skin and has many prac-

tical problems. The skin beneath the strapping becomes sweaty and rashes are common. The weight is applied to the bone indirectly via the soft tissues and these can be disrupted if too much weight is applied. The usual upper limit is 5 kg (12 lb). For these reasons, skin traction is really only suitable for children and as a temporary measure in adults until definitive treatment is instituted.

The mechanics of traction

The mechanics of traction are straightforward. Every force has an equal and opposite force; traction is no exception. The 'opposite' force to traction can be applied in three ways, described below.

Fixed traction with a splint. In the simplest form of fixed traction, the limb is rested on a splint such as the Thomas splint, originally devised by Hugh Owen Thomas (p. 125) for applying fixed traction to the lower limb, and still widely used (Fig. 9.3). The lower end of the splint has a 'V' shape to hold traction cord applied to the patient's limb either by skin traction or, as a first aid measure, by tying the patient's boot to the splint. The limb is then stretched with a Spanish windlass (nowadays usually made of two wooden tongue depressors) and the counter pressure taken by a padded leather ring at the upper end of the splint under the ischial tuberosity. The

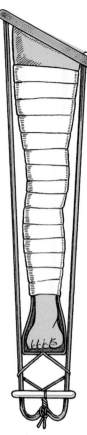

Fig. 9.3 Fixed traction with Thomas splint using a Spanish windlass.

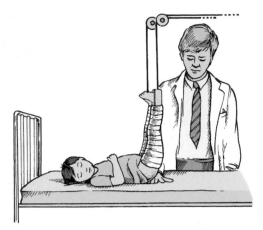

Fig. 9.4 Gallows traction. The weight of the child should be enough to hold the limb out to length. A hand can be slipped between the buttocks and sheet.

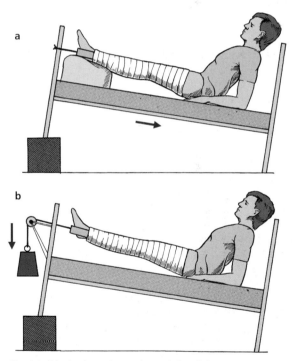

Fig. 9.5 (a) Fixed traction – the weight of the patient provides traction; (b) sliding traction – the weight of the patient still applies traction but his own weight is counterbalanced by a weight attached to a cord running over a pulley.

Thomas splint is ideal for transporting patients because it is self-contained and does not need pulleys or weights.

Fixed traction using gravity. The fundamental principle of this type of traction is to string the patient up by the injured limb and leave them hanging until the bone has joined. Gallows traction for a child under the age of 3 with fractured femur is a good example of this. Children tolerate the position surprisingly well for the 2–3 weeks necessary for the fracture to unite at this age (Fig. 9.4).

Gravity can also be applied to the limb by fixing the patient's leg to the foot of the bed, which is then raised so that the patient slides down towards the pillow (Fig. 9.5).

A similar principle is used in a hanging cast for fractures of the humerus in which a cast is applied to the forearm and suspended by a collar and cuff so that the combined weight of the arm and cast pull the humerus into line (Fig. 9.6). The arm must

hang; a sling supporting the elbow prevents the traction reaching the fracture site.

Sliding traction. Suspending the patient and tying the feet to the end of the bed restricts the patient's mobility and makes nursing difficult. This can be

125

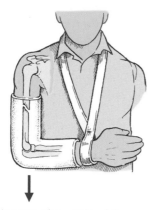

Fig. 9.6 Hanging cast. The weight of the arm and cast pulls the humeral fragments into line.

overcome by weights and pulleys but the system is complicated and needs regular adjustment.

At its simplest, sliding traction is little different from fixed traction, except that the patient can move freely in the bed, but more complex arrangements are possible. Hamilton–Russell traction uses a single cord to apply a horizontal force that is twice the vertical force because the cord, on its horizontal run, runs through a three-pulley system which gives it a velocity ratio of 2. This means that a 1 kg weight will exert a 1 kg upwards pull, but a 2 kg longitudinal pull (Fig. 9.7).

Balanced traction. It is uncomfortable to leave a broken limb lying on a bed so that the fragments rub against each other whenever the patient turns over (Fig. 9.8). Greater comfort can be achieved by resting the limb on a splint which is then suspended so that the limb is, in effect, in a gravity-free field.

In the most complicated arrangements this is done by resting the leg on a Thomas splint with a weight and pulley attached to each corner. If the weights are correctly adjusted the patient can be lifted almost with a fingertip, which makes nursing easier and avoids pressure sores. None of these weights act on the fracture, which must be controlled by a longitudinal force.

Although there are many advantages in complex systems of balanced traction, they are difficult to maintain and a simple system is often better.

Types of traction

- Skin or skeletal.
- Fixed or sliding.
- Fixed traction – may use splint or gravity.
- Sliding traction – may be balanced or not balanced.

External splints/slings/braces

Any device that holds a fracture steady is a splint and those that set hard around the limb are casts. A cast will hold a limb straight and still but cannot hold it out to length; casts are therefore unsuitable for fractures in which the limb is shortened.

To maintain the alignment of a bone, the plaster is not just wrapped around the leg and allowed to set; pressure must be applied to the cast while it sets so that the bones are held accurately by three-point pressure (Fig. 9.9).

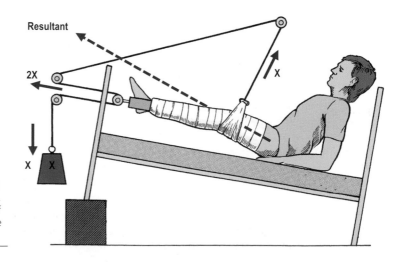

Fig. 9.7 Hamilton–Russell traction. The longitudinal traction has a velocity ratio of 2 and the vertical traction a velocity ratio of 1. The resultant force is 2.24 times the mass of the weight applied at an angle of 27° to the horizontal.

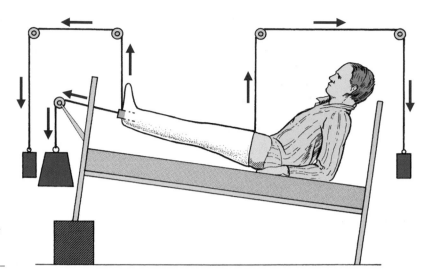

Fig. 9.8 Balanced sliding traction. One weight applies longitudinal traction and others are applied to the upper and lower ends of the limb so that it 'floats' in a gravity-free field.

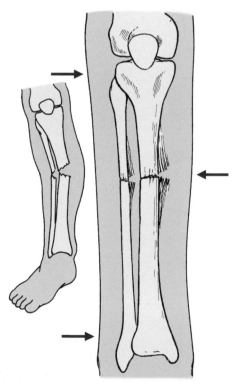

Fig. 9.9 Three-point pressure. The fracture line is closed by pressure at three points.

In most fractures it is necessary to immobilize both the joint above and the joint below the fracture.

Use

Splints do not provide rigid fixation. If applied immediately after the fracture they will become loose as the swelling of trauma subsides and muscles waste. The position of the fracture must be checked regularly and the position reviewed.

If the fracture slips there are several options:

1. The position may be accepted (Fig. 9.10).

2. The fracture may be manipulated again.

3. It may be necessary to abandon conservative treatment.

Materials

All casting bandages consist of a solid element covering a fibrous material. The solid part gives rigidity and the flexible part prevents it cracking. Reinforced concrete contains steel rods for similar reasons.

The original casting material was developed by the ancient Egyptians, who are said to have treated fractures by resting the injured limb in boxes containing Nile mud and straw which set hard and was broken away when the fracture had united. An Arab surgeon was the first to describe the use of plaster to treat fractures in AD 970, but it was not until the early part of the 20th century that plaster was widely used in Europe.

Plaster of Paris

The best known casting material is plaster of Paris, a high quality gypsum that originally came from Montmartre. Plaster of Paris bandages consist of a tough open-weave fabric coated with hemihydrated calcium sulphate powder. Book muslin or crinoline

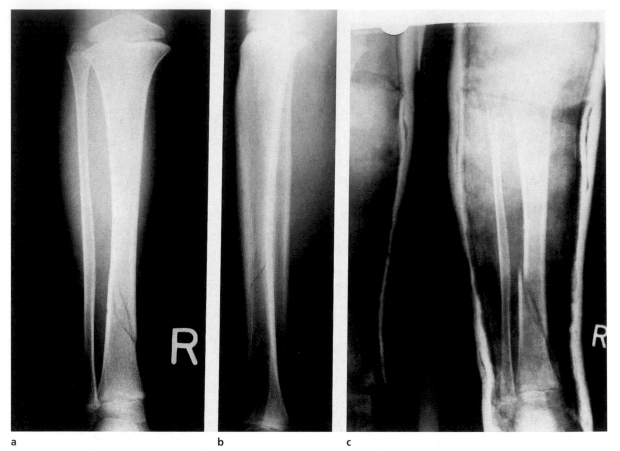

a   b   c

Fig. 9.10 Loss of fracture position: (a), (b) a spiral fracture of the tibia with minimal displacement on the day of injury; (c) the position 10 days later. The fragments have moved but the position is still acceptable.

were originally used as the fabric. When dipped in water the plaster becomes hard with crystalline hydrated calcium sulphate. The chemical reaction involved is exothermic and the plaster therefore becomes warm as it sets:

$$(CaSO_4)_2\,H_2O + 3H_2O \rightarrow 2\,(CaSO_4 \cdot 2H_2O) + heat$$

Plaster of Paris is light, comparatively soft, porous so that the limb can 'breathe', easy to remove and has stood the test of time. Its greatest disadvantages are that it disintegrates when wet and that 24–48 h are needed for it to harden enough to take the patient's weight.

Modern materials, including resins and fibreglass, are now used frequently. They are lightweight and easy to apply. Unfortunately, they are not as easy to mould as plaster of Paris and removal can be more difficult. Patients do, however, prefer them.

Applying a plaster correctly takes much practice, but the following points are particularly important (Fig. 9.11):

1. *Padding.* Apply light padding of soft wool or cotton over bony areas to avoid pressure sores, preferably over a thin layer of stockinette so that the padding will not roll up inside the cast and cause uncomfortable ridges.

2. *Water temperature.* The hotter the water, the faster the plaster sets. Cold water gives more time to apply the cast and so is recommended for beginners.

3. *Dipping.* When dipping a plaster bandage, hold it lightly so that water can penetrate to its centre. Hold it under the water until the bubbles stop and then drain it until the drips stop (Fig. 9.12). Do not wring it out like a dishcloth.

4. *Application.* Lay the bandage carefully over the limb and do not pull it tight (Fig. 9.13).

5. *The '100–90 trick'.* If a joint has to be held flexed to 90°, flex it 10° more, apply the plaster and then put the limb in the correct position (Fig. 9.14). This avoids hard wrinkles in the plaster, which can cause pressure sores at the flexure crease.

6. *Splitting the cast.* If the plaster is applied soon after injury, or at operation, split the cast and padding down to skin so that it can be spread or removed quickly in case of limb swelling.

Once the plaster is applied and set, check the following:

1. *Edges.* Check that the edges are not too sharp and do not press on the skin. If they do, bend the edges but do not cut the edge off because this loosens the plaster and makes the problem worse (Fig. 9.15).

2. *Circulation.* Check that the peripheral circulation is good, that toes and fingers will extend fully and have normal sensibility, colour and circulation. If they do not, the plaster may need splitting or removing.

3. *Advice.* Tell the patient that if the limb is painful, numb, cold or discoloured, help should be sought at once.

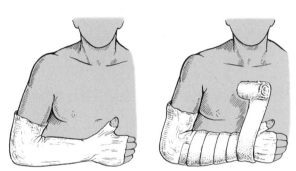

Fig. 9.11 Applying a padded plaster. Stockinette is first placed over the arm and plaster wool is rolled gently over the stockinette.

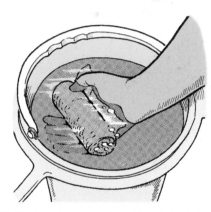

Fig. 9.12 Dipping plaster bandage. The plaster is held loosely under the water and not gripped. The end of the bandage is separated from the rest of the roll.

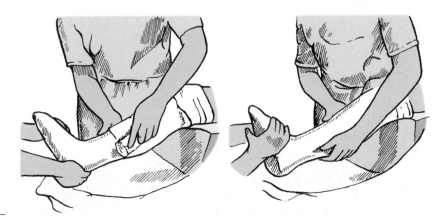

Fig. 9.13 Applying the plaster. The plaster bandage is rolled gently and carefully around the limb.

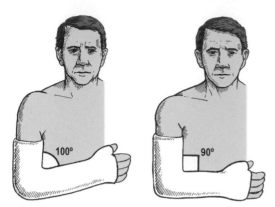

Fig. 9.14 The '100–90' trick. The plaster is applied at 100° and then straightened to 90° to avoid pressure at a joint.

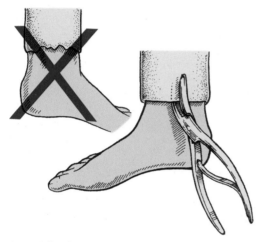

Fig. 9.15 Tight plasters. The edge should not be trimmed – this leaves a sharp ragged edge. Plaster benders should be used to ease the cast.

Removing a plaster also needs care:

1. *Saws.* If an oscillating saw is used to cut the plaster it must only be pressed 'up and down', not dragged along the length of the cast (Fig. 9.16). The saw blade can cause a nasty scratch if dragged along the skin and a blunt blade can burn. Before using the saw, test the blade on the skin of your own forearm; this will reassure the patient and remind you that the instrument is potentially dangerous.

2. *Shears.* If plaster shears are used, particularly on an unconscious patient, be certain that the shears cut plaster only and do not bruise skin (Fig. 9.17). It is distressingly easy to break the skin, especially in older patients.

3. *Advice.* Warn the patient that the limb will be stiff and that much hard work will be needed to

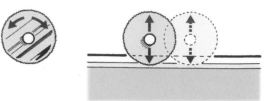

Fig. 9.16 Removing a cast with a power saw. The round blade oscillates. The plaster is cut by up and down movements at right-angles to the plaster.

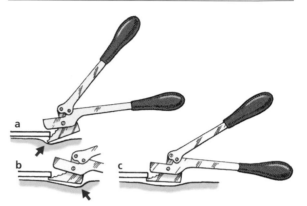

Fig. 9.17 Removing the cast with shears: (a) the tip of the shears is digging into the patient's skin; (b) the heel of the shears is digging into the patient's skin; (c) the blade of the shears is parallel with the skin and the plaster can be removed safely.

restore normal function. If this is not done the patient will be disappointed and may lose confidence.

Slings

Slings are used to support an injured arm or shoulder. There are four main types (Fig. 9.18):

- *Broad arm sling.* Made out of a triangular bandage, this sling supports the forearm and elbow and takes the weight of the upper arm.
- *Collar and cuff.* A collar and cuff does not support the elbow and allows the upper arm to hang free. This sling is used for fractures of the humerus and other injuries in which the weight of the limb will maintain alignment.
- *High sling.* A high sling holds the hand well up and is useful for hand injuries but the position is uncomfortable if there is soft tissue swelling at the elbow. Ulnar nerve damage can occur.
- *Sling and swathe.* A sling and swathe, or body bandage, is worn under the clothes. This arrangement prevents any movement of the arm and is useful after shoulder operations.

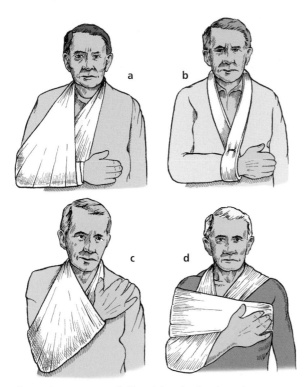

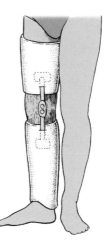

Fig. 9.19 A cast brace allowing movement of the knee.

Fig. 9.18 Four types of sling: (a) a simple triangular bandage; (b) collar and cuff; (c) high sling; (d) swathe and body bandage.

Cast braces

Cast braces are applied very closely to the limb and fitted with hinges to allow joint movement, which is important for articular cartilage nutrition (Fig. 9.19). With a cast brace patients are able to bear full weight upon their injured limbs much sooner than with conventional splints but they are difficult to apply and require special attention to detail. For the femur, for example, the cast should fit snugly around the upper part of the thigh so that the fascial sheath of the muscle can act as a hydraulic chamber to maintain length, and the hinges must be applied accurately or they will not function.

External fixation

Fractures that cannot be held reduced on traction or in a cast need to be fixed, either internally or externally. Internal fixation should not be used if the wound is severely contaminated or if there is skin loss, because of the risk of infection. External fixation must be used instead.

An external fixator is nothing more than a scaffold, or gantry, attached to threaded pins set in the bone fragments (Fig. 9.20a). At its simplest, external fixation can be applied by means of a bar secured to pins with the same acrylic cement used to fix joint prostheses, but many systems incorporating ingenious universal joints are now in general use. An older technique of external fixation was to incorporate pins into the patient's plaster but the cast did not grip the pins tightly enough to hold the fragments in position.

External fixation is used not only for long bone fractures but also for maxillofacial fractures and spinal surgery, where halopelvic traction supports the spine with bars linking the skull and pelvis.

External fixation has two great advantages:

1. It can be used in patients with skin loss or infection.
2. The position of the fragments can be easily adjusted.

Some types of external fixator provide such rigid fixation that they shield the fracture from stress and actually delay union. Other designs allow a little movement to avoid this problem, called dynamization.

More recently, 'ring fixators' have become increasingly popular (Fig. 9.20b). These utilize smooth, narrow transfixing pins attached to a circular ring. These rings can be positioned adjacent to a joint or over the diaphyseal region of the bone. The design

131

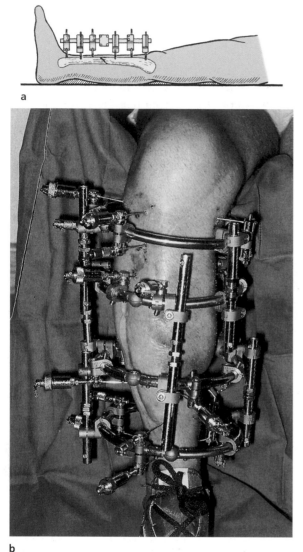

a

b

Fig. 9.20 (a) External fixation of the tibia; (b) an external ring fixator in position.

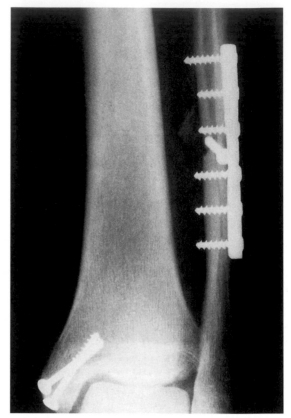

Fig. 9.21 Internal fixation of a fracture dislocation at the ankle using plate and screws.

of the systems can be complex, but accurate reduction of fractures is possible. They are particularly useful in the treatment of angular deformities and non-unions or malunions.

Internal fixation

Bone fragments can be reassembled and held in perfect position with screws, plates, wires and nails (Fig. 9.21). Although perfect anatomical reduction is important, it is not so important that every frac-

ture must be internally fixed; it is better to have a workable limb than a perfect radiograph.

The main indications for internal fixation are:

1. Fractures that cannot be controlled in any other way.
2. Patients with fractures of more than one bone.
3. Fractures in which the blood supply to the limb is jeopardized and the vessels must be protected.
4. Intra-articular, displaced fractures.

The disadvantages of internal fixation are:

1. The risk of infection at the time of operation.
2. The additional trauma of operation. A wide exposure is needed to apply screws and plates and this must devitalize some of the bone and the soft tissue. There is no virtue in replacing a healthy fracture in almost perfect position with a bone that is anatomically perfect but dead.

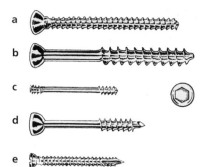

Fig. 9.22 Five types of screw: (a) cortical screw; (b) cancellous screw; (c) Herbert scaphoid screw – note the different pitch of the threads at each end; (d) malleolar screw with pointed tip; (e) self-tapping screw – note the flutes at the tip.

The following internal fixation devices are in common use.

Screws

Bone screws are different from wood screws and metal screws. Wood is a fibrous material and a wood screw is designed to cut its own thread as it is driven into a prepared hole. Because wood is fibrous and slightly soft, the tapered shank of the screw does not split the wood unless the original hole is too small. A metal screw, on the other hand, cannot find its own way through metal and must have its thread cut with a tap before it is inserted. Bone is different from wood or metal and different types of screw are used.

Two types of bone screws are commonly used but others are available for special applications (Fig. 9.22):

1. **Cortical screws**: a hole is first drilled at a chosen angle and tapped to take the screw. **Self-tapping screws** are also available but cut a less precise thread.

2. **Cancellous screws**, which have a wide thread, almost like a corkscrew, and grip soft cancellous bone.

Screws are used to compress plates against bone, or bone fragments against each other. When used to hold bone fragments together, the screw must grip only the fragment nearer the tip of the screw. If the thread engages both fragments it will hold them apart instead of pressing them together. To avoid this problem and achieve compression, either the fragment nearer the head of the screw can be overdrilled, so that the screw does not grip the bone, or a lag screw (Fig. 6.16) can be used.

Plates

Plates are used not only to hold bones in the correct position but also to compress the two bone ends together. These compression plates should always be applied on the tension side of the fracture. The tension side of a fracture is the one on which the deformity puts the soft tissue under tension. Compression can be applied in three ways:

1. First the plate is fixed to one fragment. The two ends are then pulled together with a small screw clamp, the second fragment is fixed to the plate and the clamp removed.

2. The two screws furthest from the fracture can be applied, leaving a slight gap between the plate and the bone. As the remaining screws are inserted, the gap is obliterated and there is a gradual reduction in the stress riser effect.

3. Dynamic compression plates (DCPs) can be used. DCPs are designed so that the shoulder of the screw presses against the edge of the screw hole and applies pressure at the fracture site (Fig. 9.23).

Locking plates are used to hold the bone fragments closely together. This may not be a rigid fixation, and indeed may allow a little movement of the bone ends. These fractures therefore heal with abundant callus. The advantage of this type of plate is that the screw mechanism allows strong fixation of the plate/screws to the bone; which can be particularly useful in the porotic fractures of the elderly or in cancellous bone. Newer plates are specifically designed for different anatomical sites (e.g. proximal tibia, distal tibia). The multiple bone fragments may be held individually to the plate. These can also be inserted through smaller incisions.

The disadvantages of plates are as follows:

1. Wide exposure is often needed to give access to the fracture.

2. The plate may be so large that it is difficult to close the skin over it.

3. The plate is so rigid that it causes a stress riser at each end, where fractures can occur. This can be reduced, but not eliminated, by putting the end screw through one cortex only so that there is a gradual reduction in the stress riser effect.

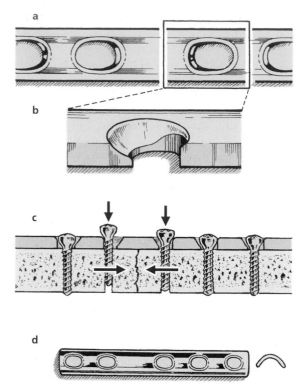

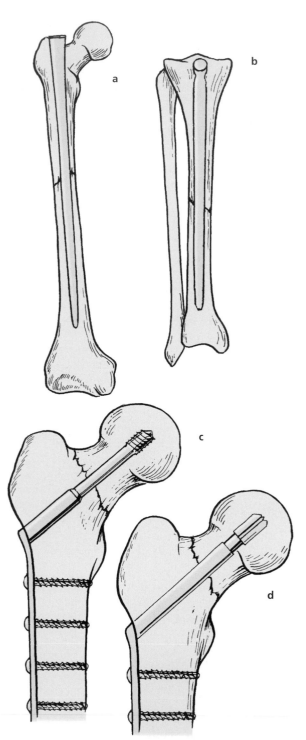

Fig. 9.23 Bone plates. (a)–(c) A dynamic compression plate (DCP). The holes are shaped so that the undersurface of the head presses against the plate and applies compression to the fracture site. (d) A semitubular plate.

4. The rigidity of the plate leads to disuse osteoporosis of the underlying bone.

5. Because of points 3 and 4, plates should be removed from the femur and tibia, even though this means another operation and the risk of fracture through one of the screw holes immediately after the plate has been removed.

Intramedullary nails

Intramedullary nails are used for fractures not only of the middle but also of the juxta-articular position of the bone. These implants have been designed to allow cross-screw function. These screws therefore hold the bone position and prevent shortening or rotation (Fig. 9.24).

Intramedullary nails have some disadvantages:

1. Because the medullary cavity varies in width and is narrowest at the centre of the bone, the shaft may need to be reamed carefully to produce a precisely machined channel to take the nail. If

Fig. 9.24 Types of internal fixation: (a), (b) intramedullary nails; (c) compression nail for fixation of the femoral neck; (d) sliding nail fixation of the femoral neck.

such a channel cannot be created, the nail, when inserted, may break the bone.

2. Although nails hold length and alignment, they are less effective for controlling rotation unless cross-screws through the nail and bone are used.

3. There is a risk of devitalizing the bone by exposing the bone and reaming the medullary cavity of each fragment. Because of this, it is preferable to insert intramedullary nails by a closed technique using an image intensifier.

Locking nails

It is possible to insert an intermedullary nail and fix the fragments of bone to the nail itself (Fig. 9.25). These nails are extremely useful for segmental fractures of the long bones, especially the femur, because they maintain length and rotation as well as alignment. In some ways they serve the same purpose as external fixators, except that they are enclosed in the bone.

In order to reduce the damage to the blood supply along the endosteal border, nails have now been designed to be inserted without the need to ream the canal. These often solid nails are guided across the fracture site and held in position with locking screws.

Wires

Wires can be used to fix fractures in three ways (Fig. 9.26):

1. *Tension band wiring*, in which the wire is applied as a loop to the outer side of the fracture so that it comes under tension when the joint is flexed. The technique is particularly useful for fractures of the patella and olecranon.

2. *Cerclage wiring*, useful in spiral fractures with minimal displacement. The technique requires very little surgical exposure.

3. *Direct fixation*. The wire holds the two fragments together like a skewer.

Wires have the following disadvantages:

1. Tension band wiring can slip; the wires may break; the wire is palpable under the skin and sometimes has to be removed.

2. Cerclage wiring does not provide rigid fixation and the wire can 'strangle' the bone, causing the tips of the fragments to break off, or even the whole bone to break transversely.

3. There is no rotational stability.

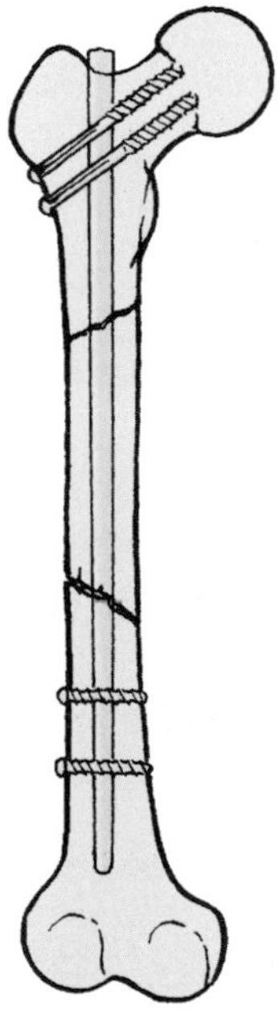

Fig. 9.25 Locking nail for a segmental fracture. Screws are passed through the bone/nail above and below the fracture to hold the bone out to length.

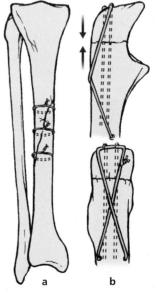

a   b

Fig. 9.26 Wire fixation of fractures: (a) cerclage wiring of the tibia; (b) tension band wiring of the olecranon.

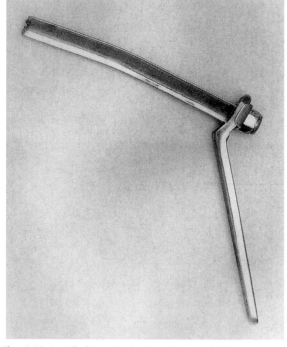

Fig. 9.27 A nail-plate. An obsolete design which was not strong enough to take the patient's full weight. This nail bent because the fracture did not unite.

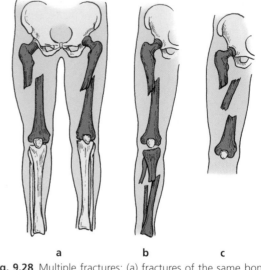

Fig. 9.28 Multiple fractures: (a) fractures of the same bone in both limbs; (b) fractures of both bones in one limb; (c) segmental fracture with two fractures of the same bone.

Nail-plates

Some fractures, particularly the extracapsular trochanteric fracture of the femur, can be treated with a nail and plate. These are now more commonly fixed with a screw and plate arrangement that allows the screw to slide within a barrel connected to the plate.

The screwnail grips the proximal fragment and the plate is screwed firmly to the femoral shaft (Fig. 9.27; p. 134). The nail has now been changed to a screw, which is easier and more precise to insert.

Selecting treatment

Selecting the right way to treat a fracture is not always easy. Some are wildly unstable and always need to be internally fixed, but some do so well with conservative management that operation need not be considered.

The selection of treatment must take into account the state of the skin, the age of the patient, the degree of bone displacement and the likelihood of the patient cooperating with treatment.

Multiple fractures need special thought (Fig. 9.28).

1. Fractures involving both bones of one limb. It is difficult to apply traction to both bones in the same limb and it is usually better to fix both bones. If this is not possible, fix one bone and treat the other conservatively.

2. Fractures of the same bone in both limbs. These are more easily managed if at least one fracture is fixed internally so that it can be left free of traction.

3. Segmental fractures, in which one bone is broken in more than one place. These are almost impossible to control unless all fractures are fixed.

When these features are considered together with the state of the skin, associated soft tissue injury and the fitness of the patient, the management of fractures is not as straightforward and mechanical as some people think.

Complications of treatment

Complications of traction

- Over-distraction.
- Loss of position.
- Pressure sores.
- Pin track infection.

Traction is not an 'easy option'. If patients are put on traction and left unattended until the fracture has united, problems are bound to occur. Setting up traction requires great attention to detail, and to maintain it requires even more. In orthopaedic hospitals with many patients on traction, there is usually a 'traction sister' responsible for checking all the traction in the hospital daily and ensuring that complications are avoided (Fig. 9.29).

Over-distraction

Pulling too hard on a fracture may cause circulatory embarrassment, stretched or damaged nerves, and hold the fragments apart so that they do not join. The amount of weight applied to a fracture must be carefully adjusted, particularly in the first 10 days, so that the bones are out to length but are not over-distracted.

Loss of position

The position of the bones must be carefully checked to be sure that they have not slipped or angulated overlapped. The fracture should be examined radiologically with portable X-rays at the patient's bedside until the callus formation has held the bone in the correct position.

Pressure sores

The skin is very vulnerable to pressure sores in the usual pressure areas and under the splint where the thigh ring or cords press the patient (Fig. 9.30). These need careful observation.

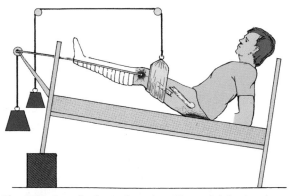

Fig. 9.29 Complications of traction. Pin track infection, loss of position, pressure sores.

Pin track infection

Although the pins of skeletal traction and external fixation are usually trouble-free, infection can occur where the pin passes through the skin and progress along the pin track. If this occurs, the skin is painful around the pin and the bone will be tender to gentle percussion. The infection should be treated by cleaning the skin carefully and giving antibiotics. This treatment should be continued until the pin is removed.

Complications of casts

- Circulatory embarrassment.
- Pressure sores.
- Undiagnosed wound infection.
- Joint stiffness.

Circulatory embarrassment

Casts are rigid boxes and limbs cannot expand inside them (Fig. 9.31). Swelling in a cast causes a similar problem to a compartment syndrome (p. 112). The blood supply to the limb is impaired, sometimes enough to cause gangrene needing amputation but more often the muscle bellies become ischaemic and heal by fibrosis, which causes a disabling contracture (p. 203).

Deformities of the toes (long flexor or long extensor muscle contractures) or finger deformities following forearm fractures are the commonest examples.

To avoid this complication, every patient with a cast is reviewed 24 h after it is applied and checked to make certain that none of the following signs are present:

1. Swelling of the digits.
2. Loss of extension of the fingers or toes.
3. Diminished sensibility.
4. Cool or dusky skin.

If any of these signs is present or there is any doubt about the circulation, the cast should be split down to the skin or removed completely. It is not enough to split the outer layer of the cast: bandages and dressings can constrict a limb, particularly if blood has made them hard.

Special vigilance is needed if there is bleeding under the cast. To tell if bleeding is continuing, draw

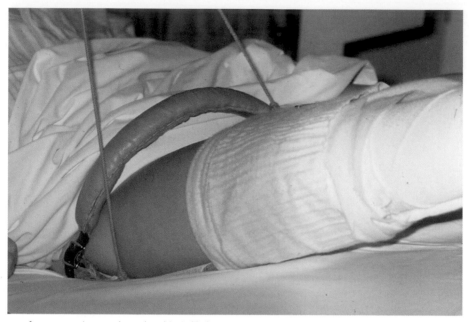

Fig. 9.30 Pressure from a traction cord on the skin is likely to cause a pressure sore.

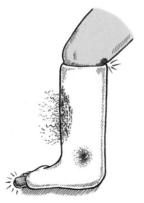

Fig. 9.31 Complications of plaster. Swelling of soft tissues, smell from infection, blood-staining and pressure on skin in flexure crease.

round the edge of the stain with a felt-tip pen and mark the line with the date and time. If the blood-stain is expanding, the plaster should be removed.

Pressure sores

A tight spot inside a cast can cause a pressure sore and any doubtful area should be inspected by 'windowing' the plaster or removing it. If a plaster is windowed, the window must be replaced and ban-

daged into position so that the underlying soft tissue does not swell and protrude through the hole in the plaster.

Infection

It is hard to be certain if there is infection under a plaster, but smell is a good guide. Do not feel embarrassed to sniff a plaster, especially one that is stained.

Patients should be discouraged from poking rulers and straightened-out wire coat hangers down the cast to scratch the skin.

Joint stiffness

The purpose of a cast is to immobilize the fracture but the neighbouring joints are also immobilized. Some patients feel they must hold the rest of the limb stiff as well and this can lead to permanent loss of motion. Patients must be urged to move every joint that is not immobilized as vigorously as possible, particularly the hand and fingers.

Patients with Colles' fracture, for example, have a tendency to leave the arm resting unused in a sling until the cast is removed, by which time there will be severe stiffness of the fingers, elbow and shoulder requiring many months of physiotherapy to restore movement.

Complications of internal fixation

- Infection.
- Skin necrosis.
- Neurovascular damage.

Infection

Infection of open fractures has already been mentioned (p. 97). Infection of closed fractures treated by internal fixation is even more serious because it is the direct result of treatment and probably introduced at operation.

Meticulous technique and prophylactic antibiotics minimize the incidence of infection but it still occurs and must be treated energetically, with removal of the implants if necessary.

Skin breakdown

Surgical exposure of the fracture involves cutting and mobilizing injured skin, which may not heal. The implants are often bulky and this can make skin closure difficult, especially if there is soft tissue swelling. If the wound breaks down, exposing both the implant and the fracture, an infected non-union is likely. This complication can lead to amputation.

Neurological and vascular damage

In some fractures exposing the fracture may involve mobilizing or retracting nerves and vessels. The swelling and bleeding of the fracture make these difficult to identify and vulnerable to injury at the time of operation.

Soft tissue injuries

Skin
Immediate primary closure

Wounds can only be closed directly by sutures, clips or adhesive tape if there is negligible skin loss, the wound is clean, and the edges come together easily without tension. The edges of the laceration must be brought neatly together, particularly if the wound will show.

Facial injuries should, ideally, be sutured by a plastic surgeon. The wounds should not be excised or debrided, especially those of the eyelids or lips, and lacerations of the lips, eyelids and nostrils must be treated by an experienced surgeon. Special care must be taken if there is the possibility of damage to the parotid or lacrymal ducts or the facial nerve.

All facial wounds should be closed as carefully as possible with fine sutures of 6/0 nylon or 5/0 absorbable material that are removed after 2 or 3 days. Wounds on the face should not be closed with deep sutures of heavy material.

Crushed tissues

If a laceration on a crushed digit or limb is sutured, the stitches will be put under a great strain and the soft tissue swelling may cause tissue necrosis (Fig. 9.32). Wounds on crushed limbs are best treated by elevation.

When the swelling has subsided, perhaps after 7–10 days, the wound can be closed with sutures if necessary. Although inexperienced surgeons or casualty officers will be tempted to close meticulously all the wounds that they see, in the case of a crushed finger or limb this can only lead to disaster.

Wound debridement

Wound debridement means the radical excision of all debris, foreign material, dead muscle and dead skin margins to leave a wound that is completely free of all contaminated tissue and foreign material. Nothing but healthy, living tissue should be visible at the conclusion of the procedure, but nerves and blood vessels should be preserved. General anaes-

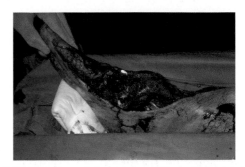

Fig. 9.32 Extensive soft tissue injury with degloving caused by a lorry wheel passing over the limb.

thesia is usually needed. To close the wound of an open fracture in the accident department under local anaesthetic is tempting, but complete debridement is almost impossible under local anaesthesia and should never be done.

High speed road traffic accidents are the commonest cause of wounds needing debridement, and tissue contaminated by road surface is difficult to clean. Bone ends that have been scraped along the tarmac have grit and dirt deeply embedded and this must be carefully removed. Skin that has been scraped along the road needs thorough scrubbing under general anaesthetic to remove all particles of dirt because any particles that remain will tattoo the skin. Never close a contaminated wound.

Delayed primary suture

In contaminated wounds immediate primary closure is not possible because of the risk of infection and delayed primary suture is necessary (Fig. 9.33). This is an established technique, derived from military surgery, and requires at least two operations:

1. The wound is debrided thoroughly and packed lightly with paraffin gauze.
2. Between 2 and 5 days later the gauze and dressings are removed and the wound closed with sutures.

Delayed secondary closure

If the defect is too large or too deep to be closed by delayed primary suture, delayed secondary closure with a split skin graft or flap may be required.

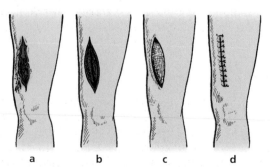

Fig. 9.33 Delayed primary suture: (a) contaminated wound; (b) the wound has been excised; (c) the wound packed; (d) the wound closed.

Closing skin defects

Methods of closing skin defects

- Relaxing incisions.
- Split skin grafts.
- Whole thickness grafts.
- Skin flaps.
- Foreign skin (xenograft).
- Free flaps.

The wound of a compound fracture must be thoroughly debrided and never closed by primary suture.

Wounds cannot be closed with sutures, clips or tape if there is any skin loss; one of the following methods must be used instead:

Relaxing incisions

In some circumstances a wound can be closed after a relaxing incision is made elsewhere to take tension off the skin in the wound area.

Split skin grafts

Split skin (partial thickness) grafts from intact areas can be applied directly to the defect. These grafts take well but the grafted area is of poor quality.

Whole thickness grafts

Full thickness grafts produce a supple grafted area, but take less reliably and leave a scar at the donor site. They are best for small defects.

Skin flaps

Flaps of skin, muscle, fascia or a combination of these can be mobilized locally or at a distance and used to cover large defects. Mobilizing the flap is difficult and is best done by plastic surgeons.

Foreign skin (xenografts)

Foreign skin, e.g. pig skin, can be used as a temporary biological dressing if there is very extensive skin loss. Xenografts are shed 1–2 weeks after application but the resulting defect is usually clean and may be grafted directly or closed by direct primary suture.

Free flaps

Free flaps of skin can be taken and their vessels anastomosed by microsurgery to vessels in the denuded area. These grafts are very successful when a good blood supply is achieved but the operation is tedious, and if the graft becomes necrotic an alternative solution must be found.

Gunshot wounds

Gunshot wounds have a bad prognosis with a high incidence of gangrene and anaerobic infection. Three types of injury are seen: (1) low velocity injuries; (2) high velocity injuries; and (3) shotgun wounds.

Low velocity injuries are caused by a heavy bullet travelling at low speed, e.g. the bullet from a Colt 45 of 'Western' fame, which could knock a man off his horse. These missiles travel at about 200 m/s and cause little soft tissue damage as long as they remain stable. If the bullet is unstable and cartwheels through soft tissue, more damage is done.

High velocity injuries are caused by missiles such as rifle bullets travelling at around 1000 m/s. They are more serious than low-velocity injuries, partly because of foreign material in the wound and partly because missiles travelling at this speed do not drill a clean hole through a limb but create a cavity behind them, which sucks soil, clothing and other harmful material into the limb. The cavitation opens up tissue planes and provides ready access for infection. The effect is rather like a small explosion within the limb.

Shotgun injuries are untidy and cause widespread soft tissue damage. Clothing, pellets and the wad from the cartridge are driven into the soft tissues by the blast and careful debridement is needed. It is unnecessary, and usually impossible, to remove all the pellets.

In civilian practice, gunshot wounds are becoming more common and must be treated by thorough debridement and delayed primary suture in the same way as battle injuries.

High speed road traffic accidents present a different problem because there is little foreign material and no cavitation from the projectile. Immediate closure is possible provided that the wound is meticulously debrided and all grit, dirt and contaminated soft tissue have been removed.

A gunshot wound is different; it must *never* be closed and debridement must be very thorough,

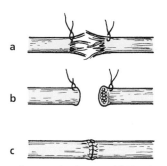

Fig. 9.34 Secondary repair of nerve: (a) the damaged nerve ends are tagged; (b) the nerve ends are trimmed at 10 days; (c) the nerve is repaired with sutures through the epineurium.

taking special care to remove fragments of clothing, soil and wadding from the wound.

Compartment syndromes

Compartment syndromes must be treated promptly and are dealt with on p. 112.

Nerves

Nerve injuries may be treated by one of the following (Fig. 9.34):

- Immediate primary suture.
- Secondary suture.
- Cable grafts.

Immediate primary suture

Because of the way in which nerves are injured (p. 42), few nerve lesions are suitable for immediate repair. Clean-cut lacerations, such as those caused by a hand going through a plate glass window, are suitable and should be repaired as carefully as possible using an operating microscope.

Secondary suture

Unless conditions are ideal, i.e. a clean and recent cut treated by an experienced surgeon in a well equipped operating theatre, nerve injuries are better treated by secondary repair, which involves two operations. At the first, the wound is cleaned and debrided, the nerve ends identified and tagged with a suture for recognition later, and the wound closed.

141

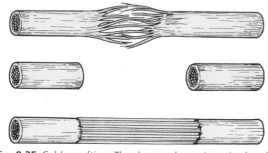

Fig. 9.35 Cable grafting. The damaged area is excised and replaced with several lengths of a smaller nerve.

At the second operation, at least 2 weeks later, the nerve ends are identified and 'freshened' by cutting away the tissue at the tip and the nerve mobilized to give enough length to bring the ends together.

Sutures are then placed in the thickened epineurium at the end of the nerve.

Cable grafting

Long defects in nerves caused by crushing or tearing must either be left untreated or bridged with a graft made of a less important nerve, such as the saphenous or sural nerve in the calf (Fig. 9.35). The results are not as good as primary suture but may be better than nothing.

Blood vessels

Cut arteries can be resutured accurately but those that are torn or crushed can be repaired only by excising the damaged segment and eliminating the gap by shortening the limb, rerouting the artery, or inserting a graft.

Veins present greater difficulty because their walls are thinner and the flow within them is so slow that clotting occurs.

Replantation of limbs

Severed limbs can be reattached to the body, although the operation is technically difficult and takes a long time.

The vascular repair is straightforward and must be adequate for the limb to be viable. Soft tissues, including muscle, skin and tendons, can be reconstructed and bones can be put back together by internal fixation. The finished limb may look very like the original but, despite initial success, the limb may have to be amputated later.

The reason for such disappointment is the inadequacy of the nerve repair (p. 141). Nerves cannot be repaired accurately and the limb may be both numb and paralysed. A prosthetic limb has more practical value to the patient than an insensitive and paralysed arm, which may be little more than a living paperweight, or a lower limb that functions, at best, as a rather heavy, unwieldy and unstable pillar.

Despite these gloomy observations, replanted limbs do sometimes work effectively and the techniques of operation are continually improving.

Case reports

These three case studies represent different methods of management of femoral shaft fractures.

Case A

A 5-year-old child was playing on a trampoline in his garden when he fell awkwardly, sustaining a closed fracture of the mid shaft of the right femur. The leg was externally rotated and the limb was shortened.

He was taken to the accident and emergency department, where it was noted that there was normal distal neurovascular supply; appropriate analgesics were given. The patient was managed by the orthopaedic team with balanced skin traction and was kept in hospital for a period of 3 weeks. During this time the position of the fracture was monitored using radiographs and the traction was adjusted accordingly to allow correction of the rotation and shortening of the limb.

At 3 weeks the patient's limb was immobilized in a hip spica cast after it was shown that there was abundant callus around the fracture. The patient was discharged from the hospital on crutches, non weight-bearing.

Case B

A 23-year-old motorcyclist was involved in a high energy road traffic accident and sustained an open comminuted fracture of the mid shaft of the right femur. At presentation it was clear that there was a 10 cm contaminated wound on the lateral side of the thigh and, indeed, a portion of the femur could be seen in the depth of the wound.

After the patient had been haemodynamically stabilized he was transferred to the operating theatre. The wound was thoroughly irrigated and all necrotic and contaminated tissue was removed. Because of the significant contamination at the wound site an external fixator was placed across the fracture to stabilize the femur.

The patient was subsequently returned to theatre on two further occasions when the wound was again debrided; it was finally closed after 4 days. The patient elected to remain with the external fixator (although an intramedullary nail was offered) and this was held in situ until the femur had healed at 3 months.

Case C

A 76-year-old lady was doing her weekly shopping when she caught her right foot on a manhole cover and fell, twisting the leg underneath her as she fell. She sustained a closed spiral supracondylar fracture of the distal right femur. There was marked angulation and displacement of the fracture fragments.

After haemodynamic stabilization and ensuring there were no other injuries while she was in the accident and emergency department, she was subsequently transferred to the care of the orthopaedic surgeons and was operated on that same evening. The femoral fracture was fixed using a locking plate, which allowed reduction of the fracture fragments and stable fixation using a plate fixed to the lateral surface of the femur.

Summary

These three femoral fractures represent very typical practice in most hospitals. Those patients with skeletal immaturity are often treated conservatively because of fear of damaging the growing physis with any surgery. Traction is a perfectly acceptable method of management as long as it is monitored carefully and the position of the fracture is maintained throughout.

Open fractures need to be treated aggressively because of the risk of potential contamination and subsequent infection. The second patient was operated on early and returned to the operating theatre on a number of occasions to ensure that all potentially necrotic tissue was removed. External stabilization of the femur allows control of the fracture fragments while soft tissue management is undertaken. Definitive fixation with a nail or plate can then be used.

Low energy injuries in the elderly can often result in quite significant fractures. Stabilization in this case was with a plate to hold the fracture fragments securely in position. Immobilization for long periods of time in traction in this group of patients is fraught with potential problems and subsequent complications. Similarly, the use of an external fixator would be unnecessary in a closed, low energy injury without soft tissue contamination.

Chapter |10|

Injuries to the face, head and spine

Be the end of this chapter you should be able to:

- Classify head and neck trauma.
- Understand the different mechanisms of injury to the cervical spine.
- Appreciate the severity of spinal injuries and decide on the degree of instability.

Facial injuries

Facial injuries are complex, dangerous and best dealt with by faciomaxillary or plastic surgeons, but they must first be recognized in the accident department.

Nose

Fractures of the nasal cartilages and nasal bone are common and leave a deformity if not correctly treated. There are several different types of fracture, and not all 'broken noses' are the same (Fig. 10.1). If a nasal fracture is suspected, hold the patient's nose gently and move it slightly. Pain or abnormal movement indicates a fracture.

Treatment

Treatment depends on the pattern of the fracture. Dislocations or displaced fractures of the nasal bones need to be repositioned accurately. If a deformity is to be avoided, treatment is best carried out by facial, ENT or plastic surgeons.

Zygoma

The zygoma can be fractured by a direct blow to the face and the injury is often missed because of soft tissue swelling. A depressed zygoma (Fig. 10.2) can be identified by inspecting the patient's face from above, bearing in mind that almost every face is slightly asymmetrical, and by palpation.

Untreated, a fractured zygoma leaves a flattened cheekbone, a depression in the floor of the orbit, which can result in diplopia, and damage to the infraorbital nerve. Always look for a fracture of the zygoma if there is a bruise over the cheekbone or a lateral subconjunctival haemorrhage.

Treatment

Once diagnosed, the fragment needs repositioning and sometimes fixation with wires or external fixation.

Orbital fractures

Orbital fractures are difficult to recognize but should be suspected if there has been direct trauma to the

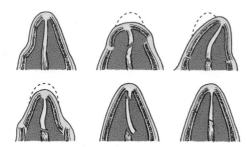

Fig. 10.1 Six types of nasal fracture. Each requires slightly different treatment and has a different prognosis.

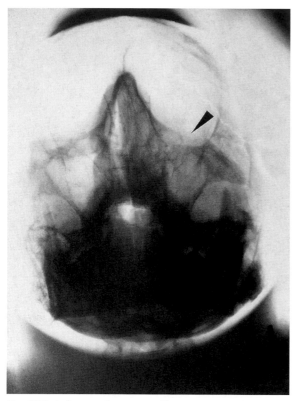

Fig. 10.2 A depressed zygoma with an opaque antrum.

orbit or eye. A 'blow-out' fracture, in which the small muscles of the eye can be caught in a fracture of the floor of the orbit, is particularly serious. Diplopia and the abnormal position of the eye should lead to the diagnosis.

Treatment

Treatment should be carried out by facial surgeons.

Mandible

Dislocations of the temporomandibular joint can follow direct or indirect trauma, or even a wide yawn. Dislocations can usually be reduced easily, but only if the mandible is intact.

The mandible can fracture through its neck, body, symphysis or ramus (Fig. 10.3), and the fracture can be recognized by tenderness when the mandible is palpated or squeezed gently, and by a deranged dental occlusion. Fractures of the mandible often happen during a fight, sometimes after drinking. Aggressive drunks seldom like their painful jaws being palpated and the fracture can be missed. Radiographs are essential if a fractured mandible is suspected (Fig. 10.4).

Soft tissue swelling round a fractured mandible can obstruct the airway. This is particularly serious if the patient vomits and lapses into unconsciousness, as inebriated patients often do.

Treatment

Faciomaxillary surgeons are usually responsible for treating these fractures, which may require internal fixation, interdental wiring (Fig. 10.5) or dental treatment.

Maxilla

Le Fort classification of maxillary fractures

Maxillary fractures were divided into three main types by Le Fort, a French surgeon of the early 20th century who broke the faces of corpses with a cudgel to study the fracture lines. His classification is as follows (Fig. 10.6):

- Le Fort 1 – through the maxilla, leaving the nose and orbits intact.
- Le Fort 2 – through the maxilla into the orbits and across the nose, leaving the middle third of the face mobile.
- Le Fort 3 – through the lateral wall of the orbit and across the nose.

All maxillary fractures require urgent attention because the middle third of the face may be unstable and can fall backwards to obstruct the airway. Tracheostomy may be needed.

Because facial injuries are, by definition, head injuries, they are often seen in unconscious patients

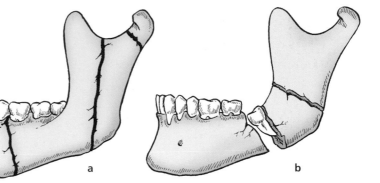

Fig. 10.3 Fractures of the mandible: (a) undisplaced fractures of the ramus, body and neck; (b) displaced fracture with impacted tooth.

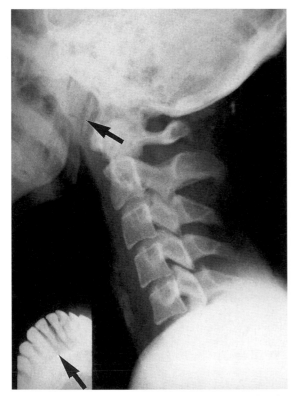

Fig. 10.4 Fracture of the mandibular ramus (*arrowed*) and the arch of the mandible caused by a blow to the point of the chin.

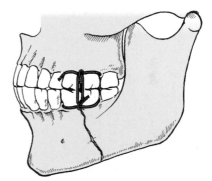

Fig. 10.5 Interdental wiring for fractured mandible.

with brain damage. Always look at the maxillary antrum on the skull radiograph of patients with head injuries; if it is opaque, it is probably full of blood and there is a maxillary fracture.

Treatment

When the airway is secure, the fracture can be treated by the appropriate specialists. External fixation to the skull is often required to hold the displaced fragments in their correct position.

Head injuries

Injuries to the head cause brain damage, the severity of which depends on the energy absorbed by the brain and not by the skull. A skull can be crushed between two fixed objects with surprisingly little brain damage; however, rapid deceleration causing nothing more than an undisplaced linear fracture may be associated with severe brain damage (Fig. 10.7).

Pathology

Trauma causes *primary* and *secondary* brain damage (Fig. 10.8).

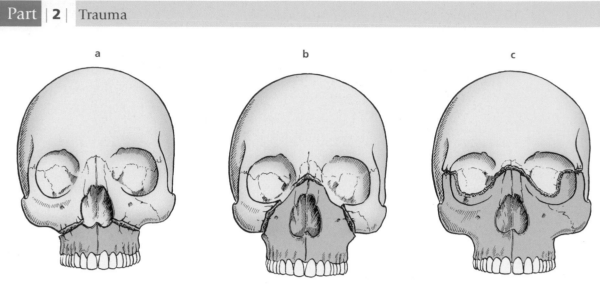

Fig. 10.6 Le Fort facial fractures: (a) Le Fort 1; (b) Le Fort 2; (c) Le Fort 3.

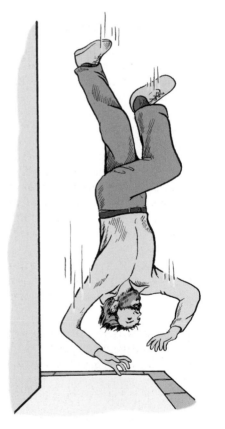

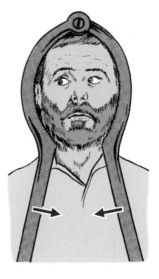

Fig. 10.7 Brain injury and head injuries. Rapid deceleration causes more cerebral damage than a crushing fracture with little deceleration.

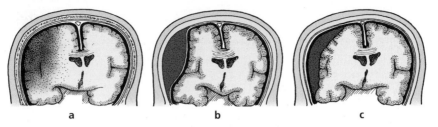

Fig. 10.8 Types of brain damage: (a) brain contusion with bleeding and oedema; (b) extradural haemorrhage; (c) subdural haemorrhage.

Primary

- Contusion or laceration caused by violent impact of the brain against the skull, either at the point of injury or directly opposite to it, a contrecoup injury.
- Penetration of the skull and direct damage to the brain.

Secondary

- Oedema of the brain.
- Extradural haemorrhage.
- Subdural haemorrhage.

Clinical presentation

From a clinical standpoint, there are three main types of brain injury: concussion, contusion and compression.

Concussion

Concussion is a transient loss of consciousness following a blow to the head. Recovery is usual. The duration of amnesia following the blow is a good guide to the severity of injury. A boxer who is knocked out in a fight has concussion.

Contusion

There is damage to cerebral tissue from localized bleeding or oedema. Recovery is slower than after concussion and may be incomplete, leaving a neurological deficit.

Compression

Compression is usually caused by bleeding into the skull. As the bleeding continues, the brain is com-

pressed and the clinical condition becomes worse. Decompression and arrest of the bleeding can be life saving.

Patients with concussion and contusion are at their worst immediately after injury and then recover. Compression causes steady deterioration instead of recovery, although there may be a lucid interval.

Management of head injuries

Distinguishing between concussion, contusion and compression depends upon careful monitoring of cerebral function. The level of consciousness and the eye signs are the most reliable clinical signs.

Level of consciousness

The level of consciousness must be recorded carefully so that any deterioration can be identified quickly. It is not enough to record that the patient is 'awake' or 'unconscious'. A fully conscious patient will be alert and oriented in time and space; i.e. will know where he or she is, what time it is, and will be able to hold a normal conversation.

At the other extreme, the patient will be unrousable and not responding to painful stimuli. Between these two extremes, the level of consciousness may be graded as follows:

- Alert and oriented.
- Drowsy.
- Reacts to movement.
- Reacts to painful stimulus.
- Unrousable.

A more accurate assessment is possible with the Glasgow coma scale (Table 10.1).

Eye signs. Raised intracranial pressure impairs the function of the iris on the side of the lesion. The size

149

Table 10.1 Glasgow coma scale

		Score
Eye opening	Spontaneous	4
	To voice	3
	To pain	2
	None	1
Verbal response	Oriented	5
	Confused	4
	Inappropriate words	3
	Incomprehensible sounds	2
	None	1
Motor response	Obeys command	6
	Localizes pain	5
	Withdraw (pain)	4
	Flexion (pain)	3
	Extension (pain)	2
	None	1
TOTAL		
	Glasgow coma scale	
	Score	
	14–15 = 5	
	11–13 = 4	
	8–10 = 3	
	5–7 = 2	
	3–4 = 1	

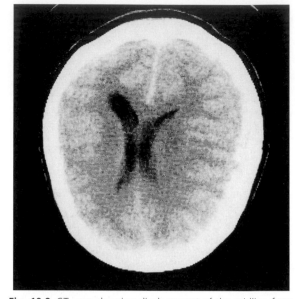

Fig. 10.9 CT scan showing displacement of the midline from cerebral oedema.

of the pupil and its reaction to light is recorded as a sign of intracranial bleeding. A fixed dilated pupil indicates an urgent problem.

Temperature. The thermoregulatory mechanism may be damaged in brain injury and the body temperature may rise. The temperature may need to be controlled by fans or tepid sponging.

Open fractures of the skull

Penetration of the skull always requires exploration by a neurological surgeon to remove dead bone, foreign matter and dead brain. Scalp wounds must not be sutured in the accident department if there is a depressed fracture under the wound.

Cerebral oedema (Fig. 10.9)

Cerebral oedema follows any major head injury and can be reduced with diuretics, such as a mannitol infusion, or by controlled hyperventilation with the patient paralysed and ventilated. This treatment is best conducted in a dedicated neurosurgical unit.

Extradural haematoma

The classic story of an extradural haematoma is the patient who walks into hospital after a minor head injury and gives a clear, sensible history. The radiograph shows a small temporal fracture. The patient is discharged home, lapses into unconsciousness and is found dead the following morning. This is a constant nightmare for those who treat head injuries. Extradural haemorrhage can be caused by damage to the middle meningeal artery. As the artery bleeds, a haematoma develops and the brain is gradually compressed. The level of consciousness slowly deteriorates until the patient becomes unrousable. If the diagnosis is made soon enough, the haematoma should be evacuated through a burr hole and the artery tied.

In days gone by, it was safer to drill burr holes than risk missing an extradural bleed but with the advent of CT scanning this complication should not take the surgeon by surprise. CT scanning is now an essential part of the management of head injuries and will show areas of brain damage as well as extradural haematomas and the position of the falx (Fig. 10.10).

Although these investigations are reliable, ligation of the middle meningeal artery can be life saving

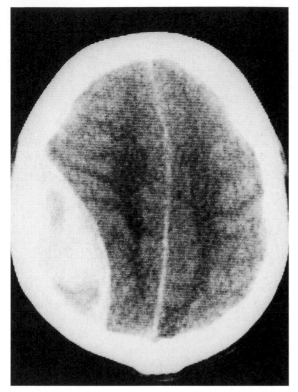

Fig. 10.10 CT scan showing an extradural haematoma, with shift of the midline to the opposite side.

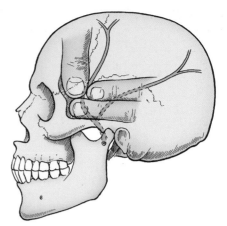

Fig. 10.11 The pterion. The middle meningeal artery crosses the pterion; it can be identified with the thumb and fingers as indicated.

and the correct site for the burr hole should be memorized by everyone who may be exposed to the treatment of patients with an extradural haematoma. The middle meningeal artery crosses the pterion, which lies two fingers above the zygoma and three fingers behind the orbit (also see Fig. 10.11). The artery can be found either by exposing the fracture and nibbling away the edges of the skull, or by making a burr hole at the pterion itself.

Subdural haemorrhage

Acute subdural haematomas usually accumulate slowly and cause more gradual loss of consciousness than an extradural haematoma. The cause is the gradual enlargement of a blood clot beneath the dura. As the clot liquefies, serum is drawn into its centre and it gradually increases in size. A chronic subdural haematoma is not a clinical emergency but any patient whose level of consciousness deteriorates in the weeks following a head injury should have a CT scan.

Post-traumatic amnesia

The fact that a patient appears alert and oriented does not exclude brain damage. It is by no means uncommon to find that patients who have been unconscious for only a few minutes are unable to recall events for several days after their accident.

The period of post-traumatic amnesia is a reliable guide to the severity of the head injury:

1. Patients with less than 24 h post-traumatic amnesia can expect complete recovery.
2. Those with a post-traumatic amnesia of 1 week usually have some permanent impairment.

CSF rhinorrhoea and otorrhoea

Cerebrospinal fluid (CSF) can leak from nose or ears if the fracture enters the subdural space. The leak usually ceases spontaneously but if it is profuse or persists for more than 2 weeks the defect in the dura may need to be patched with fascia.

Late sequelae

The long-term results of brain damage include continued neurological deficits, personality change, epilepsy, and serious physical disabilities requiring long-term care and rehabilitation.

Decisions in management

There are three very practical decisions in the management of head injury: when to request a skull radiograph, when to admit the patient and when to consult a neurosurgeon.

Skull radiograph

Indications for requesting a skull radiograph:

- Loss of consciousness or amnesia at any time.
- Abnormal neurological symptoms or signs.
- Suspected penetrating injury, swelling or scalp bruising but not a simple laceration.
- Intoxication.
- Difficulties in assessment, e.g. epilepsy, mental subnormality and the very young.

Indications for admission following head injury

Admission is indicated in the following circumstances:

- Confusion or impaired consciousness at the time of examination.
- Skull fracture.
- Abnormal neurological signs, headache or vomiting.
- Difficulties in assessment, e.g. epilepsy, mental subnormality and the very young.
- Other medical conditions, e.g. haemophilia.
- Bad social conditions or lack of responsible adult or relative.

Neurosurgical assistance

A neurosurgeon should be consulted in the following circumstances:

- Skull fracture and (1) confusion and impaired consciousness, or (2) focal neurological signs, or (3) fits.
- Confusion or neurological signs lasting more than 12 h.
- Coma continuing after resuscitation.
- Suspected open fracture of the vault or base of the skull.
- Depressed skull fracture.
- Deterioration in the level of consciousness or neurological signs.

Cervical spine injuries

A 'broken neck' has sinister connotations but not all cervical spine injuries have serious complications. Some are undisplaced and a few lucky patients sustain a potentially serious fracture without neurological damage.

Fractures of the spine are managed just as fractures elsewhere but the consequences of displacing the fragments are more serious.

Handling the patient with a cervical spine injury must be done cautiously to prevent further damage to the cervical cord. Even though the greatest damage occurs at the moment of impact, when the neck has been subjected to enough force to break bones and tear soft tissues, careless movements must be avoided.

It is very unlikely that careful handling can do more harm than the original injury if the patient is conscious and there is protective muscle spasm. Damage to the cervical cord following a spinal injury is unusual in the conscious patient.

This is not true for the unconscious patient. Many neurologically intact patients have probably been rendered paraplegic by careless handling and enthusiastic first aid.

Cervical injuries can be caused in four ways:

1. Flexion.
2. Extension.
3. Vertical compression.
4. Rotation.

Flexion injuries

Flexion is involved in the commonest and most serious cervical injuries, usually seen in the lower part of the cervical spine. The following are the commonest lesions (Fig. 10.12):

- Crush fracture of the vertebral body (Fig. 10.13).
- Rupture of the supraspinous ligament, making the spine unstable.
- Dislocation of the posterior facets.
- Dislocation with fracture of the vertebral body.

Crush fractures

Crush fractures are the result of vertical compression as well as flexion. They are stable but cause severe pain in the neck.

Treatment. Symptomatic relief with a four-post collar or cast and analgesia for approximately 6 weeks is all that is required (Fig. 10.14).

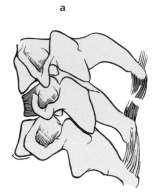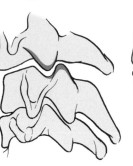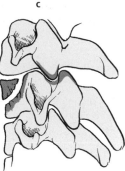

Fig. 10.12 Injuries of the cervical spine: (a) a flexion injury with crush fracture of the vertebral body and rupture of the supraspinous ligament; (b) locked facets; (c) locked facets with fracture of the vertebral body.

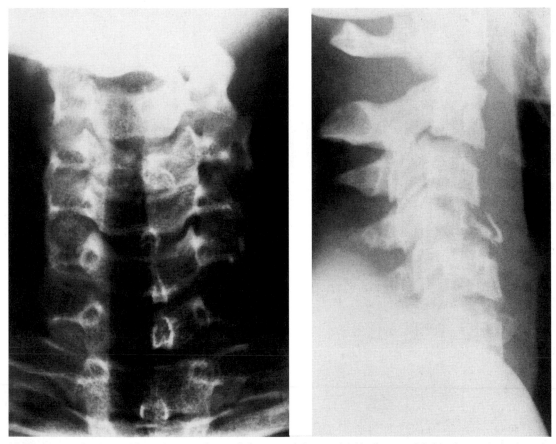

Fig. 10.13 Anteroposterior and lateral views of a crush fracture of the vertebral body. Note (1) that the cervical spines do not form a straight line and (2) the split in the body of C3 on the anteroposterior view.

Rupture of the supraspinous ligament

Violent flexion of the neck can tear the supraspinous ligament or avulse a spinous process. *The fact that the radiographs may show little bony injury is deceptive.* The posterior part of the cervical spine may be grossly unstable and neurological damage can occur if the flexion force is repeated.

Treatment. A supporting collar to hold the cervical spine in extension while the soft tissues heal is adequate.

153

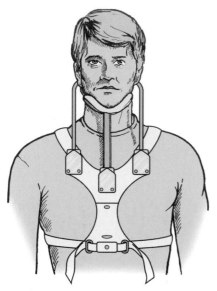

Fig. 10.14 A four-post collar.

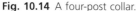

Dislocations

Forward flexion with rotation may cause one or both of the posterior facet joints to 'jump' over the edge of the facet below and dislocate (Fig. 10.15). The dislocation cannot occur without associated soft tissue injury but neurological damage is unusual after a simple facet dislocation.

Treatment. A simple dislocation can be treated either by traction or careful manipulative reduction, but this should only be done by an *experienced* surgeon with special knowledge of spinal disorders.

Fracture dislocations

Fracture dislocations in which the vertebral bodies and the facet joints are disrupted often lead to **paraplegia** and are usually caused by a fall onto the head, e.g. falling off a horse.

Treatment. The fracture must be reduced and held stable, either by traction or fixation, until it has united. Radiographs taken in flexion and extension are useful in determining the progress of bone union. *These views should not be attempted within 6 weeks of injury in case the cervical cord is damaged.*

Traction applied with a halter is a useful temporary measure but the pressure on the jaw is uncomfortable for long periods and prevents the patient eating. Skull traction, like skeletal traction in general, is

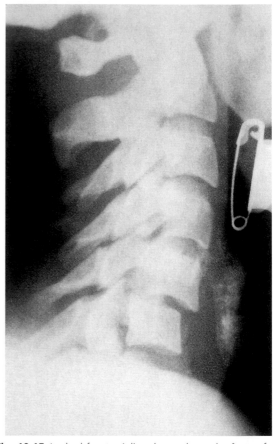

Fig. 10.15 Locked facets. A line drawn down the front of the vertebral bodies has a sharp step between C5 and C6.

much more acceptable to the patient and is applied through tongs attached to the skull.

Hyperextension must be avoided and traction should be applied in the line of the dislocated segment, not the normal line of the neck.

External fixation can be applied to the neck with a halo screwed to the outer cortex of the skull and supported on metal rods attached to a rigid 'vest' ('vest' is American for waistcoat) (Fig. 10.16). 'Halo-vest' traction is used for unstable fractures, but those which are less unstable may be treated in a firm four-post collar.

Internal fixation may be required to fix the unstable levels of the cervical spine. The operation must be carefully planned so that the exposure does not make the cervical spine completely unstable. If, for example, a hyperextension injury has occurred, the tissues in the front of the cervical spine will be damaged and exploring the spine from behind will weaken the posterior structures as well, leaving little

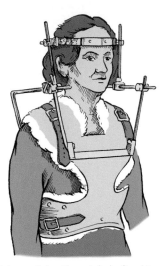

Fig. 10.16 'Halo-vest' traction. A halo fixed to the skull and attached to bars mounted on a chest piece.

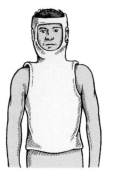

Fig. 10.17 Minerva cast.

to hold the vertebrae together and the head with no visible means of support.

Cast immobilization of the neck is also possible but is now largely historical (Fig. 10.17). A Minerva cast was used, named after the incident when the demigod Vulcan (himself reputed to have a club foot) split Jupiter's skull to relieve his headache. Minerva sprang out, fully armed, wearing a heavy metal helmet and singing triumphantly.

The cast was modelled on the helmet and was applied to the head rather like a balaclava helmet extending down onto the chest, but it was heavy and restricted movement of both chest and jaw. A four-post collar is both more effective and more comfortable.

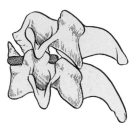

Fig. 10.18 Fracture of the vertebral body with disc prolapse. A hyperextension injury.

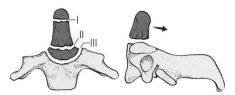

Fig. 10.19 Fracture of the odontoid process. Three types of fracture are seen, involving the base, middle and apex.

Extension injuries

Extension injuries are far more common in the upper cervical spine. The range of flexion is limited by the chin striking the chest but extension has no such natural protection.

Extension injuries are generally less serious than flexion injuries, but serious injuries can occur. The four commonest injuries are:

1. Fracture of the odontoid process.
2. Hangman's fracture.
3. Kinking of the posterior longitudinal ligament, which can damage the anterior spinal artery and cause anterior spinal artery syndrome.
4. Fracture of the vertebral body with disc prolapse (Fig. 10.18).

Fracture of the odontoid process

Fractures of the odontoid process, or dens, are difficult to diagnose and are often missed in accident departments. The fracture causes a feeling of unsteadiness in the neck and pain at the base of the skull. These symptoms should suggest the diagnosis.

There are three types of fracture (Fig. 10.19). Type II fractures, in the middle of the dens, have a roughly 50% incidence of non-union and may need atlantoaxial fusion to stabilize the neck.

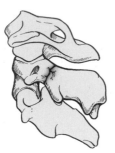

Fig. 10.20 Hangman's fracture. A fracture through the pars interarticularis of the second cervical vertebra.

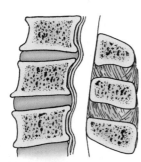

Fig. 10.21 Anterior spinal artery compression. Kinking of the posterior longitudinal ligament in an elderly patient can cause pressure on the front of the spinal cord and damage to the anterior spinal artery.

Treatment. Support in a halo-vest for up to 4 months is usually adequate but does not avoid the high incidence of non-union.

Hangman's fracture

Judicial hanging fractures the spine by distraction and hyperextension. Similar forces can be applied in falls or by patients slipping under seat-belts. The fracture usually occurs through the pedicles of C2 and is a traumatic spondylolisthesis of C2 on C3 (Fig. 10.20).

Treatment. The fracture should be managed by holding the head steady, with the minimum of traction. Too much traction can cause neurological damage: that is how hanging kills.

Anterior spinal artery syndrome

Hyperextension in the degenerate cervical spine of the elderly may kink the posterior longitudinal ligament and this can compress the anterior spinal artery (Fig. 10.21), leading to central cord damage. The result is weakness and sensory symp-

toms in the upper limbs with sparing of the lower limbs, sometimes accompanied by poor bladder control.

Treatment. Immobilization in a collar is all that can be offered.

Fracture of vertebra with disc prolapse

These lesions may cause permanent damage to the spinal cord.

Treatment. Urgent decompression and stabilization is required in cases where CT scans confirm the diagnosis.

Fractures caused by vertical compression

True axial compression is an uncommon force. Most impacts are either just in front of the axis of rotation and cause flexion, or just behind, when they cause extension. Two fractures can be caused by vertical forces.

Fracture of the atlas (Fig. 10.22)

The ring of the atlas can be disrupted by a vertical compressive force, often caused by something landing on the head or the patient falling directly onto the vertex.

Treatment. The fracture should be immobilized in a halo-vest for approximately 6 weeks, followed by a collar for another 2 weeks.

Burst fracture

Vertical compression can disrupt the vertebral bodies, and causes severe pain. The fracture must be distinguished from a wedge compression or crush fracture.

Treatment. If there is no neurological damage, a halo-vest for 6 weeks and then a collar is sufficient – as for a fracture of the atlas. If there is neurological damage, the halo-vest is still needed but the paraplegia must also be treated and rehabilitation begun as soon as possible.

Rotation injuries

Most injuries are the result of a combination of forces rather than a simple sagittal or vertical force. Rotational forces are involved in many flexion injuries, particularly those caused by falls onto the head and neck.

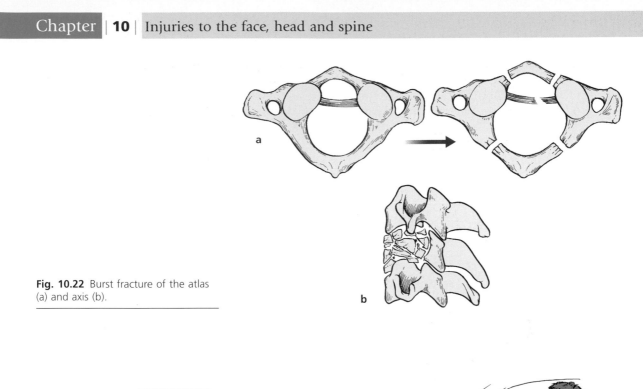

Fig. 10.22 Burst fracture of the atlas (a) and axis (b).

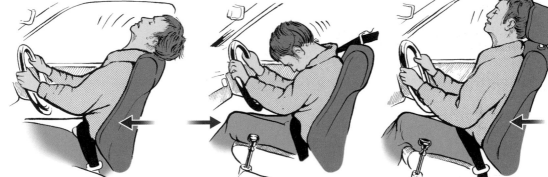

Fig. 10.23 Combined extension–flexion (whiplash) injury of the cervical spine. Movement of the head is limited by a head restraint.

Rotation with flexion is accompanied by dislocation of one facet joint, while rotation with compression may cause splits in the vertebral body. Rotation with extension, as in the extension–distraction injuries of judicial hanging, damages the posterior elements to produce complex fractures of the pedicle and pars interarticularis.

Treatment depends on the stability of the fracture and neurological involvement. Fractures with no neurological damage need a halo-vest for 6 weeks and then a collar, while those with a neurological deficit need the same fixation and early rehabilitation for the problems of paraplegia.

'Whiplash' (combined extension–flexion) injury

Combined extension–flexion injuries, often called whiplash injuries, are common in road traffic accidents.

When a vehicle is 'shunted' from behind, the head of the victim is thrown backwards and the neck hyperextended (Fig. 10.23). In severe cases the anterior longitudinal ligament may be torn and there is bleeding between the ligament and the vertebrae. This may cause enough retropharyngeal swelling to cause dysphagia a few hours after the injury. Head

157

restraints limit the range of hyperextension and minimize the effects of this injury.

In accidents where the vehicle decelerates rapidly at the moment of impact, the head is thrown forward and the cervical spine flexed. The chin will then hit the chest, which limits flexion, and there will be little damage unless the forward movement of the head is so great that there is a longitudinal distraction as well, a little like hanging. This can cause neurological damage. In the recoil from impact the victim is thrown backwards and hyperextension can occur.

Clinical features

There may be no symptoms until 6 or even 12 h after the injury, but patients involved in road traffic accidents are sometimes brought to hospital immediately after the accident before the symptoms have developed. The radiograph is usually normal and the patient may be discharged from the casualty department with a normal X-ray before the onset of symptoms. This may be difficult to explain to sceptical lawyers if the accident becomes the subject of litigation, as many do.

The leading symptoms are pain and stiffness in the neck, accompanied by aching across the shoulders and down the arms, and sometimes dysphagia. Neurological symptoms such as tingling or numbness are sometimes present but usually transient.

The prognosis is notoriously unpredictable. Ninety per cent of patients are free of symptoms within 2 years, but in a very small proportion the symptoms can last for many years. Some patients may be unable to turn the head enough to reverse a car, which may have a serious impact on everyday life and ability to work.

Unfortunately, many patients seeking compensation for their injuries without demonstrable pathology complain of identical symptoms.

Treatment

A soft supporting collar and analgesics have been advocated in the first few days after injury but the collar should be discarded as soon as possible and physiotherapy begun to restore neck movement. If this is not done, the cervical spine may remain stiff and painful.

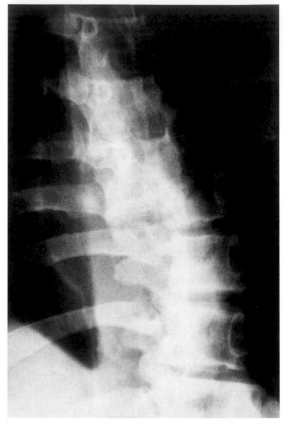

Fig. 10.24 A transverse fracture of the thoracic spine. The displacement of the fragments was accompanied by complete transection of the spinal cord.

Thoracic spine injuries

The thoracic spine has little mobility and this rigidity gives it some protection from injury. Combined flexion–extension injuries and dislocation of the facet joints do not occur in the thoracic spine. Although rarer than injuries to other parts of the spine, thoracic spine injuries are generally severe and often cause paraplegia (Fig. 10.24). There are two reasons for this:

1. The spinal canal is narrow relative to the spinal cord.

2. The displacement of the fragments at the fracture may be considerable and this damages the cord.

Types of fracture

The pattern of fracture depends on the position of the axis of flexion and the direction of the force at the time of impact. There are four main types of fracture:

1. Compression fractures.
2. Burst fractures.
3. Seat-belt (flexion–distraction) fractures.
4. Fracture dislocations.

The injury is commonest in elderly patients with porotic bone who slip and land on their bottom, but it can also occur in younger patients who fall from a height and land on their heels, an injury which also causes a crush fracture of the calcaneum. Pilots who eject from jet aircraft also suffer from this fracture because the upward force of the rockets in the ejector seat is enough to crush the vertebra.

Compression fractures

Compression, or crush, fractures occur at the thoracolumbar junction where the thoracic kyphosis ends and the lumbar lordosis begins. They are caused by a vertical force just in front of the midline of the spine which compresses the anterior lip of the affected vertebra (Figs 10.25, 10.26).

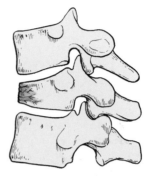

Fig. 10.25 Compression fracture of a thoracic vertebra.

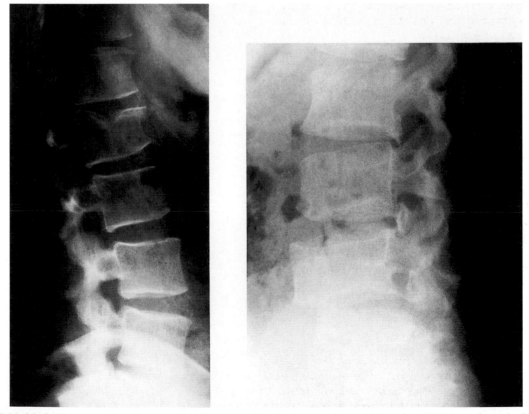

Fig. 10.26 (a), (b) Two examples of compression fractures of the lumbar vertebrae with less than 50% loss of vertebral height.

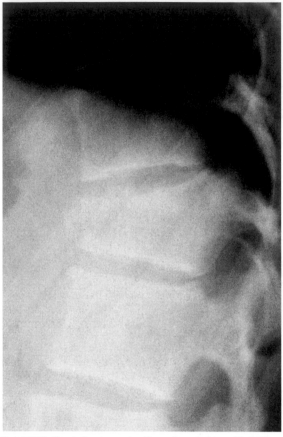

Fig. 10.27 Crush fracture of a thoracic vertebra with 50% loss of vertebral height.

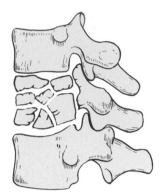

Fig. 10.28 Burst fracture of a thoracic vertebra.

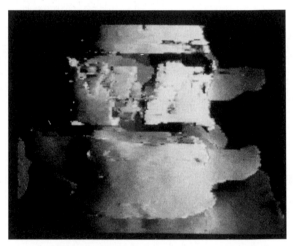

Fig. 10.29 A burst fracture of a vertebral body. By kind permission of Philips Medical Systems.

Treatment. The deformity can usually be accepted but if more than 50% of the anterior vertebral height is lost, distraction and internal fixation may be needed (Fig. 10.27). Even in slight deformities, back pain may persist for 2 or more years after injury and sometimes indefinitely.

If there is less than 50% loss of vertebral height, the patient can be mobilized rapidly within the limits of pain.

Burst fractures

A crush fracture is caused by axial compression of the anterior margin of the vertebra but a burst fracture is the result of a pure axial force. The sides of the vertebra are pushed outwards and disc material may be forced into the vertebral body or the spinal canal (Fig. 10.28). CT scans are invaluable (Figs 10.29, 10.30).

Burst fractures may be stable or unstable, depending on the pattern of the fracture. They are often associated with neurological damage from backward displacement of the vertebral body or its fragments.

Treatment. Unstable fractures can be treated by bed rest for 6 weeks, brace immobilization or operative fixation. Stable fractures can be mobilized more rapidly, as soon as pain permits.

Seat-belt fractures (flexion–distraction fractures)

Rapid deceleration in a road traffic accident throws the victim forwards against the seat-belt and may cause a flexion–distraction injury. The vertebral body may be split, and displacement can be severe.

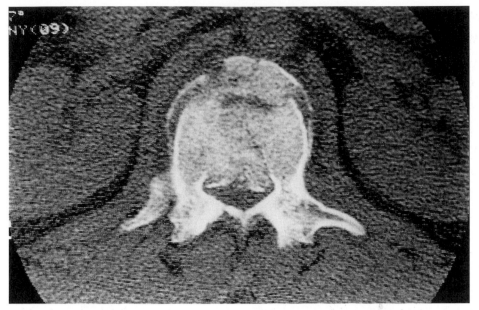

Fig. 10.30 CT scan of a burst fracture of a thoracic vertebra with bone fragments pushed backwards into the spinal canal.

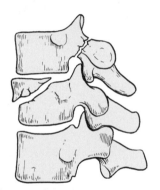

Fig. 10.31 A fracture of the thoracic spine with oblique fracture of the vertebral body and disruption of the pedicles.

Treatment. These fractures can usually be managed conservatively with bed rest for 6 weeks, followed by a plaster jacket. The patient should be nursed with the spine in extension over a pillow and the cast applied in extension.

Fracture dislocations

Combined flexion, compression and rotational forces occur in many injuries, including the fall of masonry onto the flexed spine and falls from a height (Fig. 10.31). The vertebral body is split, or the pedicles fractured and the facet joints may be dislocated. Paraplegia is usual.

Treatment. Fracture dislocations may be treated conservatively or operatively. If the patient is paraplegic, early spinal fusion allows the patient to begin rehabilitation at the earliest possible moment. The onset of paraplegia is a terrible experience for the patient and early rehabilitation helps to give a sense of purpose.

If the patient is not paraplegic, the aim of treatment should be stabilization of the spine to prevent neurological damage. Stabilization can be achieved by immobilization in bed for an extended period of time or by operative fixation to support the spine until union has occurred.

Lumbar spine injuries

Like the cervical spine, the lumbar spine has some mobility and both major and minor fractures occur.

Avulsion of the transverse processes

The transverse processes have powerful muscles attached to them and can be avulsed by violent twisting or flexing movements or by violent muscle spasm such as an epileptic fit. An avulsed transverse process is not a serious injury but the pain and muscle spasm last for 6–8 weeks.

161

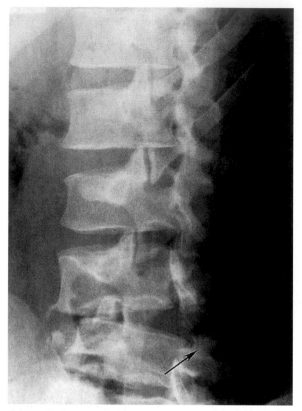

Fig. 10.32 Fracture of the pars interarticularis of L5. This is a traumatic spondylolisthesis.

Treatment. No treatment is required apart from analgesics and gradual mobilization.

Compression fractures

Compression or crush fractures at the thoracolumbar junction are described on page 159.

Flexion–rotation fractures

Twisting and rotational forces disrupt vertebrae in the lumbar spine (Fig. 10.32), as they do in the thoracic spine (p. 156), and cause neurological damage. Because the spinal cord does not extend below the first lumbar vertebra, only the lower motor neurone and sensory nerves are involved and the neurological problem is very different from the cord injuries of the cervical and thoracic spines.

Treatment. As in other situations, treatment may be conservative or operative but conservative treatment is the rule because the cauda equina is involved in this region and nerve roots are more robust than the spinal cord. Cauda equina lesions have a much better prognosis than cord lesions.

The large mass of cancellous bone and muscle makes non-union of such fractures unusual but fixation may be required to stabilize an unstable fracture (Fig. 10.33). Details of management depend upon the anatomy and the CT scan.

Paraplegia

The management of a paraplegic patient is described in many textbooks but must be included here because many paraplegic patients are admitted first to an orthopaedic ward.

Level of the lesion

It is important to establish the neurological level of the lesion. This does not correspond to the vertebral level because the spinal cord is shorter than the spinal column. Nerve roots damaged at the fracture site will have lower motor neurone lesions, and the roots leaving the cord below the fracture site will have upper motor neurone lesions (Fig. 10.34).

The degree of damage must be assessed carefully as soon as possible after injury and reassessed three times each day because the damage may worsen as the spinal cord and soft tissues swell in the days following injury.

Root escape

One of the difficulties in determining the final result is 'root escape'. The nerve roots are tougher than the spinal cord and it is possible for the cord to be crushed or severed while the roots that cross the fracture remain intact. Surviving roots may not work normally at first because of oedema, axonotmesis or neurapraxia, but recovery from these conditions is possible. The lower the lesion, the more roots are likely to escape damage.

Prognosis

The prognosis depends on the neurological findings 48 h after injury. Patients with complete cord loss at 48 h do not recover but those with some cord function may continue to improve for up to 2 years after injury.

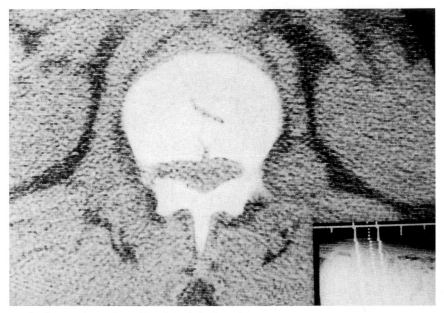

Fig. 10.33 CT scan of a fractured vertebra with minimal displacement.

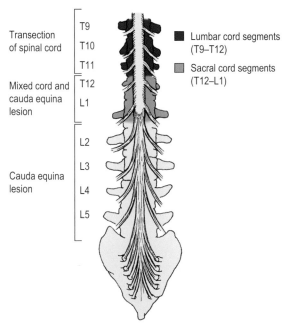

Fig. 10.34 Relationship of spinal cord nerve roots and vertebrae. The spinal cord ends at L1 and injuries below that level involve nerve roots only.

The bladder in paraplegia

There are two main types of bladder dysfunction in paraplegic patients.

Complete denervation

The completely denervated bladder distends without the patient being aware of it and retention with overflow develops. If this is not recognized, back pressure on the kidneys and renal failure may follow. Urinary infection is a serious problem and every care must be taken to prevent it by catheterization with strict sterile technique and careful management.

The automatic bladder

If the bladder retains some autonomic activity, there may be reflex spasm of the detrusor muscle and unexpected emptying of the bladder. As with the completely denervated bladder, the automatic bladder must be catheterized with full sterile precautions.

In the later stages of rehabilitation, the voiding reflex can sometimes be put to good use if it can be initiated by a simple manoeuvre such as pressure on the lower abdomen.

Skin care

Pressure sores occur quickly in areas of insensitive skin. If a paraplegic patient lies immobile for more than 2 h the skin at the point of contact with the bed dies and a pressure sore results. If weight is not taken

163

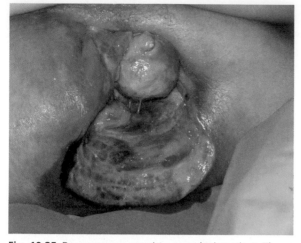

Fig. 10.35 Deep pressure sore in a paraplegic patient. The femoral head is visible.

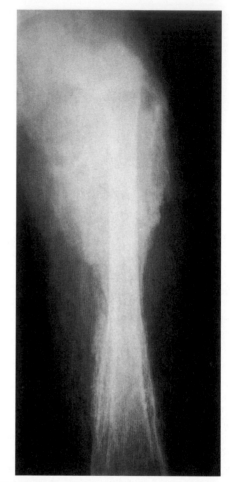

Fig. 10.36 Massive new bone formation around a fracture in a denervated limb.

off the affected area, the subcutaneous tissues also perish, until the skeleton is exposed (Fig. 10.35).

To prevent this disaster the patients must be turned regularly, at least every 2 h. This involves much heavy lifting, and in some paraplegic units a full-time 'turning team' moves around the wards, turning the patients at regular intervals.

Joint stiffness

If joints are not moved regularly, they become stiff. This is a particular problem in paraplegic patients because stiffness makes it impossible to restore movement even if recovery occurs. All the joints must therefore be put through their full range of movement every day to avoid serious contractures.

Muscle spasm is another problem. Muscles with an upper motor neurone lesion contract violently and cause severe cramp-like pain. Muscle relaxants sometimes help but surgical denervation may be required.

Fractures

For reasons that are not known, fractures in paralysed limbs throw out an unusually large mass of new bone and this may restrict joint motion (Fig. 10.36).

Rehabilitation

The rehabilitation of a paraplegic patient involves not only the body but morale as well. A clear pro-

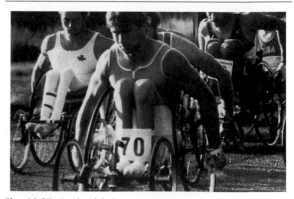

Fig. 10.37 A wheelchair race.

gramme of events is essential, and demonstrable progress is more encouraging than anything else. The prospect of a return to competitive sport is especially helpful, and wheelchair games are invaluable (Fig. 10.37).

Case reports

These case studies represent three different presentations of lumbar spine fractures.

Patient A

An 82-year-old lady fell while gardening and sustained a low injury to her lumbar spine. She was in severe pain and discomfort, but was able to walk unaided.

She attended her general practitioner who treated her conservatively with oral analgesics. An X-ray was requested and this confirmed previous osteoporotic wedge fractures of the lumbar spine and what appeared to be a potentially new fracture of the third lumbar vertebra.

Treatment in this case was conservative as there were no abnormal neurology signs and the pain was managed satisfactorily with simple oral analgesics. The patient was subsequently referred for bone density analysis and treatment for osteoporosis was instituted.

Patient B

A 32-year-old lady was thrown from a horse while eventing, and landed awkwardly in rough terrain. She had immediate significant back pain, but it was clear that she still had use of both lower limbs.

She was evacuated to the hospital after her spine was immobilized on a spinal board and a careful assessment of the back and lower limbs was performed. It was clear that there was no neural deficit and bowel and bladder control were unaffected. Plain radiographs confirmed a burst fracture of the third lumbar vertebra and subsequent CT confirmed the extensive injury, but no apparent damage to the spinal cord.

Methods of management were discussed with the patient and she elected to be treated conservatively with bed rest, subsequent brace immobilization and cautious mobilization thereafter.

She declined fixation of the fragment because of the potential risks to the spinal cord.

Patient C

A 22-year-old gentleman was involved in a high energy injury while racing his motorbike. At the scene of the accident it was clear that he had very little, if any, use of his lower limbs and he was immobilized on a spinal board then transferred immediately to the accident and emergency department of the nearest hospital.

On initial assessment it was clear that he was paraplegic. X-rays confirmed a fracture at the thoracolumbar junction with encroachment of the spinal cord by bony fragments.

After appropriate resuscitation and stabilization of the patient it was elected to fix the fracture fragments using a combination of pedicle screws and rod immobilization above and below the fracture. This allowed stabilization of the spine.

He was subsequently transferred to a spinal injuries unit, where he regained very little use of the lower limbs.

Summary

Low energy injuries in the elderly often result in osteoporotic crush-type fractures. These are rarely associated with neurological compromise and can be managed conservatively with analgesics and mobilization. As with all osteoporotic fractures they should be investigated and patients treated for osteoporosis where appropriate.

High energy injuries with significant disruption of the bone and potential instability of the spinal column can be treated conservatively or operatively. Operative stabilization of the fracture fragments allows easier rehabilitation of the patient, but may not alter the long-term history of either the neurology or the incidence of subsequent back pain.

Chapter |11|

Injuries to the trunk

By the end of this chapter you should:

- Understand the complications of rib fractures and, in particular, the injuries to the chest cavity and pleura.
- Understand the different mechanisms of injury to the pelvis and how this affects the fracture pattern and complications.
- Be aware of these complications and, in particular, vascular, neural and urogenital injuries.

Rib fractures

The severity of rib fractures depends on their number and stability. Multiple fractures which interfere with breathing have serious complications, but isolated cracks can usually be treated as severe bruises.

Isolated fractures

Fractures of a single rib can follow a direct blow or, in elderly patients, a fit of violent coughing. At the moment of fracture the patient feels sudden pain in the chest followed by pain on deep inspiration. On examination, there is well localized tenderness at the fracture site and pain on 'springing' the ribs.

It is most unwise to reassure patients that their ribs are intact just because the radiographs do not show a fracture. Radiographs only show the fracture if the X-ray beam catches it at exactly the right angle, which is rare, and for practical purposes clinical signs are more reliable than radiographs in the first week after injury.

After 2 weeks, the fracture can be recognized more easily by the rarefaction of the bone ends and callus around the fracture.

Treatment

Isolated fractures seldom require active treatment and can be regarded as 'a bad bruise'. Untreated, they are very painful for 10–14 days and moderately painful for a further 4 weeks. By 8 weeks from injury they should be pain-free, when the callus can be felt as a firm bony swelling at the fracture site.

Analgesics are essential in the first few days and an intercostal block with local anaesthetic is sometimes needed. Breathing is painful without analgesia, chest movement is limited, the underlying lung develops atelectasia, secondary infection can follow and the patients may die if they are infirm.

Strapping the chest. Once the standard treatment for all fractured ribs (Fig. 11.1), strapping relieves pain by restricting rib movement. Today, strapping is indicated only for robust, hard-working individu-

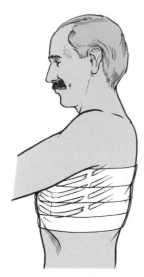

Fig. 11.1 Strapping for broken ribs.

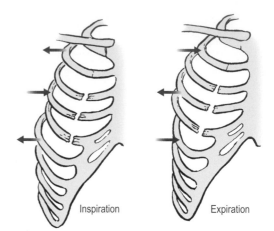

Fig. 11.2 A flail chest with paradoxical respiration. An unsupported segment of chest with ribs broken at each end moves inwards during inspiration and outwards during expiration.

als who wish to get on with their job and pretend that the injury never happened.

In dire emergencies, such as the battlefield, a pad bandaged over a flail segment reduces its excursion and minimizes the interference with inspiratory volume. A pad and bandage is also helpful if there is a penetrating wound of the pleura because it closes the opening into the pleural space.

Although valuable as an emergency measure, strapping is not good long-term treatment. Restricting thoracic movement and relying on diaphragmatic movement alone for breathing leads to lobar collapse, which predisposes to chest infection and creates further respiratory difficulties. Definitive treatment is therefore determined by the type of fracture and the stability of the chest.

Multiple fractures

Flail chest. The main function of the ribs is to act as a moving cage to suck air into the lungs as it is elevated by the chest musculature. If this rigidity is lost and part of the chest wall is free to move independently of the rest of the thorax, it will be sucked inwards when the patient attempts to inhale and blown outwards on exhalation (Fig. 11.2). This is 'paradoxical respiration'; it dramatically reduces tidal volume and can cause respiratory failure.

Flail segments are commonly caused by a direct blow to the chest rather than by a crushing injury. A blow from a horse's hoof produces a circular flail segment about 15 cm across, and a blow to the

sternum from a steering wheel can fracture all ribs on both sides to produce a flail segment that includes the mediastinum.

Crushed chest. If a chest is crushed, there will be fractured ribs on both sides of the chest. Because it is difficult to fracture more than three ribs on one side of the chest and leave the other side intact, the presence of more than three fractures on one side of a crushed chest usually means that there are fractures on the other side as well, whatever the radiographs show.

A crushed chest does not usually have paradoxical movement but pain from the fractures interferes seriously with breathing and this can also cause respiratory failure.

Treatment

Treatment of multiple rib fractures depends upon their stability.

Stable fractures. Provided the rib cage is stable and there is no flail segment, inspiration is possible. Treatment is then similar to that of an isolated fracture, but more energetic. The pain is more severe, areas of tenderness are more numerous, inhibition of inspiration is more marked and breathing and movement are more painful. Stronger analgesics or intercostal nerve blocks may be required to make breathing comfortable.

Unstable fractures. Unstable flail segments are best treated by positive pressure ventilation so that the 'bellows' function of the chest is disregarded and the

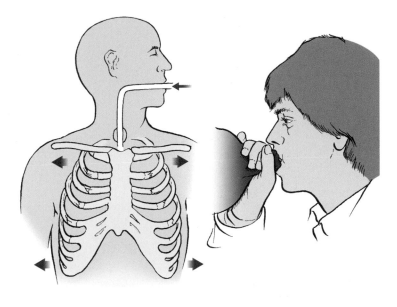

Fig. 11.3 Positive pressure respiration. If there are multiple rib fractures, the chest may be inflated passively like a paper bag.

chest inflated like a paper bag (Fig. 11.3). Strapping the flail segment is useful until the patient reaches hospital. Positive pressure ventilation can be instituted and, if necessary, maintained by tracheostomy for 2 or 3 weeks until the chest wall is stable.

The decision to ventilate a patient is made in conjunction with the thoracic surgeons and anaesthetists and the patient is best managed in the intensive therapy unit.

Pathological fractures

The ribs are a common site for metastatic deposits and pathological fractures are common. Suspected rib fractures deserve radiological examination, even though they are often undetectable.

Injuries to the costal cartilages

The costal cartilages are softer and more flexible than ribs but can be fractured by direct violence. The clinical features are similar to those of an isolated rib fracture but the pain is less severe.

The joints between the costal cartilages of the false ribs can also be injured and dislocations of these joints produce pain and tenderness which can be very slow to resolve.

Treatment

Injection with hydrocortisone acetate is sometimes helpful.

Fractures in the elderly

In the elderly, the pain from rib fractures impairs respiratory function. Pain relief in these patients is particularly important and local infiltration of the fracture with local anaesthetic or an intercostal nerve block may be required.

Injuries involving the pleural cavity

There are three types of pneumothorax (Fig. 11.4):

1. Closed
2. Open
3. Tension.

If lung and pleura are damaged, a pneumothorax, haemothorax or chylothorax may follow.

Closed pneumothorax

Most pneumothoraces consist of nothing more than a little air in the pleural cavity which will be absorbed in a few days (Fig. 11.5). Because the air in the pleural space floats upwards, a pneumothorax cannot be seen on an anteroposterior radiograph

169

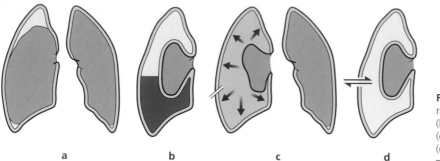

Fig. 11.4 Types of pneumothorax: (a) simple pneumothorax; (b) haemopneumothorax; (c) tension pneumothorax; (d) open pneumothorax.

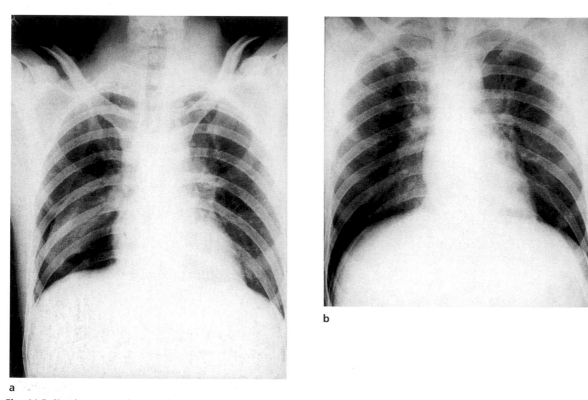

Fig. 11.5 Simple pneumothorax: (a) marked collapse and (b) very slight collapse of the right lower lobe.

unless the patient is standing or sitting upright, when it is seen above the clavicle.

If the pneumothorax is small, the only evidence may be the absence of lung markings at the apex. If a standing or sitting radiograph is not possible, a lateral radiograph may show air lying against the lateral wall of the chest.

Treatment

A pneumothorax occupying more than 25% of the hemithorax causes respiratory embarrassment and

draining may be needed, using a catheter attached to an underwater seal.

Open pneumothorax

If the skin and parietal pleura are broken, the pleural space will communicate with the outside air, which will be sucked in and out of the chest on inspiration and expiration. Respiratory embarrassment follows unless the opening is closed. Infection is an additional risk but is unusual if the lung can be kept expanded and the pleural space obliterated.

Treatment

As first aid, a pad can be placed over the opening, or the patient simply laid with the wound downwards until a chest drain can be inserted. It is not necessary to close the wound unless it is large or contaminated.

Tension pneumothorax

If the opening into the pleura is oblique it can work like a flap valve and allow air into the pleural cavity on inspiration but will not let it out on expiration (Fig. 11.6). The pleural space will then be inflated under pressure, the lung will collapse and the mediastinum will shift to the opposite side. Unless treated promptly, the patient will die within minutes. This is a tension pneumothorax.

If there is a rib fracture as well, the air will be forced out through the fracture site into the subcutaneous tissues to produce surgical emphysema, which can extend over the whole of the chest wall and into the neck (Fig. 11.7). A similar appearance is also seen after vigorous positive pressure ventilation of patients with fractured ribs.

Treatment

In patients with a tension pneumothorax the insertion of a chest drain is a life-saving procedure. A pneumothorax or chest drain pack is available in all accident departments and every doctor likely to be exposed to such a patient should know how to use it.

Emergency treatment of tension pneumothorax

1. Make a short skin incision in the fourth rib space (i.e. between the fourth and fifth ribs) in the midaxillary line on the side of the pneumothorax (Fig. 11.8).
2. Dissect right down through the intercostal muscles and pleura with scissors. Open the scissors widely to release air. The hiss of air will be felt and heard and the patient will improve dramatically.
3. Pass a chest drain through the incision and into the pleural cavity. The situation is then under control.
4. Secure the drain to the patient and connect it to an underwater seal or valve.

To push a pair of sharp scissors into a patient's chest may seem hazardous, but in a patient with a tension pneumothorax the vital structures are pushed well away from the point of entry. There is no time for a radiograph to confirm which side of the chest is involved but this is obvious clinically because the affected side contains so much air that it is tympanitic to percussion.

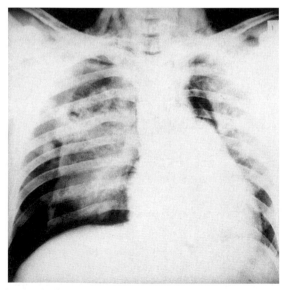

Fig. 11.6 Bilateral pneumothorax with tension pneumothorax on the right side. Note the surgical emphysema in the neck.

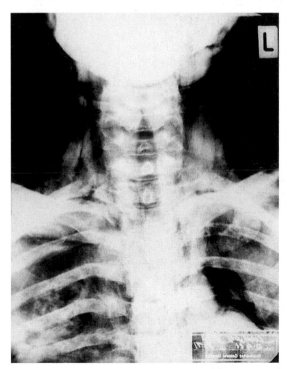

Fig. 11.7 Massive surgical emphysema caused by rupture of a main bronchus.

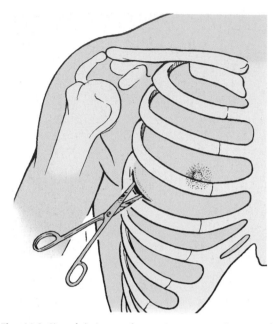

Fig. 11.8 Site of drainage of a tension pneumothorax at the fourth intercostal space in the midaxillary line. Keep the scissors close to the upper border of the lower rib.

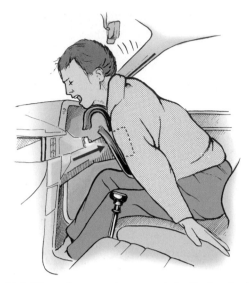

Fig. 11.9 Effect of not wearing a seat-belt. The head strikes the windscreen, the neck is hyperextended and the steering column is driven into the precordium.

Haemothorax

Bleeding into the pleural cavity will produce a more gradual deterioration than a pneumothorax. The pulse rate rises, blood pressure falls and the chest is dull to percussion; the diagnosis can be confirmed radiologically.

Treatment

Treatment is by drainage as described, or if the bleeding cannot be controlled then a thoracotomy may be required to stop the bleed.

Chylothorax

Damage to the thoracic duct can cause chyle (lymph) to run into the pleural cavity, producing a chylothorax, which causes a steady deterioration.

Treatment

Treatment is difficult and may require the attention of the thoracic surgeons to close a thoracic duct leak, but many heal spontaneously with tube drainage and parenteral nutrition. Healing may take several weeks and the patient must take nothing by mouth during this time.

Injuries to the mediastinum

The steering column of every car is aimed liked a spear at the heart of the driver and injuries to the mediastinum are a common cause of death. Despite collapsible steering columns, steering wheels contoured to fit the thorax (Fig. 11.9) and adequate seat-belts worn correctly, rapid deceleration from a head-on collision can still force the steering wheel back against the chest. The result may be a fracture of the sternum and the ribs attached to it, or rupture of the heart, aorta, a main bronchus and occasionally the oesophagus. More recently, cars fitted with 'air bags' have become more popular. When inflated these reduce the risk of direct damage to the anterior chest as well as the head and neck.

Aortic and cardiac rupture

Rupture of the heart is usually so rapidly fatal that it need concern neither the casualty officer nor the orthopaedic surgeon. A laceration or rupture of the aortic arch may leak into the mediastinum over a period of days or suddenly increase and cause exsanguination. The usual site of aortic rupture lies just distal to the left subclavian artery at the junction where the fixed and mobile parts of the aorta meet (Fig. 11.10).

To diagnose this serious injury, the width of the mediastinum should be noted on a radiograph

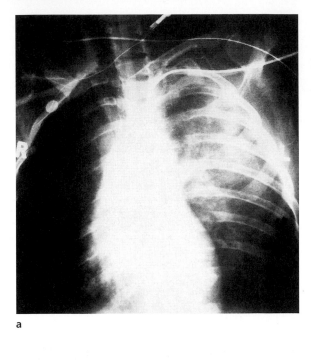 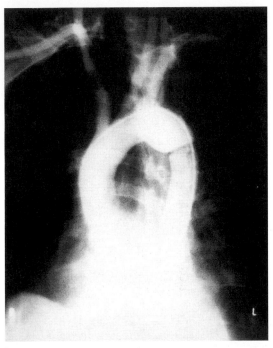

a

b

Fig. 11.10 (a) Widened mediastinum. (b) Complete transection of the aorta demonstrated by aortography. The blood is contained by the adventitia only.

(taken at 1.8 m) of every patient who has suffered a blow to the chest, particularly drivers.

Not all injuries to the heart are so serious. Cardiac contusion may cause arrhythmias, and valves can be ruptured, causing murmurs which can be heard.

Treatment

If there is any widening of the mediastinal shadow it must be assumed that this is due to haemorrhage into the mediastinum and the opinion of a thoracic surgeon obtained as a matter of urgency. A CT scan or arch arteriogram may be needed to demonstrate the lesion.

Fracture of the sternum

Fracture of the sternum can be caused either by direct trauma, which requires extreme force and is usually associated with other injuries, or by violent flexion of the thoracic spine accompanied by a wedge fracture of the thoracic spine.

Fractures of the sternum are not serious in themselves and usually unite soundly, but their presence

should alert the doctor to the possibility of a more serious injury. A flail segment including the mediastinum may be difficult to control, even by positive pressure respiration (see Fig. 11.3).

Treatment

If the fractured sternum is not properly aligned it may need reduction and wiring.

Injuries to viscera

Lung

Like other tissues, damaged lung becomes inflamed and engorged. Damaged lung does not function as well as healthy tissue and extensive lung contusion leads to respiratory failure. This, together with poor thoracic movement, pain, flail segments and pneumothorax, may precipitate respiratory failure even when the initial resuscitation has been successful.

The result, sometimes known as 'shock lung', is due to a combination of factors:

173

1. Physical trauma to lung tissue.
2. Over-transfusion, especially with saline or dextrose.
3. Poor chest movement.
4. Adult respiratory distress syndrome (ARDS).

The initial trauma causes platelet aggregation and activation of the neutrophils. The platelet aggregates occlude small vessels, leading to shunting and the release of hormones, which in turn cause bronchospasm and pulmonary hypertension. Superoxide radicals are also released by neutrophils and these act on the alveolar epithelium to increase pulmonary permeability.

Treatment

Adequate oxygenation, diuretics and positive pressure ventilation are required. *Do not over-transfuse with crystalloid solutions.*

Bronchus

Rapid deceleration can tear a bronchus, causing a massive leak into the pleural space.

Treatment

The lesion must be repaired as soon as possible by a thoracic surgeon.

Heart

Rupture of the heart is usually fatal but stab wounds are less serious. Because the heart contracts during systole, the wound is sealed at the moment of greatest pressure and blood loss is reduced. A haemopericardium follows but only causes cardiac tamponade if the pericardium is intact (Fig. 11.11). If the pericardium is ruptured or cut, as it would be with a stab wound, the cardiac tamponade decompresses itself and exsanguination is the main danger.

Treatment

Thoracotomy and repair of the injury, with pericardial drainage.

Traumatic asphyxia and compression injuries

Rapid compression of the trunk squeezes the fluid contents, both liquid and gas, within the chest and

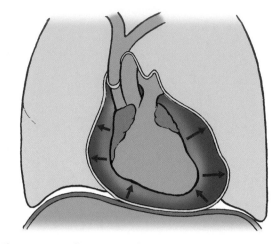

Fig. 11.11 Cardiac tamponade.

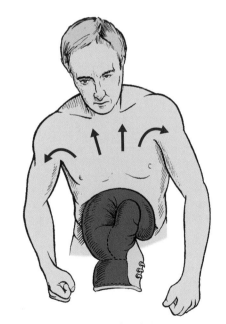

Fig. 11.12 Severe pressure on the abdomen may cause petechial haemorrhages in the face and hands.

abdomen and causes a violent surge of pressure in the peripheral vessels of the face, arms and legs. This can cause petechial haemorrhages at the periphery, ruptured bowel, and rupture of the diaphragm with bowel lying in the pleural cavity (Fig. 11.12). The petechial haemorrhages on the face, neck and arms are similar to those seen after strangulation and the condition is called traumatic asphyxia.

Treatment

No specific treatment is required apart from adequate oxygenation and repair of the intrathoracic and intra-abdominal injuries.

Beware of abdominal trauma!

Small wounds or bruises may be the only sign of:
- Ruptured spleen.
- Ruptured liver.
- Ruptured gut.

Ruptured spleen

The spleen is a very vascular structure and remarkable for its trouble-free performance. The main affliction of the spleen is rupture; this can be followed by bleeding into the peritoneal cavity, which can be life-threatening and need surgery for its control. The injury that damages the spleen need not be violent: a blow to the left hypochondrium on the edge of a desk is quite sufficient, although more vigorous blunt trauma is usually involved.

Because the spleen has no sensory fibres, the patient does not experience pain but shows the signs of blood loss with a rapid pulse, falling blood pressure and pallor. The abdomen may be normal apart from diminished bowel sounds and there may be no other abnormality on clinical examination, but unless treated promptly the patient is likely to die from haemorrhage.

Some ruptured spleens behave in an even more treacherous manner. If the capsule remains intact it will limit the extent of the haemorrhage, but in some patients the capsule may rupture 24 h after injury. Detecting small amounts of intraperitoneal blood is therefore important, and abdominal paracentesis, with a few hundred millilitres of warmed saline run into the peritoneal space, drained out and inspected for blood, may be needed to make the diagnosis.

MRI is helpful but difficult to arrange as an emergency procedure on an ill patient. Laparoscopy is also helpful.

Treatment

Urgent laparatomy and splenectomy are life-saving measures. The abdominal surgeons should be asked to see any patient in whom a ruptured spleen is suspected.

Ruptured liver

Rupture of the liver, which is larger than the spleen and just as vascular, can also cause intraperitoneal haemorrhage. The commonest causes are rapid deceleration injuries and blunt trauma, usually sustained in road traffic accidents and accompanied by chest injuries. The liver cannot be removed but bleeding must be controlled, which is difficult because the liver is so soft and friable.

Treatment

Laparatomy is required to control bleeding by suturing individual vessels, packing, or selective ligation of the hepatic vessels. Dead and doubtful tissue must be excised to avoid sepsis.

Ruptured gut

Although the bowel and stomach can be ruptured by direct trauma, great force is required. Radiographs will often demonstrate gas in the peritoneal cavity on a sitting or standing film because the gas rises. The presence of gas under the diaphragm in an injured patient always indicates rupture of the stomach or bowel.

Treatment

Laparatomy and repair or resection of the affected bowel.

Stab wounds

Any stab wounds between the nipple line and the pubis can cause serious intra-abdominal damage. The length of the wound is no guide to the length of the blade and quite serious lesions, even perforation of the aorta, can be caused by a very narrow blade or glass sliver.

Treatment

Most wounds need formal exploration, including laparotomy, but careful exploration sometimes shows that the wound has not entered the peritoneum.

Retroperitoneal haematoma

The retroperitoneal space is large and includes the aorta, vena cava, kidney, psoas muscles and parts of

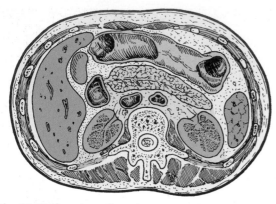

Fig. 11.13 The retroperitoneal space.

the autonomic nervous system (Fig. 11.13). Haemorrhage into the space can follow damage to any of these structures, and is seen after fractures of the lumbar vertebrae or avulsion of the transverse processes.

A retroperitoneal haematoma not only causes a painful restriction of lumbar movement but also interferes with the autonomic nervous system and may cause paralytic ileus.

Treatment

No specific treatment is required but the patient must not eat or drink until bowel function has returned.

Kidneys

Trauma to the lumbar region may cause renal injury, followed by an accumulation of urine and blood in the retroperitoneal space. Damage to the upper urinary tract should be suspected if there is haematuria and the opinion of a urologist obtained. An excretion urogram will usually be required.

Treatment

Treatment is best in the hands of urologists and depends on the site and extent of the lesion. Suture, partial nephrectomy or total nephrectomy may be needed.

Pelvic injuries

Like fractures of the ribs, fractures of the pelvis are of varying severity. Patients can bleed to death from

pelvic fractures if the iliac vessels are torn, and some fractures destroy the hip joint while others are little more serious than a bad bruise.

Pelvic fractures have a well-deserved reputation for being missed. The pelvis is easily fractured in crushing injuries and a serious fracture with an unstable pelvis should always be suspected after any compression injury. A pelvic X-ray is mandatory in the assessment of the acutely injured patient who has signs of cardiovascular instability.

In general, fractures can be divided into:

1. Avulsion.
2. Single bone.
3. Complex.
4. Acetabulum.

Avulsion

Avulsion fractures of the origin of the adductors, rectus femoris and sartorius muscles are seen in young fit athletes.

Treatment

The treatment is based on the severity of the injury and the degree of displacement. At times, large fragments will need to be reduced and held with internal fixation, i.e. a screw.

Single bone

These injuries are common in elderly patients with porotic bone or where there has been a well localized area of trauma. Fractures include pubic rami (Figs 11.14, 11.15) and the wing of the ilium. Pubic rami fractures often occur in pairs and can be trivial in nature. Occasionally, however, there can be associated injury to bladder or urethra.

Treatment

Early mobilization in uncomplicated injuries is recommended. Patients will be in severe pain for the first few days but should be mobile in about a week.

Wing of the ilium

The main function of the wing of the ilium is to provide a firm foundation for muscle attachment and the protection of the pelvic contents. A fracture is caused by a direct blow or a crush injury.

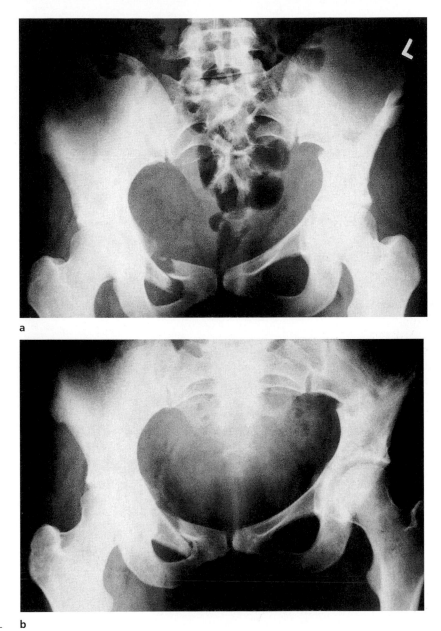

Fig. 11.14 (a) Fracture of the right pubic rami and a fracture of the left ilium combined with a fracture extending into the left acetabulum, immediately after injury. (b) The same fracture 12 weeks later. Note the remodelling of the pubic rami.

Treatment. As there is excellent muscle attachment, the blood supply is good. These fractures heal rapidly but may be very painful for the first few weeks.

Complex

The pelvis can be considered to be a ring structure. It is uncommon to be able to break the true ring in a single place, and fractures can therefore be multiple. There are three main fracture patterns, depending on the mechanism of the injury. These are:

1. Anterior/posterior compression (open book).
2. Side compression.
3. Vertical compression.

Anterior/posterior compression

Anterior/posterior compressions can involve not only the pubic diastasis but also fractures of the

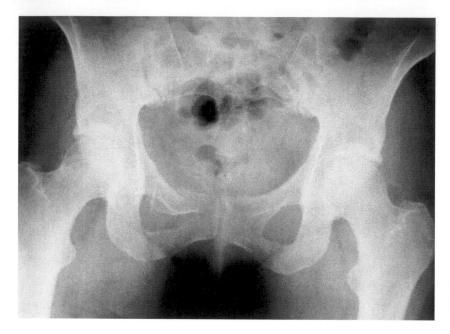

Fig. 11.15 Fracture of the upper and lower pubic rami on the right side.

pubic rami and/or sacroiliac joints, ilium or sacral body. This injury can cause catastrophic blood loss from tearing of the iliac vessels.

Treatment. Minor injuries can be treated with bed rest and gradual mobilization. More major injuries may need the reduction of the fracture – i.e. 'closing the book'. This can be accomplished by a pelvic sling, or internal or external fixator. In those cases with significant blood loss, early rapid application of an external fixation (Fig. 11.16) can be life-saving. This may be necessary in the emergency room.

External compression

These are caused by a blow to the side of the pelvis or greater trochanter. The side of the injury is rotated inwards, resulting in fractures of the pubis or ilium, disruption of the sacroiliac joint or fracture of the sacrum.

Treatment. Minor injuries can be left and patients treated conservatively with bed rest until the pain has settled. They can be mobilized with the aid of crutches until the fracture has consolidated (>6 weeks). More major injuries may require open reduction and internal fixation of the fracture fragments.

Vertical compression

These are often associated with a fall from a height. There is disruption not only of the anterior part of

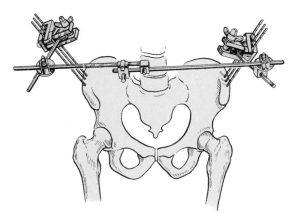

Fig. 11.16 External fixation of a pelvic fracture.

the ring but also of the sacrum, sacroiliac joint or ilium. Neurological damage can occur due to the shearing injury and damage to the sacral plexus.

Treatment. Reduction of the hemipelvis is necessary in order to stabilize the pelvis. This can be achieved by traction, or external or internal fixation.

Acetabulum

Fractures of the acetabulum disrupt the hip joint (Fig. 11.17). Major disruption will often lead to osteoarthritic degeneration in the long term. The major goal of treatment is to limit the chance of this

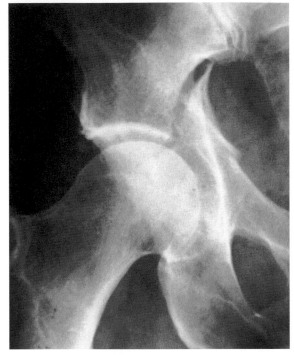

Fig. 11.17 Plain radiograph of a fractured acetabulum.

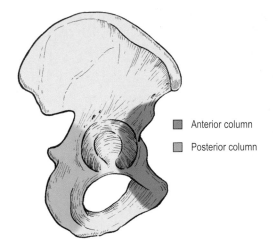

Anterior column

Posterior column

Fig. 11.18 The anterior and posterior columns of the pelvis.

and to retain early active movement of the hip joint.

Accurate assessment of the fracture is necessary in order to formulate an appropriate treatment plan. Plain radiographs do not give sufficient detail of the acetabulum to classify the type of fracture or the degree of displacement of the fracture fragments. Specialized X-rays (Judet views) or CT scans are required. Fractures can be classified according to their location in the acetabulum. There are anterior or posterior column fractures, or a combination of both (Fig. 11.18).

Treatment

In those that are undisplaced, early rapid movement is essential in order to regain the mobility of the hip joint (Fig. 11.19). Initially, patients can be treated in bed for the first few days to allow the pain to settle, then they should be mobilized with a non-weight-bearing regimen for a minimum of 6 weeks.

In those fractures that are significantly displaced, there is a need to reduce the fracture fragments and this is best achieved by open reduction and internal fixation. Undoubtedly, some fractures are

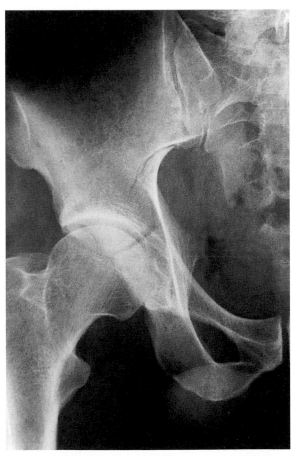

Fig. 11.19 Fracture of the right ilium extending into the acetabulum with minimal displacement.

so convoluted that this is impossible and then patients may be treated with traction and early active mobilization while on traction.

Damage to the bladder and urethra/rectum

Bladder

Direct trauma to the pelvis can rupture the bladder, particularly if it is full at the time of injury. The injury to the bladder will usually be extraperitoneal unless there is an associated penetrating wound of the abdomen.

Urethra

The urethra can be damaged in any major injury of the pelvis and urethral damage should always be suspected. If there is a discharge of blood from the urethra or a boggy swelling in the perineum a urologist is required.

Treatment

The urologists should be involved at an early stage and a catheter should not be passed until they have been consulted.

Rectum

The rectum can also be damaged and a rectal examination is always recommended. This will assess not only the rectum but also the urogenital tract.

Posterior dislocation of the hip

Posterior dislocation of the hip is common in head-on road traffic accidents in which the hip and knee are both flexed (Fig. 11.20). This dislocation should be suspected in any patient involved in such an injury. The impact is transmitted via the patella, patellofemoral joint, femur and hip joint to the posterior lip of the acetabulum, which is a thin bone and not designed for such impact (Figs 11.21, 11.22).

The injury is often associated with fracture of the patella, rupture of the posterior cruciate ligament and fracture of the femur (Fig. 11.23).

Until the dislocation is reduced, the femoral head lies behind the pelvis and the leg is internally rotated and shortened (p. 182).

There may also be a segmental or 'slice' fracture of the femoral head. The fragment may become jammed in the hip joint and prevent reduction or, worse, the sciatic nerve may be caught between the femoral head fragment and damaged when the hip is reduced (Fig. 11.24).

Complications

Posterior dislocation of the hip has a high incidence of complications (Fig. 11.25).

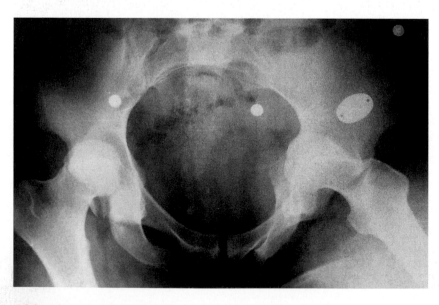

Fig. 11.20 Bilateral posterior dislocation of the hips with a fracture of the posterior lip on the right.

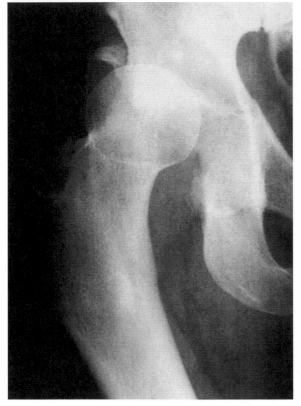

Fig. 11.21 Posterior fracture dislocation of the hip.

Complications of posterior dislocation of the hip

- *Damage to the sciatic nerve*. The lateral part of the sciatic nerve, responsible for dorsiflexion of the foot, lies immediately behind the hip and is often damaged in posterior fracture dislocation.
- *Aseptic necrosis of the femoral head*. Aseptic necrosis of the femoral head occurs in about 20% of patients with this injury but the incidence is less if the hip is reduced soon after injury. Aseptic necrosis may not be apparent until 2 years or, in exceptional cases, 8 years later. This is important when assessing the long-term prognosis of the injury, necessary for legal purposes if the fracture occurred in a road traffic accident.
- *Osteoarthritis*. If the femoral head has been damaged or there is aseptic necrosis, osteoarthritis is almost inevitable.
- *Ectopic ossification* can occur round a dislocated hip, reducing joint movement and causing pain.

Treatment

The dislocation should be reduced as soon as possible and certainly within the first 4–6 h post-injury. Reduction is usually easy, but be careful if there is an associated fracture of the femoral head or neurological damage. *Always record the neurological function*

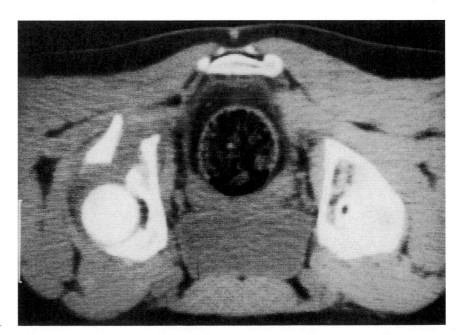

Fig. 11.22 CT scan of the pelvis showing a displaced fracture of the posterior lip of the acetabulum.

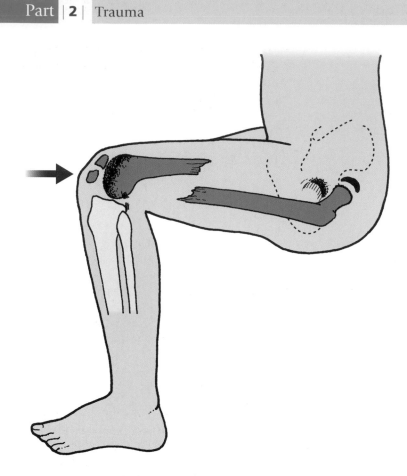

Fig. 11.23 Injuries caused by a blow to the patella with the hip and knee flexed: (i) fracture of the patella; (ii) damage to the articular surface of the femur; (iii) ruptured posterior cruciate ligament; (iv) fractured femur; (v) fracture dislocation of hip.

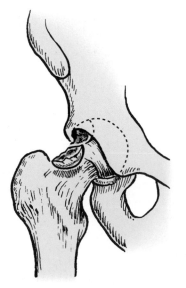

Fig. 11.24 Osteochondral fracture of the femoral head. This lesion often accompanies a dislocation of the hip.

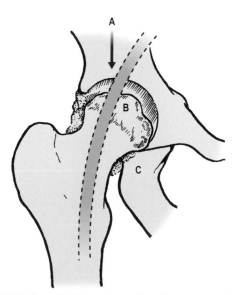

Fig. 11.25 Complications of posterior dislocation of the hip: (A) damage to the sciatic nerve; (B) aseptic necrosis of the femoral head; (C) ectopic ossification around the hip.

before and after reduction. If reduction is not easy, open reduction is needed to avoid damage to the sciatic nerve.

Definitive management depends on the stability of the reduction. If the hip is stable and the acetabular fragment is small, bed rest for 2–3 weeks with early mobilization is sufficient.

If the fracture is unstable but the fragments are in good position, bed rest for 6–8 weeks is advisable. If there is a large single fragment or a fragment in poor position and the hip is unstable, the fragment should be replaced and internally fixed.

Anterior dislocation of the hip

Anterior dislocation is rare but may follow violent abduction, although such a force is more likely to fracture the femur.

Complications

Complications include aseptic necrosis of the femoral head and osteoarthritis.

Treatment

Treatment is by closed reduction.

Sacral fractures

Sacral fractures are uncommon and usually associated with fractures of the pelvis.

Treatment

Treatment depends upon the associated pelvic fractures but internal fixation is hazardous and seldom needed.

Fractures of the coccyx

Fractures of the coccyx result from a direct blow to the bottom from a fall onto the coccyx. They are exceedingly painful.

Treatment

No specific treatment is required apart from analgesics and a soft cushion. The pain may be very slow to resolve and can lead to lasting disability.

Case reports

The management of pelvic injuries can be difficult. The following two cases highlight some of these difficulties.

Patient A

A 30-year-old pedestrian was involved in a road traffic accident when hit by a car travelling at speed. The mechanism of injury was unknown and the patient was brought to the accident and emergency department conscious and haemodynamically unstable with a painful abdomen.

The initial clinical review confirmed a normal Glasgow coma scale, increased respiratory rate, blood pressure of 110/40 and tachycardia. On palpation the abdomen was tender, maximally in the suprapubic area. There was marked bruising of the scrotum and blood at the external meatus. Both legs lay in slight external rotation and there was an abrasion over the skin of the lower abdomen.

Despite vigorous fluid rehydration with crystalloids and colloids the patient remained haemodynamically unstable. Radiographs were obtained of the cervical spine, abdomen and pelvis. The pelvic X-rays confirmed wide diastases of the pelvis. A CT of the abdomen confirmed no liver or splenic injury but fluid within the pelvis and the diastases.

The urologists reviewed the patient and confirmed the urethra had been disrupted but the patient did not have a large bladder at that time. Because the patient remained haemodynamically unstable a traction sling was applied around the pelvis to attempt to 'close the open book'. This failed to alter the haemodynamic state and the patient was then taken to theatre and an external fixator applied across the front of the pelvis to stabilize it.

Stabilizing the pelvis in such cases reduces the intrapelvic volume and tamponades the posterior arterial and venous structures, thereby causing haemostasis.

Patient B

An 18-year-old student, depressed by a poor examination performance, jumped from a three-storey building, landing predominantly on the right leg. He sustained injuries to the leg and pelvis.

When reviewed in the casualty department it was noted that he had bruising of the right heel, no pain within the knee, but pain with all movements of the right hip and low back pain.

Radiographic review confirmed a fractured calcaneum, a vertical sheer fracture of the right hemipelvis with a disruption of both posterior and anterior columns, but no thoracolumbar injury.

Cardiovascular status remained satisfactory and the patient remained haemodynamically stable. The patient was treated with bed rest and traction to allow the hemipelvis to heal and subsequently made a good recovery.

Moral

When assessing a pelvic fracture it is important to remember the mechanism of injury. Different types of fracture are associated with different complications. 'Open book' injuries are often associated with urological complications and patients may have significant hypovolaemia. Urgent surgery may be required to stabilize the pelvis to restore the haemodynamic state.

Lateral compression or vertical sheer fractures may not have the same morbidity but, because of the severity of the injury to the pelvis and the associated injuries to other parts of the skeleton, may have a more long-term effect with prolonged patient pain, immobility and dysfunction.

Chapter 12

Injuries to the upper limb

By the end of this chapter you should be able to:

- Remember your anatomy of the brachial plexus. This will help with the diagnosis and exact site of neural injury.
- Make a diagnosis of and know how to reduce a dislocated shoulder.
- Diagnose a fracture of the shoulder girdle and be aware of injuries to the surrounding nerves.
- Differentiate between the different common fractures of the elbow and forearm.

Brachial plexus lesions

Brachial plexus lesions are serious and tragic. The most frequent victims are young men thrown from their motorcycles who may become unemployable as a result of their injuries.

Closed injuries

Closed injuries can occur in two ways:

1. By violent lateral flexion of the neck with depression of the shoulder or forced abduction of the arm.
2. At birth, although this is now rare in developed countries. This is associated with obstructed or difficult deliveries.

Open injuries

In the past, cavalrymen wielding sabres disabled the enemy by cutting the upper cords of the brachial plexus of opposing infantry. Today, open injuries still occur and are just as devastating but they are more often caused by falling objects such as glass or steel.

Patterns of brachial plexus lesion

- Supraclavicular lesions, which can be (1) preganglionic or (2) postganglionic.
- Infraclavicular lesions.

Supraclavicular lesions

Trauma

Blows to the shoulder and head cause violent lateral flexion of the cervical spine and depression of the shoulder. This tears the upper part of the brachial plexus. In the UK about 90% of these injuries occur in motorcyclists landing on the head and shoulder (Fig. 12.1).

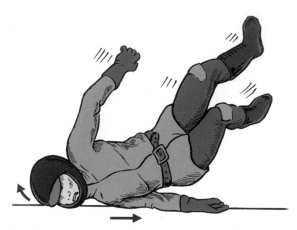

Fig. 12.1 Traction injury of the brachial plexus. Violent abduction of the neck and shoulder can tear the upper cords of the brachial plexus.

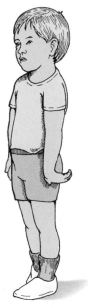

Fig. 12.2 The position of the hand in Erb's palsy.

Obstetric palsy

If the upper cords of the plexus are damaged at birth, the supinator, deltoid, wrist extensors and elbow flexors will be weak, causing a 'waiter's tip' position of the arm (Fig. 12.2). This condition is known as Erb's palsy, a term which is often applied to the same pattern of neurological deficit in the adult.

Infraclavicular lesions

Trauma

Injuries in which the arm is violently abducted can tear the lower part of the brachial plexus. The commonest mechanism is anterior dislocation of the shoulder, but the lesion can also be caused by a fall from a height in which the hand is caught so that the full weight is taken by the arm.

Birth trauma

The end result of damage to the lower cords of the brachial plexus at birth is a Klumpke's palsy, which consists of a weakness of the finger flexors and intrinsics.

Assessment

The first step in management is to define the anatomy of the lesion. The roots, trunks or branches of the brachial plexus can be torn or the roots avulsed from the spinal cord. Each lesion has a different prognosis and the site of the lesion must be identified by a careful neurological examination.

The anatomy of the brachial plexus is so variable that trying to identify the exact site of the lesion using a map of the brachial plexus is most unreliable, but it does give a rough idea of the extent of the lesion (Fig. 12.3). In general terms, the more distal the lesion, the better the prognosis.

It is important to decide whether the lesion lies between the spinal cord and the dorsal root ganglion (preganglionic) or distal to the ganglion (postganglionic). *Preganglionic lesions never recover, postganglionic lesions sometimes do.*

One way of determining the exact site of the lesion clinically is to assess muscle function. The first branches to leave the brachial plexus are the motor nerves to the rhomboids and levator scapulae. If the patient has power in these muscles and can elevate the scapula, the lesion must be distal to the origin of these nerves from the plexus and the prognosis will be better than for a patient who cannot elevate the scapula.

A useful approach is to look at the activity of the autonomic nervous system. If a Horner's syndrome is present, the lesion must be close to the cord and the prognosis is poor (Fig. 12.4). Axonal reflexes involving the triple response or sweating can also be used. If axonal reflexes are present but the function of the dorsal root ganglion

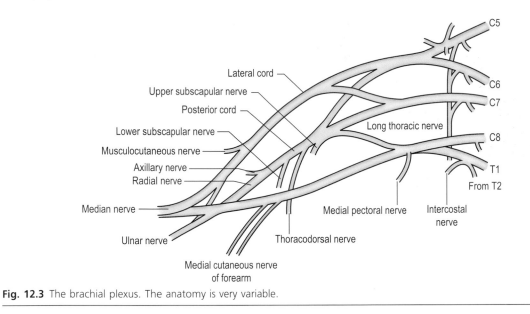

Fig. 12.3 The brachial plexus. The anatomy is very variable.

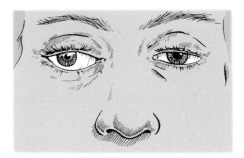

Fig. 12.4 Horner's syndrome, with drooping eyelid, small pupil, slight protrusion of the eyeball and no sweating of the surrounding skin.

is absent, the lesion must be preganglionic and close to the cord.

Investigations are less useful than clinical examination. The most useful investigation is the EMG, which can identify accurately the roots involved. Radiculography will show if the roots are still attached to the spinal cord and may demonstrate traumatic meningocoeles along the roots, but reveals little else. CT scanning does not give much information about the peripheral nerves, although MRI may prove helpful.

Treatment

If the roots are torn out of the spinal cord, nothing can be done to restore continuity. If the lesions are distal to the ganglion or there is a clean cut across the nerve, microsurgical repair may be possible. Cable grafting of defects in the supraclavicular part of the plexus is practised but the results are unpredictable, and a few patients eventually request amputation to rid themselves of their heavy, useless arm (p. 86).

Artificial limbs are available but many patients find them an encumbrance and do not wear them.

Management of brachial plexus lesions

1. Identify the site of the lesion by careful neurological examination and EMG.
2. Decide if the lesion is preganglionic or postganglionic.
3. Preganglionic lesions (Horner's syndrome, absent axonal reflex) cannot be repaired.
4. Postganglionic lesions have a better prognosis: the more distal, the better the outlook.
5. Surgical repair or grafting is sometimes possible for clean cuts and distal lesions.

Injuries to the clavicle

A fractured clavicle is one of the commonest of all fractures. Clavicular injuries include (Fig. 12.5):

1. Fracture of the midshaft of the clavicle.
2. Fracture of the outer end of the clavicle.
3. Acromioclavicular separation.
4. Sternoclavicular dislocation.

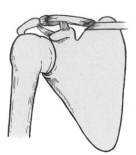

Fig. 12.5 Sites of fracture of the clavicle.

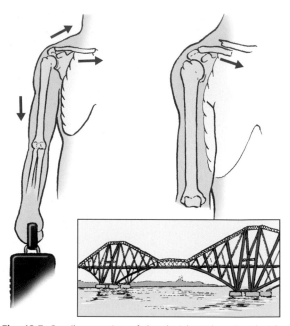

Fig. 12.7 Cantilever action of the clavicle. When the clavicle is broken, the shoulder is not supported and moves downwards and medially.

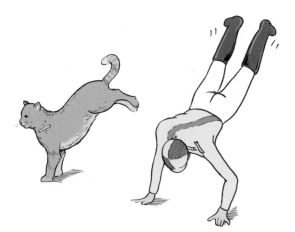

Fig. 12.6 Falls on the outstretched arm. The cat does not fracture its clavicle because the sternum and humerus are not linked as in humans.

Fracture of the midshaft of the clavicle

The usual force that breaks a clavicle is a violent upwards and backwards thrust caused by landing on the outstretched hand or a direct blow to the point of the shoulder. This can happen after being thrown from a horse or going over the handlebars of a bicycle. The domestic cat does not have this problem because its clavicles are free at both ends (Fig. 12.6). Humans have clavicles firmly attached to the sternum medially and the acromion and coracoid laterally by ligaments that are stronger than the bone. The clavicle therefore fractures instead of moving to absorb the impact.

The cat's clavicle is adapted for landing on the forelegs but the forearms of humans are adapted for carrying weights. The human clavicle acts as a strut to hold the shoulder and arm away from the body, like a cantilever (Fig. 12.7). This function is only possible if the bone is intact; when the clavicle is broken the weight of the arm makes the fragments overlap and go on to malunion (Fig. 12.8).

In adults, a fractured clavicle takes about 6 weeks to become solid, although function returns after about 3 weeks. In children the fracture will be solid after only 2 or 3 weeks. If the fracture is comminuted, it will usually unite more quickly than a simple transverse fracture because there is more callus to 'glue' the bone ends together.

Complications

Complications are often seen after this injury (Fig. 12.9).

Malunion. Because the fragments are displaced by the weight of the arm, malunion is unavoidable. Internal fixation with a contoured plate may give better anatomical results but the surgery has risks (neurovascular, skin etc.)

Damage to vessels. Splinters of bone can rupture the great vessels or the lung at the time of injury. It is said that Sir Robert Peel (the founder of the Metropolitan Police Force) died from this complication after being thrown by his horse.

Non-union is unusual and seldom causes symptoms. Internal fixation and grafting are required on the rare occasions when it does cause symptoms.

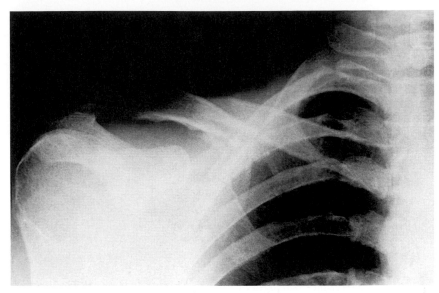

Fig. 12.8 Malunion of the clavicle with overriding bone fragments.

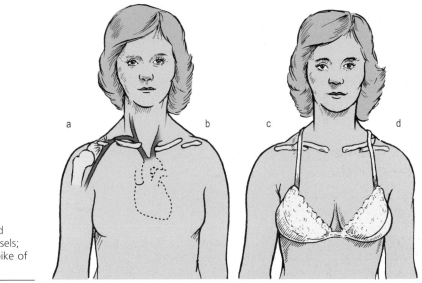

Fig. 12.9 Complications of fractured clavicle: (a) damage to the great vessels; (b) non-union; (c) malunion; (d) a spike of bone.

Deformity. Large spicules of bone around the fracture site can produce an unsightly appearance, as well as an unwelcome pressure area, and may need removing (Fig. 12.10).

The callus at the fracture site also produces a visible lump that interferes with the shoulder straps of bras and backpacks. The lump is particularly alarming to the parents of children with a greenstick fracture of the clavicle. The clavicle looks normal immediately after injury and the swelling may be mistaken for a malignant tumour. In time, the swelling diminishes as the bone remodels and the surrounding bone enlarges.

Treatment

A sling to support the weight of the arm relieves pain at the fracture site, but the sling must not rub against the fracture. The sling can be removed after

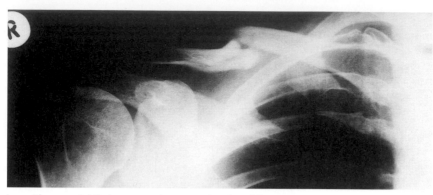

Fig. 12.10 Malunion with an unsightly bony prominence at the site of fracture.

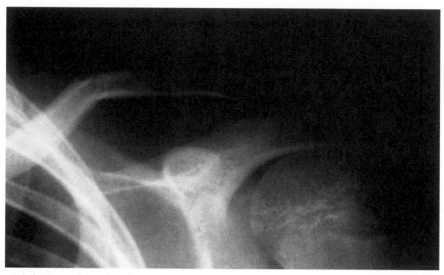

Fig. 12.11 Greenstick fracture of the clavicle.

10 days if pain permits. Greenstick fractures require very little support (Fig. 12.11).

A firm support such as a figure-of-eight bandage to pull the shoulders backwards also helps to relieve pain but it must be readjusted every few days (Fig. 12.12). The function of a figure-of-eight bandage is to support the fracture and not to reduce it. Harnesses and braces that attempt to reduce the fracture by pulling the shoulder blades backwards are doomed to failure: the arm weighs several kilograms and anything that exerts such a force on the shoulder is bound to cause pressure sores in the soft axillary skin, even without the sweat that is inevitable under a bulky dressing.

Internal fixation is seldom required for fractures of the clavicle.

Fractures of the outer end of the clavicle

Fractures of the outer end of the clavicle lie lateral to the coracoclavicular ligament and the distal fragment remains attached to the acromion. Fractures may involve the acromioclavicular joint and may be displaced or undisplaced.

Thus, the fractures can be classified as displaced or undisplaced and articular or non-articular.

Treatment

Undisplaced non-articular fractures are treated conservatively with a sling, analgesics and early mobilization.

Displaced non-articular fractures have a high incidence of malunion and non-union when treated conservatively. Like displaced fractures that enter the joint, they should be treated by open reduction and fixation.

Complications

The fragment may fail to unite, causing a painful non-union. Excision of the un-united fragment may be needed if this occurs.

Acromioclavicular separation

The acromioclavicular joint is a plane joint between the end of the clavicle and the acromion. It contains a fibrocartilaginous disc and is easily disrupted by a fall onto the point of the shoulder (Fig. 12.13). The

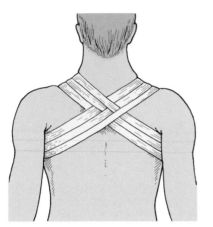

Fig. 12.12 Figure-of-eight bandage for fractured clavicle.

injury is sometimes called a 'separated' or 'sprung' shoulder and occurs in rugby football, riding accidents and ice hockey if the shoulder is struck against the boards around the rink. The lesion is usually a simple dislocation of the joint but a fragment of the clavicle sometimes remains attached to the acromion.

Clinical examination will show tenderness of the acromioclavicular joint and a step at the joint, best seen when the arm is allowed to hang. The step can be eliminated by lifting the arm and the elbow while holding the clavicle down.

Grading and treatment

There are six grades of acromioclavicular separation. The grade determines the treatment:

1. Sprain with no displacement. Analgesics and symptomatic treatment only.

2. Subluxation. Treatment consists of analgesia and, if necessary, a sling to support the elbow.

3. Dislocation. Complete separation of the joint usually requires internal fixation.

4. Dislocation with perforation of the overlying deltotrapezius fascia. Open reduction with internal fixation and repair of the fascia may be needed.

5. Lesions described in (4) above with the addition of posterior dislocation. Open reduction and internal fixation is required for this serious injury.

6. Subcoracoid dislocation. Open reduction and internal fixation is required for this serious injury, which involves the scapula.

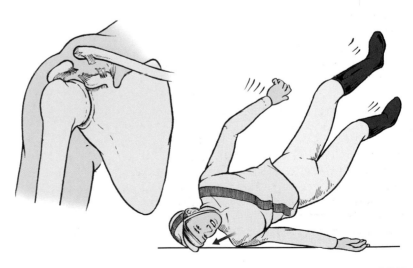

Fig. 12.13 Fracture of the acromioclavicular joint. Falling onto the point of the shoulder can rupture the coracoclavicular ligament.

Sternoclavicular dislocation

The sternoclavicular joint lies medial to the stout costoclavicular ligament that acts as a pivot for the clavicle, which see-saws about this point. When the outer end of the clavicle is raised, the medial end moves downwards, and vice versa – confirm this by putting a finger on the medial end of the clavicle and moving the shoulder.

Treatment

If the injury is seen early, which is unusual, acute repair may be required. The decision to operate depends on the age and fitness of the patient and the severity of the injury. Left untreated, recurrent subluxation can occur. Soft tissue repair is difficult and the patient may prefer to accept the minor disability of recurrent subluxation instead.

Fractures of the scapula

Fractures of the acromion

The acromion can be broken by direct trauma or by violent abduction of the shoulder (Fig. 12.14). It is

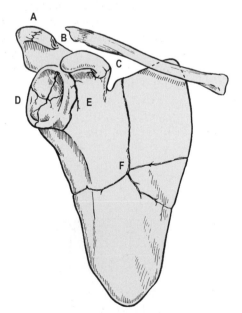

Fig. 12.14 Sites of fracture of the scapula: (A) acromion; (B) fracture dislocation of the acromioclavicular joint; (C) coracoid; (D) glenoid; (E) neck of scapula; (F) blade of scapula.

easy to confuse the normal apophysis of the acromion in the growing skeleton with a fracture, and many a normal acromioclavicular joint has been 'treated' in a sling for this reason.

Treatment

Acromioclavicular injuries with little separation and intact coracoclavicular ligaments require no treatment. Rest in a sling is sufficient unless there is gross displacement of the fragments, when internal fixation may be needed to stabilize the joint.

The blade of the scapula

The blade of the scapula, like the wing of the ilium, functions mainly as an attachment for muscles. It can be fractured by direct trauma, causing pain, bruising and soft tissue swelling.

Treatment

Treatment is by support in a sling, analgesics and early mobilization. A good result is usual, but the shoulder girdle may be weaker than before because of muscle damage.

The glenoid

The glenoid can be fractured by a direct blow to the shoulder from the lateral side, comparable with the force which causes a fracture of the floor of the acetabulum.

Treatment

Unless there is gross displacement of the fragments, treatment is by early mobilization. Because the glenoid is not a weight-bearing joint, exact anatomical restitution of the joint surfaces is less important than early mobilization.

Dislocation of the shoulder

The shoulder is mechanically unstable. The head of the humerus is held against the glenoid by a cowl of muscles that pull the round head of the humerus up against the small flat glenoid, which faces downwards. The cowl of muscles is complete everywhere except below, in the axilla, where there is nothing to hold the humeral head against the glenoid.

Bearing this intrinsic instability in mind, it is remarkable that dislocation is not more common.

> ### There are five types of shoulder dislocation:
>
> 1. Anterior dislocation.
> 2. Posterior dislocation.
> 3. Luxatio erecta, or true inferior dislocation.
> 4. Fracture dislocations.
> 5. Multidirectional.

Anterior dislocation

Anterior dislocation is by far the commonest pattern and is the result of the head of humerus slipping off the front of the glenoid when the arm is abducted and externally rotated (Fig. 12.15). The shoulder can also dislocate during grand mal attacks or electro-convulsive therapy and may then pass unnoticed for some days.

Once off the glenoid, the head slips medially when the arm is lowered, producing the characteristic profile of a dislocated shoulder. Because the head of the humerus is not lying in its normal position, the shoulder has a flatter appearance than usual and the elbow points outwards. If the tip of the acromion and the lateral epicondyle can be joined by a straight line (Hamilton's ruler test), the shoulder is dislocated (see Fig. 2.13).

This appearance, together with the observation that the patient is holding the injured arm in the other hand, makes it possible to diagnose a dislocated shoulder from the far end of the accident department. A similar flattened contour is also seen in patients with wasted deltoid muscles and in dis-placed fractures of the surgical neck, but in these patients the humeral head is still in its normal position and the 'ruler test' is negative.

Radiographic examination of a dislocated shoulder is not easy (Fig. 12.16). It is difficult to position the patient accurately and the usual lateral film in abduction is impossible, but an axial view will reveal the dislocation. A lateral scapula view is excellent. Fractures of the humeral head should be looked for specifically, or they will be missed and a fracture dislocation will be treated as a simple dislocation, with potentially serious clinical and medicolegal consequences.

Complications

> ### Complications of anterior dislocation of the shoulder
>
> • Damage to the circumflex axillary nerve.
> • Arterial damage.
> • Irreducibility.
> • Joint stiffness.
> • Recurrent dislocation.

Neurological damage. Damage to the axillary nerve as it runs round the neck of the humerus (Fig. 12.17) causes partial or complete paralysis of the deltoid. When damage is suspected, the axillary nerve should be examined with an EMG 3 weeks after injury and again 3 weeks later. If there is no change between the two examinations, the nerve should be explored and, if necessary, repaired.

Brachial plexus injuries also occur if there has been a violent abduction strain.

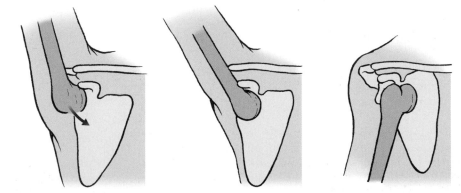

Fig. 12.15 Mechanism of anterior dislocation of the humerus, beginning with abduction and extension.

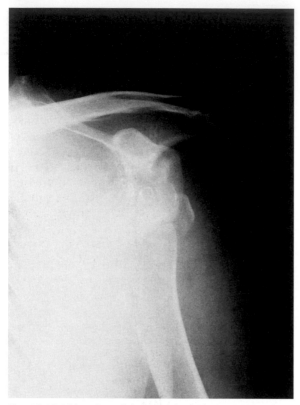

Fig. 12.16 Dislocation of the shoulder with separation of the greater tuberosity.

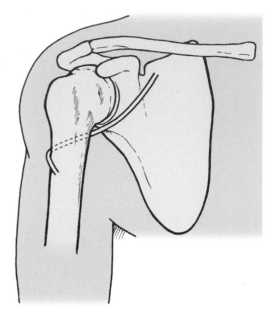

Fig. 12.17 To show the relationship of the circumflex humeral nerve to the deltoid and the surgical neck of the humerus.

The results of dislocation in the presence of neurological damage are often poor.

Arterial injury. The axillary artery can be damaged by traction at the time of injury or by pressure from the humeral head. The radial pulse should be checked and its presence recorded.

Irreducibility. The humeral head sometimes 'buttonholes' through the subscapularis, making reduction impossible. Open reduction is then necessary.

If the shoulder is not reduced within a few days of dislocation, reduction may then be impossible. This is a particular problem in elderly patients in whom the shoulder can be dislocated with trivial trauma. Open reduction is a difficult and uncertain operation and it may be better left dislocated in an elderly patient who places little demand on the shoulder.

Joint stiffness. Because the shoulder depends upon muscle and soft tissue for stability, adhesions or fibrosis in the rotator cuff can cause serious loss of movement. Physiotherapy is important to prevent this.

Recurrent dislocation. Once dislocated, the shoulder is liable to do so again and may require stabilization. Adequate treatment of the initial dislocation is therefore important.

Treatment

First, examine the shoulder radiologically, however obvious the diagnosis may be. Attempts to reduce the shoulder before radiographs are available are ill advised and may be dangerous if there is an associated fracture.

The humeral head must be reduced but, before attempting reduction, test the function of the axillary nerve, which runs around the surgical neck of the humerus. This nerve can be damaged either at the moment of dislocation or during reduction. Because the nerve is so vulnerable, it is important to test the function of the nerve and record it before reduction is attempted.

Motor function cannot be tested adequately but the area of sensory supply of the circumflex nerve, over the outer side of the deltoid, is easily tested. If there is any abnormality it should be clearly recorded and special care taken when the shoulder is reduced. If this is not done, any subsequent circumflex nerve dysfunction may be attributed to the reduction rather than the injury.

194

There are four ways to reduce the humeral head:

1. Manipulation under general anaesthetic (MUA).
2. Hanging-arm technique.
3. Hippocratic method.
4. Kocher's method.

Manipulation under general anaesthetic (MUA). If there is no fracture of the humeral head, the shoulder can be reduced easily under general anaesthesia if required. No complicated manipulations are necessary; the arm can be pulled gently and the head pushed back over the lip of the glenoid.

Hanging-arm technique. An alternative is to place the patient face down on a couch and allow the arm to hang freely without the patient holding on to the leg of the couch or supporting the arm in any way (Fig. 12.18). The weight of the arm will then achieve reduction but intravenous pethidine or valium may be needed to achieve adequate relaxation. This technique avoids general anaesthesia and the 4 h or so discomfort that is necessary if the patient has a full stomach and has to wait for general anaesthetic.

Hippocratic method. In days gone by, the shoulder had to be reduced without full muscle relaxation and, for many years, Hippocrates' technique was used. The Hippocratic technique involved laying the patient on the floor, lifting and pulling the arm upwards and pushing the humeral head back into its correct position with the unbooted forefoot (Fig. 12.19).

Kocher's method was less spectacular and consisted of a slow external rotation of the arm to relax the spasm of the subscapularis muscle (Fig. 12.20). When full external rotation had been achieved, the humeral head could be easily replaced. This method was considered to have been first described by Kocher in the 19th century until, in 1970, an Egyptian surgeon noted that some of the paintings on the pyramids depicted injuries occurring while they were being built, together with their treatment. One such illustration unmistakably demonstrated Kocher's manoeuvre (Fig. 12.21). The unknown artist therefore preceded both Kocher and Hippocrates in his description of manipulative reduction. If only he had published his work in a reputable journal, he would have received the proper recognition for his discovery!

Aftercare. Whichever technique is used, the arm should be brought across the body and bandaged in

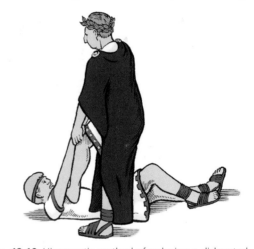

Fig. 12.19 Hippocratic method of reducing a dislocated shoulder with the unbooted foot in the axilla.

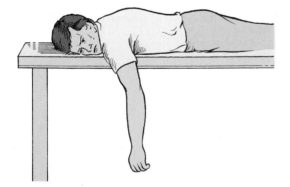

Fig. 12.18 Hanging-arm technique for reducing dislocation of the shoulder.

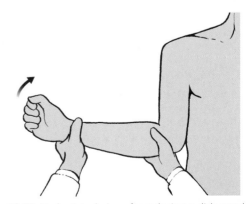

Fig. 12.20 Kocher's technique for reducing a dislocated shoulder.

195

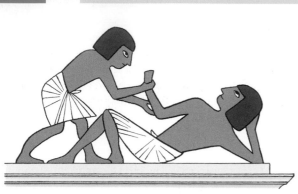

Fig. 12.21 Original illustration of Kocher's method in an Egyptian wall painting.

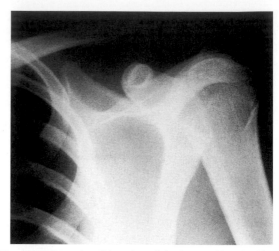

Fig. 12.22 Posterior dislocation of the humeral head with the 'light bulb' sign.

that position for 3 weeks, when the shoulder can be mobilized. Treating without immobilization runs the risk of recurrent dislocation (p. 365).

Posterior dislocation

Posterior dislocations are much less common than anterior dislocations and are often caused by a direct blow to the shoulder in internal rotation or after an epileptic seizure. Posterior dislocation can become recurrent, particularly if the patient has generalized ligamentous laxity. Some patients can dislocate the shoulder posteriorly at will as a 'party trick'.

Posterior dislocations often escape diagnosis and the lesion may be missed on the radiographs but the characteristic 'light bulb' appearance (Fig. 12.22), caused by internal rotation of the humerus, should suggest the diagnosis.

Treatment

Reduction is easily done by pulling the arm gently forwards and externally rotating it, but the reduction is often unstable. Aftercare is the same as for anterior dislocation.

Luxatio erecta

In exceptional circumstances, the humeral head becomes jammed below the glenoid with the arm pointing directly upwards, presenting a spectacular appearance sometimes mistaken for hysteria. This is a true inferior dislocation, in contrast to anterior dislocation in which the head only slips downwards after it has dislocated anteriorly.

The humeral head lies against the vessels and can cause ischaemia, and the rotator cuff is always damaged.

Treatment

Reduction can be difficult but once achieved immobilization is not required.

Fracture dislocations

Most fractures associated with dislocations of the shoulder involve the humeral head and are dealt with on page 197. The greater tuberosity may also be separated.

Rupture of the supraspinatus tendon

The supraspinatus tendon can be ruptured without a fracture. This injury is comparatively common in older patients with degenerate tendons and is usually seen in the orthopaedic clinic rather than an accident department, but sudden ruptures of the supraspinatus can also occur in young people after a violent injury.

Clinically, there is both bruising and tenderness around the supraspinatus muscle and weakness of abduction.

Treatment

Surgical repair is advisable in acute tears in young or active patients. Rehabilitation is prolonged.

Fractures of the upper end of the humerus

Avulsion of the greater tuberosity

The greater tuberosity, to which the supraspinatus tendon is attached, can be avulsed in a fall onto the shoulder in older patients. The fragment will usually unite in a good position but sometimes the supraspinatus tendon pulls it away from the bone. The fragment may then become wedged in the space between the acromion and the humeral head, obstructing shoulder movement (Fig. 12.23).

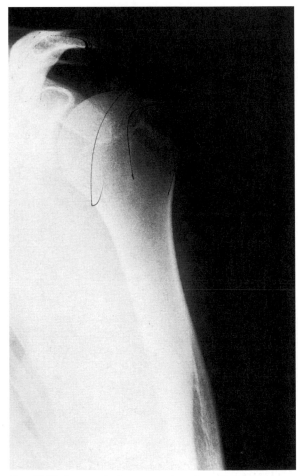

Fig. 12.23 Fragment of greater tuberosity with attached supraspinatus tendon caught in the joint between the humeral head and the acromion.

Treatment

Treatment is by support to the shoulder until the pain has settled, followed by physiotherapy 3–4 weeks later when the fragment has reattached. If the fragment is jammed in the joint, operation is needed to reduce and fix it.

Fractures of the surgical neck of the humerus

Fractures of the surgical neck occur in adults from a fall on the outstretched arm. The fractures can be displaced or impacted, stable or unstable, and are classified according to the site and number of the fragments.

Impacted fractures are more common and are visible as a line of dense bone on the radiograph (Fig. 12.24). Displaced fractures are less common but potentially more serious because the sharp bone ends can damage vessels or nerves. They may also go on to non-union and avascular collapse of the humeral head.

Treatment

Support to the limb in a sling or collar and cuff for 4–6 weeks, depending on the stability of the fracture, is often all that is required in undisplaced fractures. Mobilization can then be commenced and rehabilitation begun when pain allows.

Extensive bleeding and bruising around the fracture is usual but not of serious significance, though it may track down to the elbow and produce a spectacular discoloration. This should not delay mobilization.

Impacted fractures can be mobilized after 2 weeks, but the fragments can become disimpacted unless some protection is given until then.

Undisplaced or minimally displaced fractures almost always unite because the fracture is surrounded by muscle, and remodelling is good at the shoulder (Fig. 12.25). *Fractures that are displaced or severely angulated* may need operative intervention. In the young patient the fracture should be reduced and fixed with internal fixation. In the elderly it may be more judicious to proceed to a hemiarthroplasty, especially in four-part fractures (see Fig. 12.26).

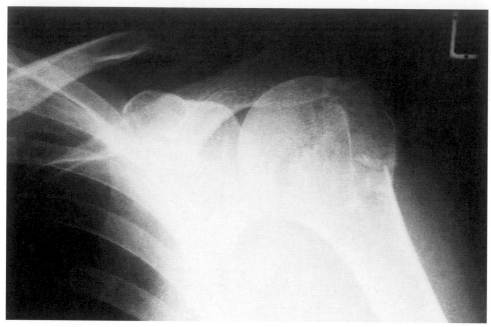

Fig. 12.24 Fracture of the humeral head with impacted fracture of the neck.

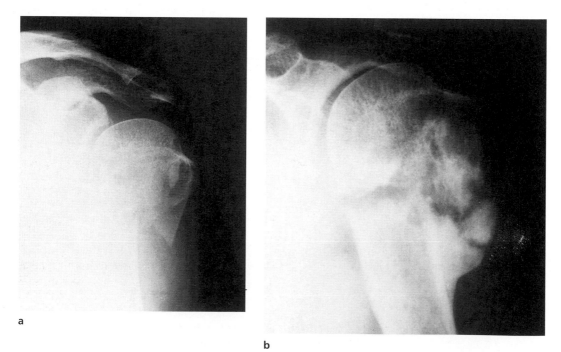

a

b

Fig. 12.25 (a) Displaced fracture of the neck of the humerus; (b) the fracture remodelled well to give good function.

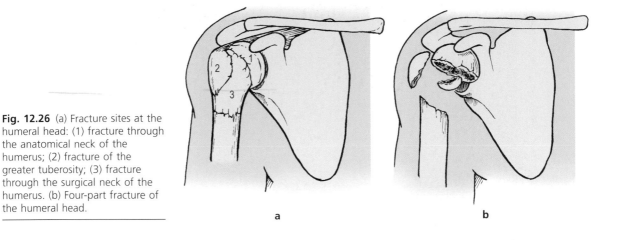

Fig. 12.26 (a) Fracture sites at the humeral head: (1) fracture through the anatomical neck of the humerus; (2) fracture of the greater tuberosity; (3) fracture through the surgical neck of the humerus. (b) Four-part fracture of the humeral head.

a

b

Proximal epiphyseal separation

Separation of the upper humeral epiphysis is a common injury in children and is one of the injuries seen in non-accidental injury.

Treatment

Treatment is by rest in a sling. In children under the age of 12 any deformity will correct by remodelling and manipulation is hardly ever required.

Fracture dislocations of the shoulder

Fractures of the humeral head with several fragments are usually accompanied by a dislocation (Fig. 12.26). Fracture dislocations of the humeral head present several problems:

1. The fragment may obstruct reduction and make open reduction necessary.
2. The reduction will be very unstable.
3. Soft tissue damage and haemorrhage into and around the shoulder lead to joint stiffness.
4. Avascular necrosis of the humeral head can follow fractures through the anatomical neck.

Treatment

Closed reduction is difficult. Open reduction may be needed in younger patients but in older patients it is preferable to accept some loss of function and institute early movement.

Severe fracture dislocations may need prosthetic replacement of the humeral head.

Humeral shaft

Fractures of the humerus can be spiral, transverse, segmented or pathological.

Spiral fractures

Twisting injuries of an arm produce a spiral fracture of the humerus (Fig. 12.27).

Transverse fractures

Transverse fractures of the humerus are caused by direct trauma or a fall onto the arm.

Pathological fractures

The humerus is a common site for metastases and pathological fractures are often seen.

Complications (Fig. 12.28)

Neurovascular damage

The fragments are shaped like spikes and can damage the radial nerve or the vessels, as well as muscle, as they wind around the bone.

Brachioradialis is a useful guide to neurological function. If there is a neurological deficit involving brachioradialis and no clinical or electrical sign of recovery after 6 weeks, the radial nerve should be explored. In the longer term, flexor tendons may need to be transferred to restore extensor function.

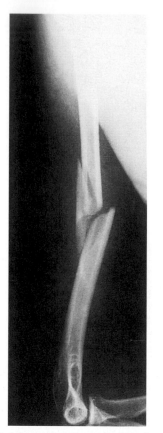

Fig. 12.27 Spiral fracture of the shaft of the humerus.

Malunion

Malunion may occur because the deltoid can abduct the upper fragment without opposition from other muscles or the weight of the arm.

Non-union

Soft tissue, including the radial nerve and triceps, can be caught between the bone ends and lead to non-union.

Treatment

Soft tissue usually holds the fragments in good position and conservative treatment is generally successful (Fig. 12.29). Either a U-slab or a hanging cast will protect the humeral shaft from additional trauma and, provided that it is supported by a collar and cuff and not a sling, the weight of the cast applies traction to the fracture site.

Some degree of malalignment is acceptable in the upper limb because it does not bear weight and

because of the excellent range of glenohumeral motion. If the position is unacceptable, internal fixation with an intramedullary nail or plate is simple and straightforward.

If the fracture is in the distal humerus, brachialis may be pulled into the fracture line. Unless this problem is recognized and treated by open reduction, with or without internal fixation, the fracture will not unite.

For pathological fractures, internal fixation is effective and allows early mobilization and restoration of function.

Fractures at the elbow (Fig. 12.30)

Supracondylar fracture of the humerus

Supracondylar fractures of the humerus occur in children who fall on the outstretched arm (Fig. 12.31). Treatment is difficult and the fracture is notorious for its complications.

Complications

Complications of supracondylar fractures of the humerus in children
1. Vascular damage.
2. Compartment syndrome.
3. Volkmann's ischaemic contracture.
4. Median nerve damage.
5. Malunion.
6. Myositis ossificans.

Vascular problems. At the moment of greatest displacement the distal fragment and the forearm are pushed backwards, pulling the brachial artery and median nerve violently against the sharp lower end of the upper fragment (Fig. 12.32). The circulation must therefore be checked carefully and recorded, with special attention to the five 'P's:

1. Pulselessness.

2. Pallor.

3. Pain.

4. Paraesthesiae.

5. Paralysis.

The skin will be cool if the circulation is interrupted and there will be loss of passive finger extension

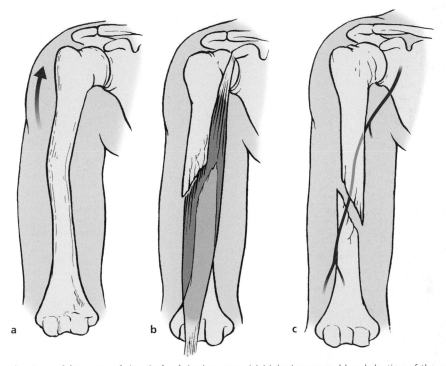

Fig. 12.28 Complications of fractures of the shaft of the humerus. (a) Malunion caused by abduction of the proximal fragment. (b) Soft tissue interposition. The biceps is lying between the muscle fragments. (c) Neural damage. The radial nerve has become caught between the bone fragments.

because of oedema in the flexor compartment. If these signs are present before or after reduction, the following steps should be taken:

1. The splint and dressings should be removed, down to skin.
2. The elbow should be extended slightly, even if this loses the reduction.
3. If the circulation still does not improve, the brachial artery must be explored at the elbow. If the artery is in spasm, it can be painted with papaverine to relax the smooth muscle of the arterial wall. If this is ineffective, as it almost always is, the artery must be opened, intimal tears corrected, and a vein patch applied if necessary.

Compartment syndrome. The median nerve and radial artery can both be compressed by swelling within the anterior compartment of the forearm. If there are paraesthesiae in the median distribution with loss of finger extension, a fasciotomy is probably needed.

Note: Compartment syndromes can occur even if the radial pulse is present!

Volkmann's ischaemic contracture is the end result of muscle necrosis caused by occlusion of the micro-circulation from any cause. Untreated vascular insufficiency following a supracondylar fracture, perhaps aggravated by a compartment syndrome, is one cause. Masses of fibrous tissue replace patches of necrotic muscle in the flexor compartment and these contract, pulling the fingers into flexion and the wrist into flexion and pronation (Fig. 12.33). The result is disabling.

Median nerve damage. The median nerve, like the brachial artery, is vulnerable at the fracture site. Because the nerve is tough it is seldom divided and function usually recovers. The anterior interosseous branch to the deep muscles is more likely to be affected than the superficial branch, which continues as the median nerve into the hand.

Malunion. Unless a good position is achieved, an unsightly malunion is likely, with the medial epicondyle pushed backwards and medially. The result is, at best, a slight loss of carrying angle, and at worst a 'gunstock' deformity (see Fig. 2.16). Corrective osteotomy may be required when growth is complete.

Myositis ossificans can follow any fracture in the region of the elbow, including a supracondylar fracture.

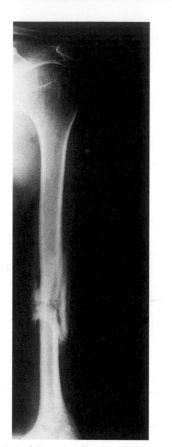

Fig. 12.29 Union of the spiral fracture shown in Figure 12.27, achieved with a hanging cast.

Treatment

Undisplaced fractures can be treated in a backslab with the elbow flexed for 3 weeks. Unstable fractures are more difficult. The fractured surfaces are small and do not 'fit' together neatly. The distal fragment has many powerful muscle groups attached to it, which can displace the fragments after reduction.

Reduction is achieved by a gentle longitudinal pull with the forearm in the midprone position. Once reduced, the elbow is flexed beyond a right angle, a plaster backslab applied and the arm supported in a collar and cuff. This position can usually be maintained but if flexing the elbow beyond 90° interferes with the blood supply it must be extended until the pulse returns. If this loses reduction, the arm should be suspended and Dunlop traction (Fig. 12.34) applied.

Percutaneous 'K' wiring or open fixation with wires may be needed, not only to reduce difficult

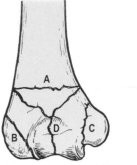

Fig. 12.30 Fracture lines at the elbow: (A) supracondylar fracture; (B) lateral epicondyle; (C) medial epicondyle; (D) Y-shaped fracture.

fragments but also to hold them in the reduced position. These wires can be removed after 3–4 weeks.

Medial epicondyle

In children, the medial epicondyle and its growth plate can be pulled off the humerus by valgus forces. The fracture is made more treacherous because it happens before the epicondyle has ossified; unless the radiographs of the two elbows are compared carefully, the lesion may be missed. The fragment can also be pulled into the joint space, where it interferes with joint movement.

Untreated, the fragment usually joins with fibrous tissue, but function may be good.

Complications (Fig. 12.35)

Ulnar nerve palsy. The valgus strain that causes the fracture can also stretch the ulnar nerve.

Growth arrest. If the growth of the epicondyle is impaired or the fracture is not reduced, a varus deformity at the elbow (cubitus varum) follows.

Treatment

The fragment should be accurately reduced, openly if necessary, and secured with a Kirschner wire for extra stability. The wire must be removed later.

Lateral condyle

Avulsion of the lateral condyle is commonest between the ages of 3 and 5. If the fragment is small and involves just the capitellum, it may turn through 180° and make closed reduction impossible.

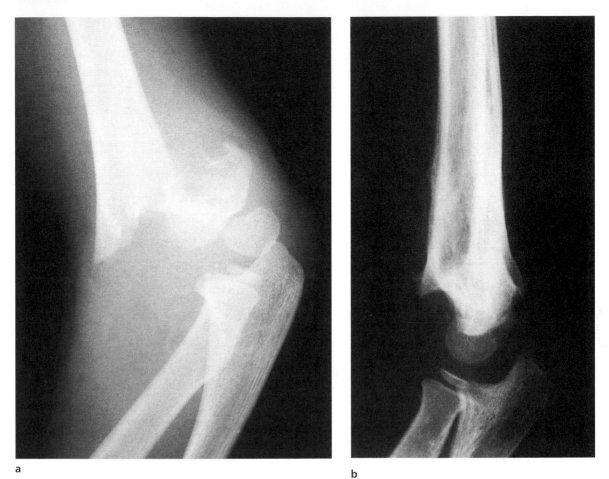

a

b

Fig. 12.31 (a) Supracondylar fracture of the humerus. (b) The same fracture 5 months later showing union and early remodelling.

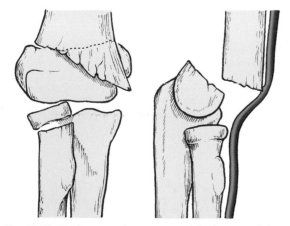

Fig. 12.32 Displacement in a supracondylar fracture of the humerus showing how the brachial artery can be damaged.

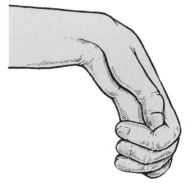

Fig. 12.33 The position of the hand in Volkmann's ischaemic contracture.

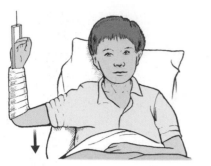

Fig. 12.34 Dunlop traction for supracondylar fracture of the humerus.

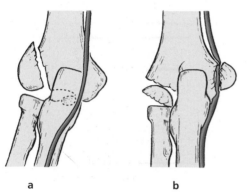

a

b

Fig. 12.35 Fracture of the epicondyle: (a) the capitellum may be completely displaced; (b) complications include a fragment of medial epicondyle caught in the medial joint space, non-union of the capitellum and tardy ulnar palsy.

Complications

If the fragment does not unite, or there is growth arrest from damage to the epiphyseal plate or mal-union, a **valgus** deformity of the lower end of the humerus follows. This stretches the ulnar nerve and causes a tardy ulnar palsy (p. 387). Non-union can occur, even if the fragment is undisplaced, and the injury must always be taken seriously.

Treatment

The fragment should be accurately reduced, by manipulation if possible, but open reduction may be necessary to replace the fragment and hold it with a Kirschner wire.

Pulled elbow

If children under 4 years of age are lifted by their hands the radial head can slip partly out of the annular ligament. The child will experience pain, will not use the arm, and the radiographs will be normal.

Treatment

The subluxation can be reduced by longitudinal pressure of the radius against the humerus with the elbow flexed. The forearm can then be alternately pronated and supinated and the radial head will pop back into position with dramatic relief of pain.

Fractures into the elbow joint

The lower end of the adult humerus can be fractured by direct trauma to produce a comminuted fracture that enters the elbow joint.

Complications

Like any fracture involving a joint, this injury is followed by loss of joint movement and late osteoarthritis.

Treatment

Exact anatomical restitution is not required unless there is gross displacement of the fragments. Conservative management with early mobilization may produce a better result than open reduction and internal fixation.

If there is gross displacement of the fragments with complete disintegration of the elbow it may be necessary to reassemble the bones and fix them internally (Fig. 12.36). The operation is difficult and the results are not always good.

Dislocations of the elbow

Although the elbow is a mechanically stable joint, it can be dislocated by a fall on the outstretched arm in almost full extension (Fig. 12.37). The lower end of the humerus will then slide forward over the coronoid process, which may be fractured (Fig. 12.38).

Complications

Joint stiffness. Full restoration of movement is unusual and a permanent loss of 15–20° of extension is almost inevitable.

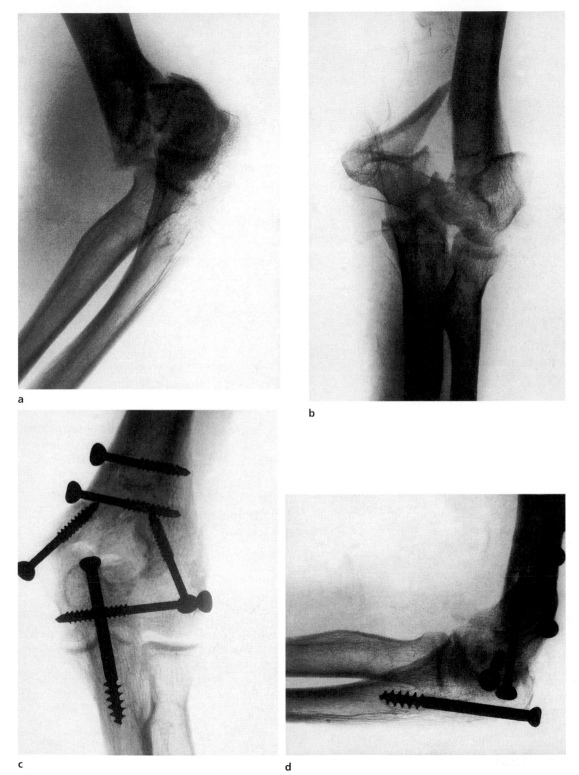

a

b

c   d

Fig. 12.36 Comminuted fracture of the lower end of the humerus: (a), (b) position of the fragments; (c), (d) position after internal fixation.

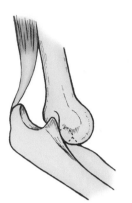

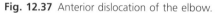

Fig. 12.37 Anterior dislocation of the elbow.

Ectopic ossification. New bone can grow as a solid mass in the soft tissues around the elbow, particularly if the patient also has a cerebral injury or the fracture has been manipulated several times. An alternative pattern of ectopic ossification is a large antler of bone attached to the lower end of the humerus with the spikes wrapped tightly round vessels and nerves.

The fragment can be removed and some movement restored, but the operation is technically difficult and the bone can reappear.

Recurrent dislocation can occur but is very rare.

Treatment

The dislocation can be reduced by a longitudinal pull in slight flexion and the reduction is usually stable. The arm should be rested in a collar and cuff for 2 weeks and mobilized gently.

Olecranon

The olecranon is easily fractured in direct falls onto the point of the elbow because the lower end of the humerus acts like a chisel and splits the olecranon at its narrowest point (Fig. 12.39). Avulsion injuries due to the pull of the triceps muscle are also common.

Treatment

Unless the fragments are undisplaced, which is unusual, internal fixation is needed, using either a screw or tension band wiring (Fig. 12.40). Rigid splintage is unnecessary if the fixation is secure.

Comminuted fractures in which the fragments cannot be reassembled and fixed can be treated by excision of the olecranon, especially in the elderly.

Injuries to the radius and ulna

Fractures of the radial head and neck

The radial head is easily fractured by a fall onto the outstretched arm and three main types of fracture are seen (Fig. 12.41).

Treatment

Treatment varies according to the type of fracture.

Undisplaced fractures and those with little displacement need blood aspirating from the joint, a soft supporting bandage and early mobilization.

Displaced fractures through the radial neck with more than 30° of angulation cause a painful restriction of pronation and supination if left untreated. The displacement should be corrected, by open reduction if necessary.

Comminuted fractures. Grossly displaced or comminuted fractures of the radial head are best treated by radial head excision and early mobilization. Prosthetic replacement of the radial head has been tried but excision is usually preferred.

Dislocation of the radial head with fracture of the ulna (Monteggia fracture)

Dislocation of the radial head accompanied by a fracture of the ulna is called a Monteggia fracture. It is a trap to catch the unwary (Fig. 12.42). Unless both components of the injury are recognized, which is not always easy, one of them will go untreated and a bad result will follow. Before treating a dislocated radial head or fractured ulna, always check that it is not one half of a Monteggia fracture.

If the ulnar fracture is very high, near the elbow joint, it may be mistaken for a fractured olecranon (Fig. 12.43). The consequences of this error can be very serious indeed.

Treatment

The ulnar fracture is so unstable that it must be internally fixed. Conservative treatment may succeed

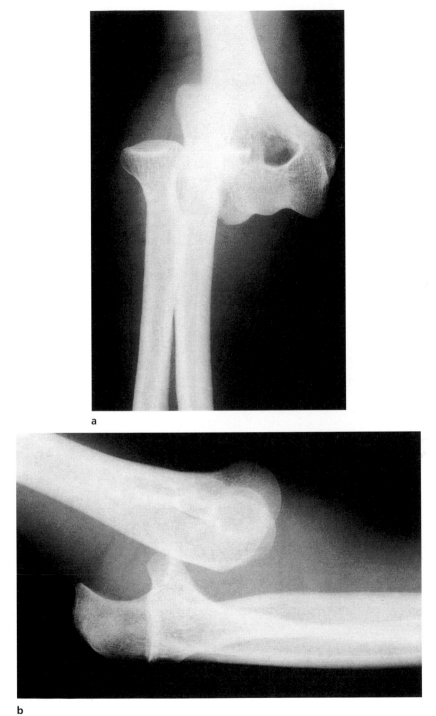

a

b

Fig. 12.38 (a), (b) Anterior dislocation of the elbow.

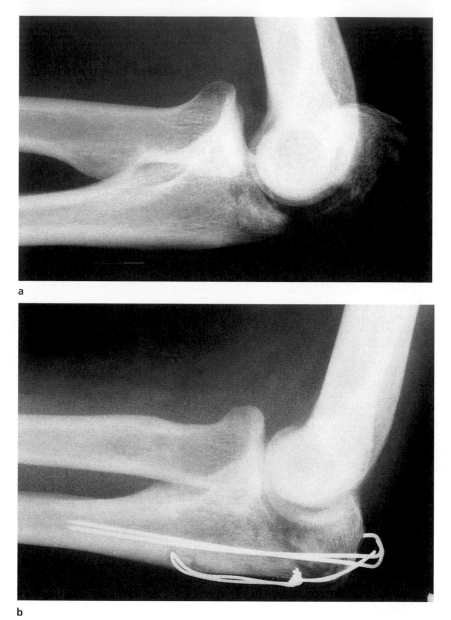

a

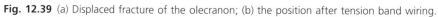

b

Fig. 12.39 (a) Displaced fracture of the olecranon; (b) the position after tension band wiring.

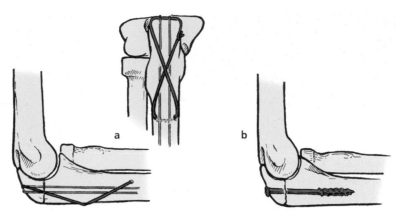

Fig. 12.40 Methods of fixation of fractures of the olecranon: (a) tension band wiring; (b) screwing.

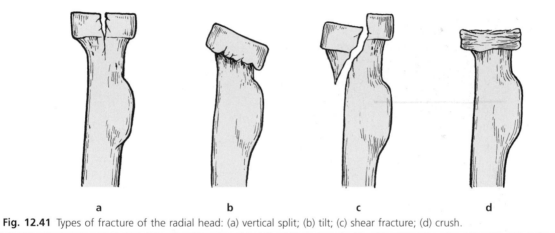

Fig. 12.41 Types of fracture of the radial head: (a) vertical split; (b) tilt; (c) shear fracture; (d) crush.

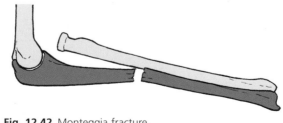

Fig. 12.42 Monteggia fracture.

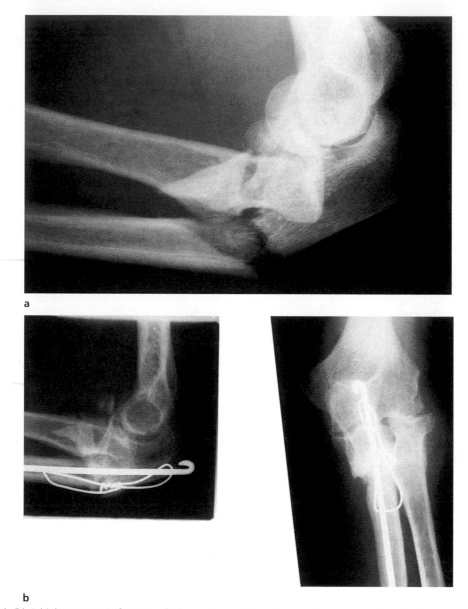

a

b

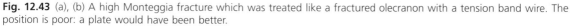

Fig. 12.43 (a), (b) A high Monteggia fracture which was treated like a fractured olecranon with a tension band wire. The position is poor: a plate would have been better.

in children but the position must be checked frequently to be certain that the fragments have not slipped.

Fracture of the radius and ulna

The radius and ulna are easily broken by a twisting injury. The fracture line separates the pronators from the supinators. Both muscle groups act unopposed and produce a nasty rotational deformity that is easily missed on a two-dimensional radiograph, which shows only the angulation and length of the bones but not their rotational relationship. If rotation is present, the radiographs will show a lateral view of the elbow and an antero-posterior view of the forearm on the same film and this sign should be looked for specifically (Fig. 12.44).

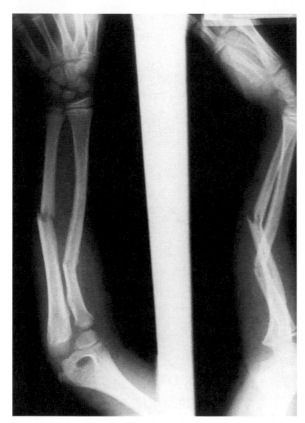

Fig. 12.44 Fracture of the radius and ulna to show displacement. This is a greenstick fracture and some bony continuity remains.

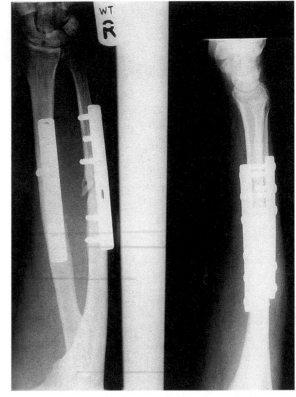

Fig. 12.45 Plating of a fracture of the radius and ulna.

Complications

Complications are common after fractures of the radius and ulna.

Malunion. Unless the rotational deformity is corrected, a malunion will follow and the patient will be unable to supinate the forearm, which makes it difficult to wash the face or collect change when shopping.

Compartment syndromes and vascular damage are common.

Non-union is common, particularly if rotation has not been controlled.

Cross-union. Some fractures unite with cross-union between the two bones, which makes pronation and supination impossible.

Treatment

These fractures are so unstable that conservative treatment is seldom successful in adults, and inter-nal fixation may even be required in children to achieve stability.

Conservative. A well applied cast can sometimes correct and hold the rotational deformity by bringing the distal fragment round to meet the proximal, which is held in unopposed supination. The cast must include both the upper arm and the hand, which is held in supination, but in this position the longitudinal position may slip and open reduction is then required.

Operative. Open reduction and internal fixation is the treatment of choice for most of these fractures (Fig. 12.45) but external fixation is needed if the wounds are contaminated. Plates and screws or intramedullary nails are generally used.

Isolated fracture of the ulna

The subcutaneous margin of the ulna is vulnerable to direct trauma and easily cracked by a direct blow when protecting the face from an impact or from missiles such as cricket balls.

Treatment

Treatment varies according to the amount of displacement.

Undisplaced fractures. Although these fractures look deceptively straightforward on the radiograph, they should be treated with great suspicion and immobilized in a full arm cast with the elbow flexed. If this is not done the fracture will be exposed to rotational stresses and non-union can follow.

Displaced fractures. The rotational element makes displaced fractures almost impossible to immobilize and they are best treated by internal fixation with a plate.

Isolated fracture of the radius

The radius can be fractured by direct trauma. Because the radiohumeral joint reduces rotational strains on the fracture, non-union is less common than in isolated fractures of the ulna.

Treatment

Treatment varies according to the amount of displacement.

Undisplaced fractures. Although these fractures look deceptively straightforward on the radiograph, like isolated fractures of the ulna, they should be treated with great suspicion and immobilized in a full arm cast with the elbow flexed.

Displaced fractures. The rotational element makes displaced fractures difficult to immobilize and they are best treated by internal fixation.

Fractured radius with dislocation of the distal radioulnar joint (Galeazzi fracture)

A fall on the outstretched hand can cause an isolated fracture of the radius with subluxation of the inferior radioulnar joint (Fig. 12.46). This is a Galeazzi

fracture and is quite different from a Colles' fracture (p. 213).

In many ways, the Galeazzi and Monteggia fractures are mirror images. The Monteggia involves dislocation of the superior radioulnar joint and fracture of the ulna, the Galeazzi a fracture of the radius and dislocation of the inferior radioulnar joint. Both slip after an initial good result, both are mistaken for other fractures, and both may need internal fixation. Beware of both!

The reason for the similarity is simple: if one forearm bone shortens, the other can only support it if it is stable, and in both fractures the 'intact' bone is dislocated at one end.

Complications

Malunion is common. Because the distal fragment has no longitudinal stability, the fracture is unstable and is notorious for slipping in plaster after an initial good position.

Treatment

The fracture is best treated by internal fixation of the radius (Fig. 12.47). It must not be treated in a short forearm cast as if it were a Colles' fracture, for which it may be mistaken.

Monteggia versus Galeazzi

- Monteggia – fractured ulna, dislocated proximal radioulnar joint.
- Galeazzi – fractured radius, dislocated distal radioulnar joint.
- Beware of both!

Crush injuries of the forearm

The forearm is frequently crushed between heavy objects or rollers. Even if no bone is broken, these injuries are serious because of soft tissue swelling inside the closed fascial compartments of the forearm.

Treatment

The arm must be elevated, the circulation watched carefully and any loss of extension of the wrist and fingers treated seriously. If in any doubt, a wide fasciotomy of the fascial compartment of the forearm

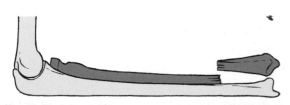

Fig. 12.46 Galeazzi fracture.

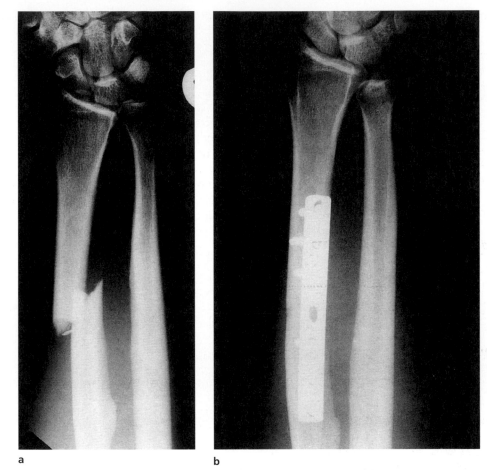

a   b

Fig. 12.47 A Galeazzi fracture: (a) before internal fixation; (b) after fixation with a plate and screws.

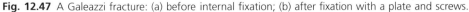

is needed to prevent the complications of a compartment syndrome.

Fractures at the lower end of the radius

Colles' fracture

The Colles' fracture, described by Abraham Colles (1773–1843), who was Professor of Surgery in Dublin, is probably the commonest fracture seen in fracture clinics and general practice (Fig. 12.48).

The fracture that Colles described:

1. Was within 1 inch (2.5 cm) of the wrist joint.
2. Had dorsal angulation of the distal fragment.
3. Had dorsal displacement of the fragment.
4. Was associated with a fracture of the ulnar styloid.

Colles' fracture is most often caused by a fall on the outstretched arm in patients over 50, usually women.

Deformity. The obvious deformity of a Colles' fracture is the classical 'dinner fork' of backward angulation but the deformity has five separate elements (Fig. 12.49):

1. Backward angulation.
2. Backward displacement.
3. Radial deviation.
4. Supination.
5. Proximal impaction.

In gross deformities the distal radioulnar joint may be dislocated.

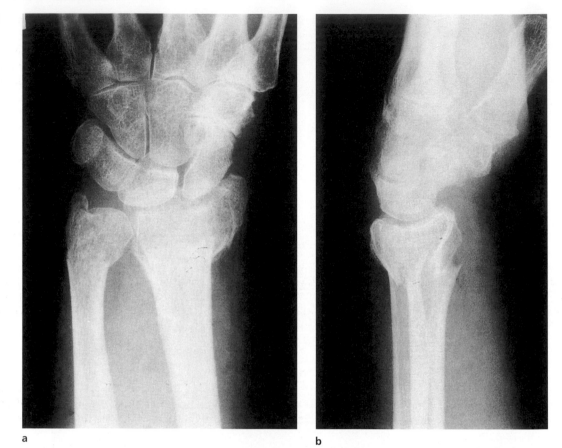

Fig. 12.48 (a), (b) Colles' fracture.

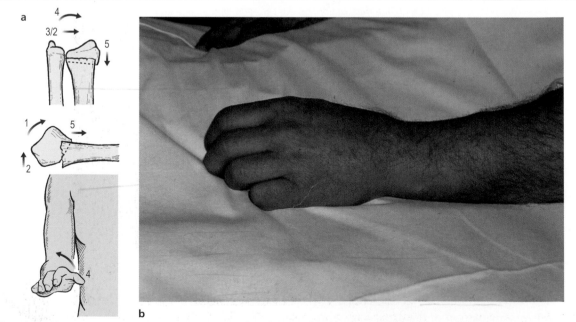

Fig. 12.49 (a) Displacement of the fragments in a Colles' fracture. (b) The 'dinner fork' deformity of Colles' fracture.

Complications

Complications are regrettably frequent after such a common and apparently straightforward injury. Most complications occur not from neglect, but simply because there is no treatment that is truly effective.

Complications of Colles' fracture

- Sudeck's atrophy.
- Median nerve injury.
- Rupture of extensor pollicis longus.
- Malunion.

Sudeck's atrophy. The hand becomes stiff, blue and cold in this variety of reflex sympathetic dystrophy, caused by a disturbance of the sensory and the autonomic supply of bone and blood vessels. The condition is particularly common if the patient is allowed to rest the hand without moving the fingers and can be prevented by ensuring that the patient keeps the fingers moving. Sometimes the condition involves the shoulder as well and is then called the 'shoulder–hand syndrome'.

Treatment is difficult and requires much patience, physiotherapy and reassurance. Because of this fearful complication, it is vitally important to ensure that the patients really do keep their fingers and shoulder moving after a Colles' fracture.

Median nerve damage. The median nerve runs right across the site of a Colles' fracture and may be compressed by the bruising and bleeding around it. Median nerve symptoms usually settle by the time the fracture is united but decompression is sometimes required.

Rupture of the extensor pollicis longus tendon. The extensor pollicis longus tendon runs across the fracture site at the dorsum of the wrist and may be worn through by movement across the sharp edge of the broken bone, producing an 'attrition rupture'.

The problem is also seen in fractures with very slight displacement and may be due to ischaemia rather than attrition. If a patient reports that the thumb has dropped following a Colles' fracture, the tendon has ruptured and must be repaired.

Malunion. Because the fracture is unstable and the bone is crushed, malunion is common (Fig. 12.50). The disability from a malunion is unpredictable and many patients manage well despite a marked and unsightly deformity.

Treatment

Left untreated, the fracture will unite with backward angulation, a loss of supination, weakness of grip and loss of ulnar deviation. The functional result is often surprisingly good.

Displaced fractures. The fracture can be manipulated into good position by pulling the hand distally

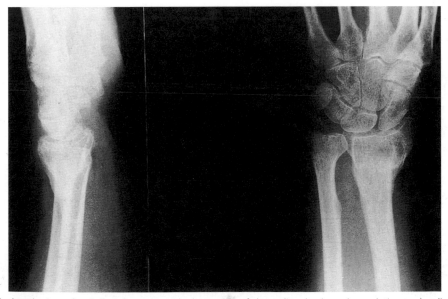

Fig. 12.50 Typical malunion of a Colles' fracture, with shortening of the radius, backward angulation and radial rotation of the radial fragment and non-union of the ulnar fragment.

to disimpact the fracture, flexing the wrist and pulling the hand round into ulnar deviation. Reducing the fracture in this way is easy but holding the position is not. Because the fragment is impacted, the bone on the dorsum of the radius is crushed and a hole is left in the dorsum of the radius when the fracture is reduced. This leaves the distal fragment unsupported dorsally and the deformity recurs as the swelling subsides.

Once reduced, a plaster is applied from the elbow to the metacarpophalangeal joints, which lie in the line of the proximal skin crease in the palm and not at the base of the fingers. *The fingers and the thumb must be left free* so that they can move freely.

The fracture should be inspected the next day to be sure that there is no undue swelling and that the patient is moving the fingers, arm and shoulder.

The patient is then seen between 7 and 10 days later and a radiograph taken to check the position. If the fragments have slipped, a further manipulation may be required. If the patient is not using the hand and shoulder at this stage, physiotherapy should be instituted at once.

The cast is retained for a total of 4 weeks, by which time there should be full movement in the fingers, thumb, elbow and shoulder. Physiotherapy or occupational therapy may be needed if the patient is reluctant to use the hand.

Impacted fractures in good position. A fracture will sometimes impact in acceptable position with little backward angulation. Such fractures need not be manipulated, but it is wise to apply a cast for 2 weeks to prevent accidental displacement.

Operations for malunion

Operation is sometimes needed to restore supination, or to relieve pain. Three procedures are available:

1. *Baldwin's procedure*, in which a 2 cm long segment of ulna is excised with its periosteum, leaving the distal 2 cm of the ulna intact. This allows the head of the ulna to move proximally and improves supination as well as the appearance of the wrist.

2. *Excision of the lower end of the ulna* improves the appearance but disturbs the stability of the wrist.

3. *Corrective osteotomy* is a more extensive procedure, sometimes needed if backward angulation of the radius is the main problem.

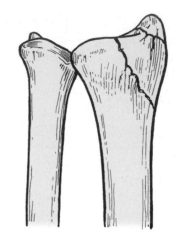

Fig. 12.51 Fractures of the radial styloid.

Colles' fracture in children

Do not make the diagnosis of a Colles' fracture in a child; it does not occur. If a 'dinner fork' deformity is present, the likely diagnosis is a fracture separation of the radial epiphysis or a greenstick fracture of the radius at its distal end (p. 219) (Fig. 12.52).

Fractures of the radial styloid

The radial styloid can fracture in falls on the outstretched arm and this is commoner in the firm bone of young adults than the soft bone of the elderly (Fig. 12.51). The fracture usually heals well without lasting disability. The size of the fragment and the degree of displacement vary.

Treatment

The majority of these fractures need no reduction and a cast for 4 weeks is enough. Large displaced fragments must be reduced and internally fixed if manipulation is unsuccessful.

Fractures of the lower end of the radius and ulna

Transverse fractures across one or both bones of the forearm, with backward angulation, are seen after falls on the outstretched arm in young patients (Fig. 12.53).

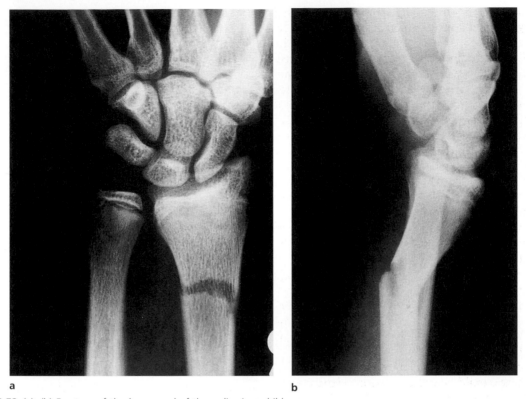

a   b

Fig. 12.52 (a), (b) Fracture of the lower end of the radius in a child.

Treatment

Manipulative reduction is usually easy and a cast for 4 weeks is sufficient. If the fracture is impacted with minimal displacement, 2 weeks immobilization is sufficient, provided that the patient is careful to avoid stressing the fracture for a further 4 weeks.

Smith's fracture and Barton's fracture

Colles' successor in the post of Professor of Surgery at Dublin was R.W. Smith, who is said to have performed the post-mortem examination on his predecessor. Smith also described the fracture of the lower end of the radius now known as a Smith's, or reverse Colles' fracture (Fig. 12.54a), which occurs if the victim lands with the wrist in flexion. Smith's fracture is very unstable and will cause a disabling flexion deformity at the wrist if not treated correctly.

In some patients, the fracture line enters the joint so that the anterior lip of the radius is displaced proximally with the hand (Fig. 12.54b). This is not a Smith's fracture but a Barton's fracture, first described by John Rhea Barton of Philadelphia, a founding father of American orthopaedic surgery.

Treatment

Both these fractures must be distinguished carefully from a Colles' fracture and treated in a forearm cast with the hand supinated and the wrist in full extension. If a good position cannot be achieved and maintained, the fracture must be reduced openly and secured with a small buttress plate attached to the volar aspect of the radius (Fig. 12.55).

If this is not done, a disabling malunion and flexion deformity follows and arthrodesis may be needed.

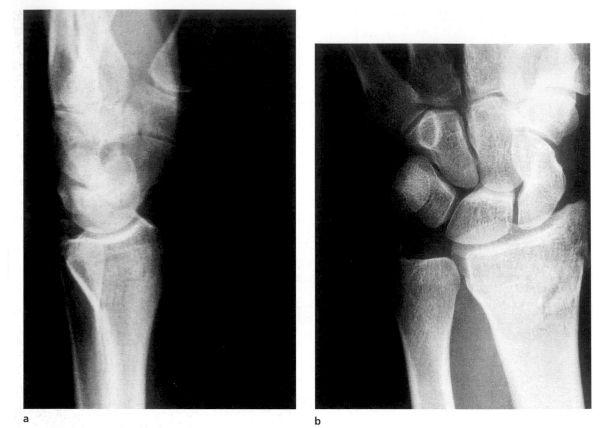

a   b

Fig. 12.53 (a), (b) Impacted fracture of the lower end of the radius with minimal displacement.

Fractures in children

Epiphyseal separations

Fracture separations of the epiphyses occur only in children and must be reduced carefully if serious deformities are to be avoided (Fig. 12.56).

The injuries occur at the wrist, elbow and shoulder. Any injury can cause a fracture separation but they can be caused by a child being swung or thrown by the arms. If a child has more than one such fracture, the possibility of non-accidental injury should be considered.

Complications

Epiphyseal arrest is the principal complication of epiphyseal injuries but aseptic necrosis of the epiphysis is also seen.

Treatment

Accurate reduction and great gentleness are required. Closed reduction is usually successful but, if the epiphysis is fractured as well as dislocated, open reduction may be needed.

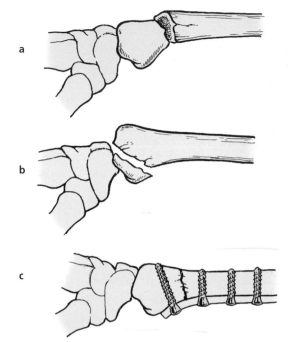

Fig. 12.54 (a) Smith's fracture; (b) Barton's fracture, which enters the joint; (c) internal fixation of Smith's fracture.

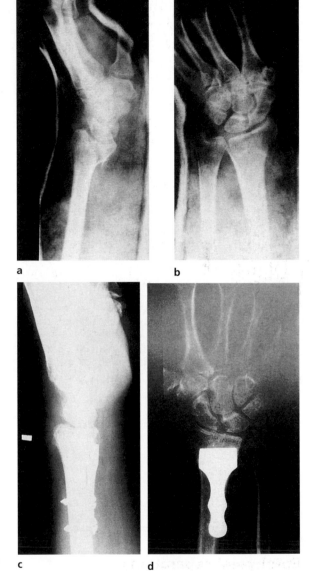

Fig. 12.55 Internal fixation of Barton's fracture: (a), (b) position before operation. The hand is in full extension but the position cannot be controlled; (c), (d) the position is satisfactory after insertion of an Ellis plate.

Greenstick fractures

Greenstick fractures occur only in childhood and are a mixed blessing. Although bony continuity is maintained and a good result can be expected, the fracture cannot be manipulated into perfect position because the bone springs back slightly. The similarity to a 'green stick' is close (p. 99).

Complications

The appearance of a greenstick fracture after removal from the cast can be alarming to the parents. The arm is not entirely straight and the parents need firm reassurance that this is normal and that the limb will remodel. Angular deformities of up to 30° in the plane of the nearest joint usually remodel perfectly but rotational deformities do not.

Treatment

If both cortices are buckled but intact, a light protective plaster for 2–3 weeks is all that is needed. These fractures cannot be manipulated into perfect position and some imperfection must be accepted.

It is impossible to overcorrect a greenstick fracture, even with three-point pressure. Provided the

219

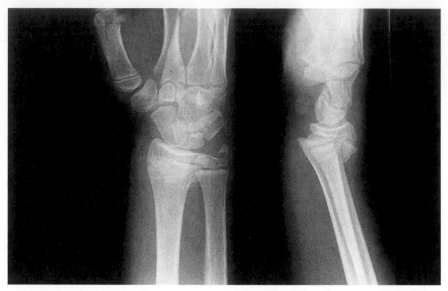

Fig. 12.56 Anteroposterior and lateral view of a type 2 Harris and Salter fracture separation of the lower radial epiphysis with a fracture of the ulnar styloid.

child does not fall again before the fracture is solid, an excellent result will be achieved whatever is done.

If one cortex is broken, a deformity can develop and correction may be needed. The cast should be retained for 3 weeks.

Supracondylar fractures of the humerus, fractures of the medial epicondyle, lateral condyle and pulled elbow are dealt with elsewhere (pp. 200, 202 and 204).

Chapter |13|

Hand injuries

By the end of this chapter you should be able to:

- Differentiate different levels of flexor tendon injury and the zone of injury. You should understand the effects of injury in each zone and how function is affected.
- Recognize levels of extensor tendon injury.
- Diagnose carpal and phalanges bone fractures and be aware of poor healing in scaphoid fractures, etc.
- Be aware of the vital importance of correct hand rehabilitation to maximize function.

The hand is a complex structure and even a slight disturbance in one part can have serious effects on its function as a whole. Because the hand is so important to work, leisure and everyday living, hand injuries demand special care and attention.

Hand injuries can involve:

- Nerves.
- Bones.
- Joints.
- Tendons.
- Skin and soft tissue.
- Blood vessels.

Nerves

The different types of nerve lesion and their management are described on pages 109, 141 (Fig. 13.1).

Median nerve

The median nerve may be cut cleanly across at the wrist or palm by sharp objects or by falls through windows.

Treatment

These injuries are ideal for immediate repair; i.e. within 24 h of injury. The results are generally good, particularly in children, but complete recovery *never* occurs. The flexor tendons are usually injured at the same time and accurate repair of all the structures involved can be very difficult.

Ulnar nerve

The ulnar nerve can also be damaged in this way but it lies deeper than the median nerve and is protected by the tendon of flexor carpi ulnaris.

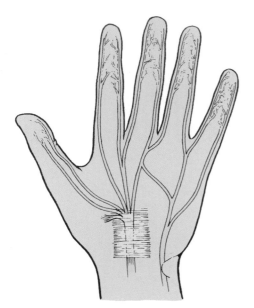

Fig. 13.1 Nerve supply to the palm of the hand. Note the position of the digital nerves and the median and ulnar nerves at the wrist, and the median nerve passing beneath the transverse carpal ligaments.

Treatment

As with the median nerve, the results of repair are acceptable but never perfect.

Digital nerves

The palmar digital nerves are very vulnerable and are cut if the patient grips a blade or a sharp object. The digital artery is usually damaged at the same time. Because the volar digital nerve supplies the pulp of the finger, injuries to it can seriously impair function.

Treatment

The cutaneous nerves on the dorsum of the finger, distal to the middle of the middle phalanx, are too small to repair. On the palmar surface the nerve is large enough to repair as far distally as the distal interphalangeal joint. Lesions proximal to these points should be repaired under magnification.

Crushed nerves and dirty wounds

Contaminated or untidy nerve lesions are not suitable for immediate repair.

Treatment

The ends of the nerve can be tagged with a marking suture and the nerve repaired when the wound has healed. The end of the nerve will then have a firm fibrous cap of epineurium, which must be removed before it can be repaired. The nerve must also be mobilized proximally and distally to give extra length.

Flexor tendons

Anatomy

The flexor tendons run part of their course through synovial and fibrous sheaths. The fibrous sheaths, which are lined with synovium, run from the distal interphalangeal (d.i.p.) joints to the distal palmar skin crease and prevent the tendon 'bowstringing' when the finger is flexed.

The synovial sheaths of the thumb and little fingers extend proximally through the carpal tunnel. The three central digits (index, middle and ring) have a separate flexor sheath in the fingers. There is also a sheath in the palm which extends proximal to the wrist (Fig. 13.2).

Sites of flexor tendon injury

Zone I : distal to d.i.p. joint.
Zone II : in the fingers.
Zone III : in the palm.
Zone IV : in the carpal tunnel.
Zone V : in the forearm.

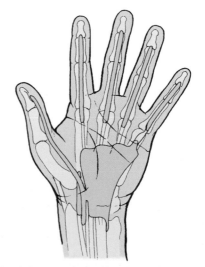

Fig. 13.2 Tendon sheaths in the palm and wrist.

This anatomy is important because it determines the management of the injuries at different levels. Tendons repaired inside a fibrous sheath do not slide smoothly and suture lines should lie outside the sheath whenever possible. If this cannot be done, the tendon must be replaced with a graft running from the distal phalanx to the palm so that there is no suture line within the synovial sheath. Repair is technically possible within the sheath but it must be done very precisely and meticulously.

Because of these complexities, flexor tendon injuries should be treated only by experienced surgeons.

Zone I: Lesions distal to the tendon sheath

Injuries distal to the d.i.p. joint lie outside the sheath.

Treatment

Zone I lesions can be treated by (1) tendon advancement, or (2) arthrodesis of the d.i.p. joint.

The cut end of the tendon can be advanced and reinserted on the distal phalanx. This may cause a slight flexion deformity.

In the thumb the advancement can be done in the forearm because the flexor pollicis longus has no connection with other flexors and its tendon can be separated from the muscle belly in the forearm and moved distally.

The results of surgery are better in the thumb than the fingers.

Early movement, active or passive, is important after any tendon repair and several devices are available to encourage this.

Zone II: Injuries in the fingers

Management of flexor injuries in the fingers depends on the tendons involved and the site of injury (Fig. 13.3). The first step is to decide which tendon has been damaged.

Profundus and superficialis action can be distinguished by asking the patient to flex the distal phalanx with the middle phalanx held still (see Fig. 2.26). Only flexor profundus will do this because superficialis does not extend beyond the middle phalanx (Fig. 13.4).

To assess superficialis, hold all the fingers down except the one that is to be tested and ask the patient

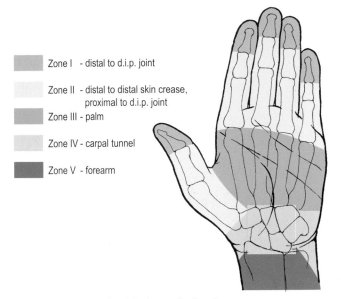

Zone I - distal to d.i.p. joint

Zone II - distal to distal skin crease, proximal to d.i.p. joint

Zone III - palm

Zone IV - carpal tunnel

Zone V - forearm

Fig. 13.3 Flexor tendon injuries to the hand.

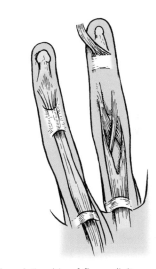

Fig. 13.4 The relationship of flexor digitorum profundus and superficialis.

to flex that finger. If the finger flexes at the proximal interphalangeal (p.i.p.) joint, superficialis is intact. Test this on your own hand.

Treatment

Division of superficialis alone. If superficialis is divided alone it is best to excise the redundant portion of its tendon and rely on flexor profundus for finger flexion, thus avoiding the problems of adhesions and stiffness. Alternatively, the lesion can be ignored.

Division of superficialis and profundus. If the tendons are cut opposite the proximal or middle phalanx they can be treated either by meticulous primary repair by an experienced surgeon or by replacing the tendon with an autograft of another tendon, such as palmaris longus or plantaris. If both tendons are cut, both should be repaired.

Division of profundus alone. If the tendon is divided within 1 cm of its insertion the tendon can be pulled up, or 'advanced', and the cut end attached to the distal phalanx.

Zone III: Injuries in the palm

Division of the flexor tendons in the palm is less serious than division in the fingers because the repair can be done outside the fibrous or synovial sheaths.

Treatment

The tendons should be repaired meticulously by an experienced hand surgeon and early mobilization instituted.

Zone IV: Injuries in the carpal tunnel

Eleven flexor tendons (flexor digitorum superficialis (4), flexor digitorum profundus (4), flexor pollicis longus, flexor carpi ulnaris and flexor carpi radialis) cross the volar aspect of the wrist (Fig. 13.5). If all these are divided, there will be 22 cut tendon ends. If the median nerve is divided as well, there will be 24 structures, which must be carefully identified, and if each pair is joined there will be 12 suture lines very close together. However carefully repaired, the tendons and nerves may stick together and form a solid mass which restricts movement at the wrist.

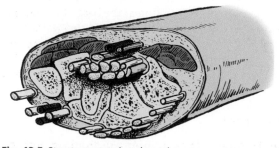

Fig. 13.5 Structures crossing the wrist.

Treatment

The problem can be simplified by discarding those tendons that are not absolutely necessary. The flexor superficialis, for example, can be sacrificed if flexor profundus is working. Finger flexion will still be full and the risk of adhesions between superficialis and profundus outweigh the improvement of function that might be obtained by repairing both.

Zone V: Injuries in the forearm

Injuries in the forearm lie outside any sheath and can be accurately repaired more easily than elsewhere.

Treatment

The tendon ends are accurately identified and repaired, and early mobilization begun.

Contaminated wounds and crushing injuries

If the wound is untidy and dirty it must be debrided and all dead tissue removed. If the wound is untidy but clean it is sometimes better to excise the tendon and replace it with a Silastic rod, which can itself be replaced with a graft when the wound has healed.

If the wound is contaminated, a clean and well-healed wound must be obtained before definitive treatment is undertaken.

Aftercare

The hand should be mobilized actively and passively as soon as pain and swelling permit.

Extensor tendons

Anatomy

Because the extensor tendons only have a synovial sheath where they cross the wrist, the problems encountered in repairing flexor tendons in the fingers do not arise. The tendons are easily identified, repair is straightforward and the fingers can be mobilized after 3 or 4 weeks.

If the tendons are divided on the dorsum of the hand they cannot contract for more than a few millimetres because they are restricted by linking fibrous bands. Even without repair some extensor function will eventually return (Fig. 13.6).

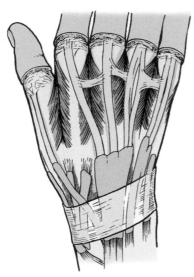

Fig. 13.6 Anatomy of the extensor tendons to show the tendon sheaths and extensor hoods.

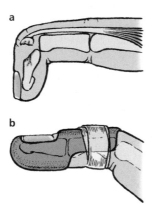

Fig. 13.7 (a) A mallet finger with avulsion of the extensor tendon from the distal phalanx; (b) a mallet finger splint holding the d.i.p. joint extended.

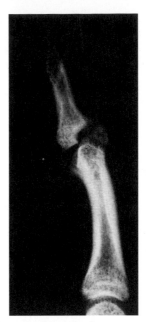

Fig. 13.8 Radiograph of a mallet finger.

Treatment

Tendons divided on the dorsum of the hand should be repaired and the fingers splinted in extension for 3 weeks.

Mallet finger

Violent flexion injuries to, or lacerations across the back of, the d.i.p. joint can avulse or divide the insertion of the extensor digitorum longus at the base of the distal phalanx (Figs 13.7a, 13.8).

Untreated, the lesion causes the distal phalanx to droop and leaves a 'mallet' finger deformity. The condition is inconvenient but function improves without treatment and it is exceptional for the patient to be seriously troubled by the injury 12 months later.

Treatment

Although the results are acceptable without treatment, splintage can produce a better result. The finger should be immobilized for 6 weeks in a mallet finger splint which holds the d.i.p. joint hyperextended but allows movement at the p.i.p. joint (Fig. 13.7b). Some loss of active extension may persist.

Boutonnière lesion

The central slip of the extensor expansion can be detached from its insertion at the base of the middle phalanx by a cut or by violent muscle contraction. This allows the two lateral slips to fall sideways and the p.i.p. joint to protrude between the two, which produces a characteristic deformity and may impair function (Fig. 13.9).

Treatment

The lesion should be splinted with the finger straight, but the results are imperfect. If the final disability

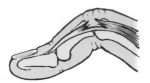

Fig. 13.9 A boutonnière lesion of the p.i.p. joint.

justifies it, the two slips can be approximated to restore extension but flexion may be lost.

Blood vessels

Injuries at the wrist

Damage to the radial or ulnar arteries at the wrist causes severe arterial bleeding, which can be controlled by firm pressure and elevation.

Treatment

If both radial and ulnar arteries are ligated, ischaemia of the hand may result, and at least one, preferably the radial, should remain intact. If both treatment arteries are damaged, arterial repair is required.

Note: Be *very* careful when applying artery forceps near the wrist: arteries, nerves and tendons can all be damaged very easily.

Injuries in the palm

The deep palmar arch can be cut by penetrating injuries and causes serious bleeding.

Treatment

Bleeding must be stopped to avoid a large palmar haematoma and skin necrosis.

Skin and subcutaneous tissue

Crushing injuries

Fingers can be crushed so hard that the skin bursts. These injuries must be treated by elevation of the arm and hand and the wounds must never be sutured. Although it is technically possible to close the wounds soon after injury, the sutures prevent the soft tissues from swelling and a stiff or dead digit will follow.

Treatment

The wound should be cleaned, lightly dressed and the hand elevated. After 48 h the swelling will begin to subside and the skin edges will come together on their own. Delayed primary suture is sometimes needed.

Degloving injuries

If the hand is caught in machinery, the skin of the hand and fingers can be peeled off like a glove (Fig. 13.10). This is a serious lesion and cannot be treated by rolling the skin back into place. The lesion can be caused by a ring.

Treatment

The skin defect must be grafted by an experienced surgeon, either by removing the subcutaneous fat from the degloved skin and applying it as a free graft or by taking a graft from elsewhere. If paratenon is stripped from the tendons, flap cover is required. Alternatively, the ring finger can be amputated and its skin used to cover the defect.

Grindstone injuries

Accidental contact with a grindstone removes skin, subcutaneous tissue and bone (Fig. 13.11). The wound is contaminated and the loss of tissue can be irreparable.

Treatment

Treatment depends on the lesion but, if the knuckle is involved, arthrodesis or amputation may be preferable to a protracted series of reconstructive procedures.

Injection injuries

Although rare, the injuries caused by high pressure injection devices such as high pressure water nozzles, paint sprays and grease guns can cause serious problems. These implements can force grease or water through the skin and into the subcutaneous tissues without any opening in the skin itself. The irritation in the soft tissues can lead to tissue necrosis and the integrity of the skin is misleading.

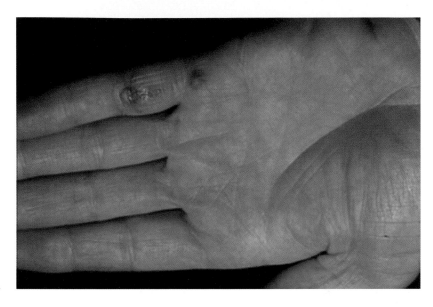

Fig. 13.10 Injury to the little finger caused by a ring. This type of injury can cause degloving. Note the small flap of skin at the p.i.p. joint.

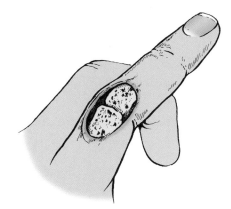

Fig. 13.11 A grindstone injury of the hand with destruction of the extensor tendon and exposure of the joint surface.

Treatment

The hand must be explored and all extraneous material removed. If this is not done the ensuing inflammation, particularly if complicated by infection, may lead to amputation.

Skin

Skin incisions or lacerations that cross skin creases on the flexor aspect of joints may shorten when they heal and form a tight fibrous contracture that holds the joint flexed. While there is no choice in the position of a laceration, incisions used to repair tendons and nerves must not cross skin creases transversely.

Treatment

The wound should be carefully cleaned, but never use spirit to clean a wound on the hand. The spirit will damage exposed nerve tissue and cause an intense inflammatory response in the flexor tendon sheath that restricts flexor tendon movement. Aqueous solutions of chlorhexidine or cetrimide are preferable and the detergent action of these agents is an added advantage.

Once cleaned, the wound edges can be brought lightly together with fine sutures and the hand elevated until swelling has subsided.

Human bites

Genuine human bites are uncommon away from the rugby field but knuckles are often injured against teeth – a 'fight bite'. Injuries caused in this way often fail to heal and become badly infected with a cocktail of exotic organisms.

Treatment

The wound should be cleaned, excised and enlarged, and left unsutured, and adequate antibiotics given.

Fractures and dislocations

The management of fractures in the hand, like the management of fractures elsewhere, follows the principle that stable fractures should be mobilized soon, whereas unstable fractures should be stabi-

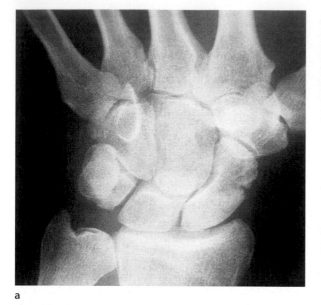

a

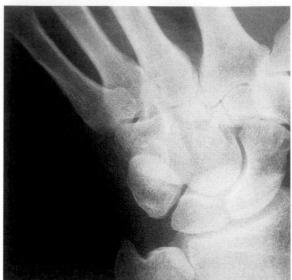

b

Fig. 13.12 (a), (b) Fracture of the waist of the scaphoid.

lized and then mobilized. Early mobilization is even more important in the hand than elsewhere.

Waist of the scaphoid

Mechanism

The carpal bones are arranged in two rows, proximal and distal. The scaphoid bridges the two rows and is exposed to stresses not encountered by the other carpal bones.

Violent hyperextension of the wrist will crack the waist of the scaphoid across its narrowest point and any force that hyperextends the wrist will do this. In days past, this was called a 'chauffeur's fracture' because a common cause was the starting handle of a petrol engine being flung backwards if the engine backfired while the handle was held incorrectly.

Fracture of the waist of the scaphoid is a treacherous fracture for several reasons:

1. It is not easily seen on initial radiographs, even if several views are taken (Fig. 13.12).

2. The fracture can go on to non-union, especially if it is not immobilized (Fig. 13.13).

3. Because the blood supply to the proximal pole of the bone enters by the distal pole in most people, the proximal fragment can be devitalized, which leads to aseptic necrosis of the scaphoid and osteoarthritis of the wrist.

4. There are very few reliable clinical signs.

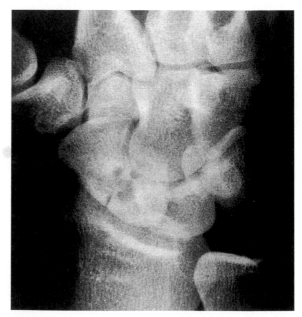

Fig. 13.13 Non-union of the scaphoid.

Physical signs

There is no deformity, crepitus or bruising around a fractured scaphoid. The only physical signs are tenderness in the anatomical snuff-box with swelling, weakness of pinch and pain on hyperextension. Even these signs are not always present.

To avoid missing this evil fracture certain precautions must be taken:

1. When the scaphoid is examined radiologically, two views are not enough. Four views must be taken at different angles, including oblique views.
2. Any patient with tenderness in the anatomical snuff-box, even with normal radiographs, should be assumed to have a fractured scaphoid and a scaphoid cast applied. The scaphoid views should be repeated out of plaster at 10 days, when the fracture line may be more easily seen because of decalcification along its length.
3. The diagnosis of 'sprained wrist' or 'sprained thumb' should not be permitted until a scaphoid fracture has been considered and excluded.

Treatment

A cast should be applied to immobilize the joint above and the joints below the fracture, i.e. the wrist, carpometacarpal and first metacarpophalangeal joints, and retained for a minimum of 6 weeks. The cast must hold the thumb roughly *opposite the ring finger* and not in wide abduction because that interferes with function and displaces the fragments.

If the fracture is not united by 12 weeks, internal fixation and grafting should be considered.

Tubercle of the scaphoid

The scaphoid has a small bony tubercle which can be avulsed. Fracture of the tubercle of the scaphoid is benign but unfortunately far less common than a fracture through the waist.

Treatment

Immobilization of the scaphoid is advisable for pain relief.

Fractures of the triquetral

Violent hyperextension of the wrist can separate a flake of bone from the triquetral.

Treatment

The fracture is little more than a soft tissue injury and need not be immobilized.

Carpal dislocations

Injuries to the carpus cause serious problems and they are frequently missed in the accident department, which makes the consequences even more serious. Like scaphoid fractures, they have a deservedly treacherous reputation.

Many types of instability occur but the commonest are: (1) perilunate dislocation, (2) trans-scaphoid perilunate dislocation and (3) other types of carpal instability.

Perilunate dislocation

Violent hyperextension pushes the carpus off the back of the radius but the lunate usually remains attached to the radius. The lesion is easily missed on a simple anteroposterior radiograph but is obvious on the lateral (Fig. 13.14). The median nerve may be damaged and the consequences of missing this lesion are serious.

Dislocation of the lunate is the same injury as perilunate dislocation except that, as the soft tissues pull the hand forwards from the hyperextension that causes the dislocation, the lunate is pushed forwards from its normal position so that it lies in front of the other carpal bones.

Treatment. The dislocation must be reduced accurately and held reduced for at least 4 weeks. Open reduction is sometimes needed.

Trans-scaphoid perilunate dislocation

This dislocation is the same as a dislocation of the lunate except that the fracture line passes through the waist of the scaphoid, leaving the proximal pole of the scaphoid attached to the lunate. Many patterns of fracture exist, some involving the radius as well.

Treatment. The fracture must be reduced carefully; open operation may be needed to replace the lunate. If the scaphoid is fractured, the carpus must be stabilized by internal fixation.

Other carpal instabilities

Instability of the carpus without a fracture is extremely difficult to diagnose at the time of injury, but becomes apparent later when the patient experiences pain or weakness of the carpus under stress.

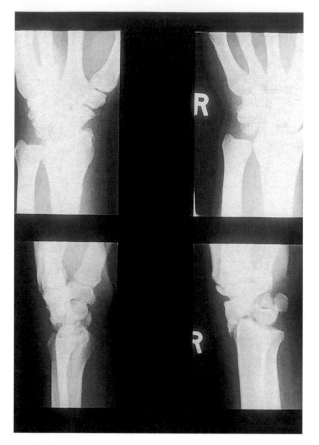

Fig. 13.14 A perilunate fracture dislocation of the carpus accompanied by fracture of the triquetral and the lower end of the radius.

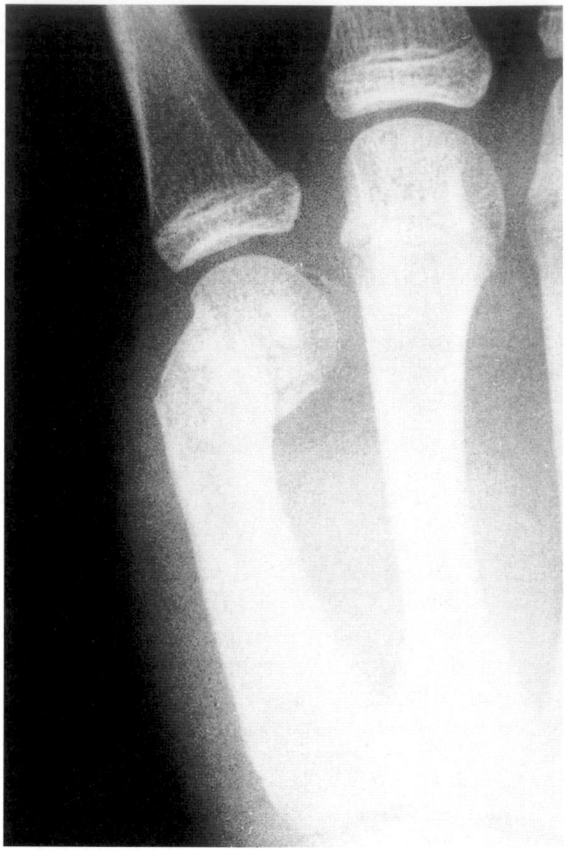

Fig. 13.15 Displaced fracture of the fifth metacarpal neck caused by punching.

The classification and management of these lesions is complex and beyond the scope of this book.

Metacarpal injuries

The fifth metacarpal is broken more often than the others. There are three types of fracture: (1) fractures of the neck, (2) oblique fractures, and (3) transverse comminuted fractures.

Fifth metacarpal neck fracture

The metacarpals are often broken by injuries to the head of the bones with the fingers flexed; i.e. punching with the fist. The fifth metacarpal is almost invariably broken in this way, whatever the patient's account of events (Fig. 13.15).

Treatment. The fracture results in a flexion and rotational deformity. Only rotation need be corrected and this can be done by holding the little finger lightly against the ring finger with elastic strapping and encouraging early flexion.

The fracture may unite with the metacarpal head drooping slightly below the line of the other knuckles and with a slight extensor lag of the little finger, which recovers. Neither causes noticeable disability.

Oblique fractures of the fifth metacarpal

Oblique fractures of the shaft are caused by the little finger being held and twisted. A nasty rotational deformity may be present.

Treatment. Rotation must be corrected carefully and the position maintained by holding the little finger against the ring finger.

Comminuted transverse fractures of the fifth metacarpal

Sideways blows to the edge of the hand will fracture the fifth metacarpal near its centre. This injury is often caused by crushing injuries to the hand, or karate practice, and leads to severe swelling of the hand, with an abduction deformity of the finger.

Treatment. The fracture should be reduced and the little finger held to the ring finger. A small plaster slab can be applied to the side of the hand to protect the fracture site from further trauma.

First metacarpal – Bennett's fracture

The first metacarpal can be broken with the fracture line extending into the carpometacarpal joint to produce a Bennett's fracture, which is often the result of punching (Fig. 13.16). If a boxer 'sprains' his thumb, he probably has a Bennett's fracture. The fracture is unstable for three reasons:

1. The proximal fragment consists of a small triangular segment attached to the trapezium.
2. The fracture line is oblique.
3. The distal fragment has many strong muscles attached to it and these pull the thumb proximally.

Treatment. If left untreated, malunion is inevitable, but the functional result is not always bad.

The fracture should be reduced and, if necessary, held with a percutaneous pin or screw (Fig. 13.16).

First metacarpal – transverse fracture

Transverse fractures produce malalignment of the shaft (Figs 13.17, 13.18).

Treatment. Unless the fragments are impacted, the fracture should be reduced and held in a scaphoid cast.

Multiple metarcarpal fractures

Multiple metacarpal fractures are caused by twisting and crushing injuries.

If more than one metacarpal is broken and the fragments are displaced, the alignment of the metacarpals must be restored with Kirschner wires passed through the intact metacarpals or a small bone plate. If this is not done, the distortion of the metacarpal arch can seriously interfere with finger function.

Metacarpophalangeal dislocations

The metacarpophalangeal joints can be dislocated by hyperextension and rotational strains. The injury is uncommon.

Treatment. Radiologically, these dislocations look deceptively easy to reduce but the metacarpal head sometimes 'buttonholes' through the volar tissues and becomes irreducible. Open reduction is then required.

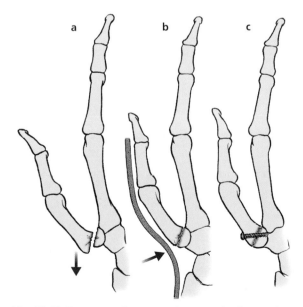

Fig. 13.16 Treatment of Bennett's fracture. The fracture is unstable because of unopposed muscle action (a); it can be held by cast pressure (b) or screw fixation (c).

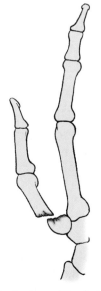

Fig. 13.17 Transverse fracture of the first metacarpal.

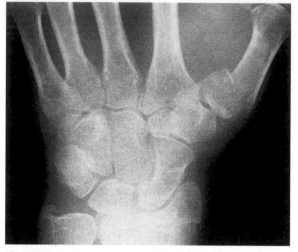

Fig. 13.18 Transverse fracture of the first metacarpal at its base. This is not a Bennett's fracture.

Gamekeeper's (poacher's) thumb

The medial collateral ligament of the first metacarpophalangeal joint is easily torn by any violent abduction injury. The lesion is called a gamekeeper's or poacher's thumb because of the method used to break the neck of game, particularly rabbits. This story is not entirely accurate. Those who break animals' necks in this way stretch their own ligaments gradually rather than break them suddenly (Fig. 13.19).

The lesion is also caused by falls, particularly on dry ski slopes, where the hand may slide down the surface until the thumb catches on an irregularity or in a pole strap. The ligament can be either torn directly across or avulsed with a flake of bone.

Treatment. Left untreated the thumb is unstable and cannot resist the force on the index finger in a pinch grip. Cast immobilization or surgical repair of the lesion is often required but there may be some residual disability.

Phalanges

The phalanges are fractured most often by twisting or angular forces (Fig. 13.20). Angulation is easily corrected but rotational deformities from spiral fractures are more difficult.

The bone usually unites soundly, the most urgent problem being the preservation of normal movement between tendon and bone.

Treatment. The simplest and most effective treatment for stable phalangeal fractures is to hold the

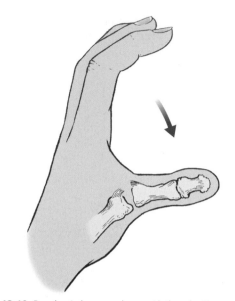

Fig. 13.19 Poacher's (or gamekeeper's) thumb. The medial collateral ligament of the first metacarpophalangeal joint is torn.

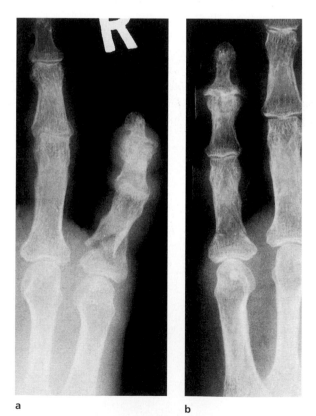

a   b

Fig. 13.20 (a) Spiral fracture of the proximal phalanx of the little finger; (b) satisfactory position achieved by strapping the little finger to the adjacent ring finger.

damaged finger against its neighbour and encourage flexion, which is impossible if there is a rotational deformity (Fig. 13.21).

The fingers should be held lightly together with elastic strapping to allow room for the swelling that is bound to follow a fracture, and a small layer of felt or other absorbable material placed between the two fingers to absorb sweat and avoid skin irritation.

Unstable fractures sometimes need internal fixation (Fig. 13.22).

Juxta-epiphyseal fracture separations

The phalanges are 'long bones' and can sustain fracture separations of the epiphysis just like those of the femur and tibia (Fig. 13.23).

Treatment. The fracture should be reduced and early mobilization commenced. Residual deformity will be corrected well by remodelling.

Interphalangeal fracture dislocations

Violent hyperextension of the thumb or fingers can avulse a fragment of the middle phalanx which remains attached to the proximal phalanx by the volar plate (Fig. 13.24). This is not a straightforward injury and may lead to a very stiff digit from scarring and fibrosis around the front of the interphalangeal joint.

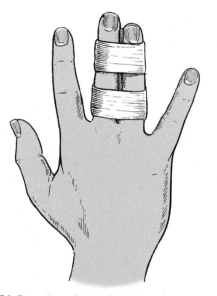

Fig. 13.21 Strapping adjacent fingers.

Treatment. If the avulsed fragment includes more than one-third of the articular surface, the fracture will be unstable and fixation with a pin may be needed. If the fragment involves less than one-third of the articular surface, the finger should be immobilized in flexion.

Phalangeal dislocation

The interphalangeal joints of the thumb and fingers dislocate and reduce easily. The dislocation may have reduced spontaneously, or have been reduced by longitudinal traction, before the patient reaches hospital.

Some swelling is inevitable around every dislocation but there is so little subcutaneous fat around the interphalangeal joints that any additional soft tissue is easily visible. For this reason, patients should be advised that the swelling of a dislocated finger will continue to subside for as long as 2 years after the injury but will never subside completely. Any rings worn on the affected finger which do not fit at the end of this time will need to be enlarged.

Treatment. Rigid immobilization is not required but the finger should be held loosely against its neighbour and early mobilization begun. The strapping can be removed after approximately 2 weeks.

Reduction is not always easy. If the head of the phalanx slips through a defect in the capsule, reduction is impossible and open reduction will be needed, as for metacarpophalangeal dislocations (Fig. 13.25).

Intra-articular fractures

The phalanges can break through their condyles to produce a very unstable intra-articular fracture.

Treatment. Like unstable fractures anywhere else, accurate reduction is important. Fixation with a percutaneous wire may be needed.

Amputations

Fingertips

Amputation of the fingertip is a regrettably common industrial accident, although guards on machines in sawmills and sheet metal works have reduced the incidence considerably.

The aim of treatment should be a mobile finger with innervated skin and a useful tip. If the fingertip lacks sensibility or, worse, is exquisitely tender, it

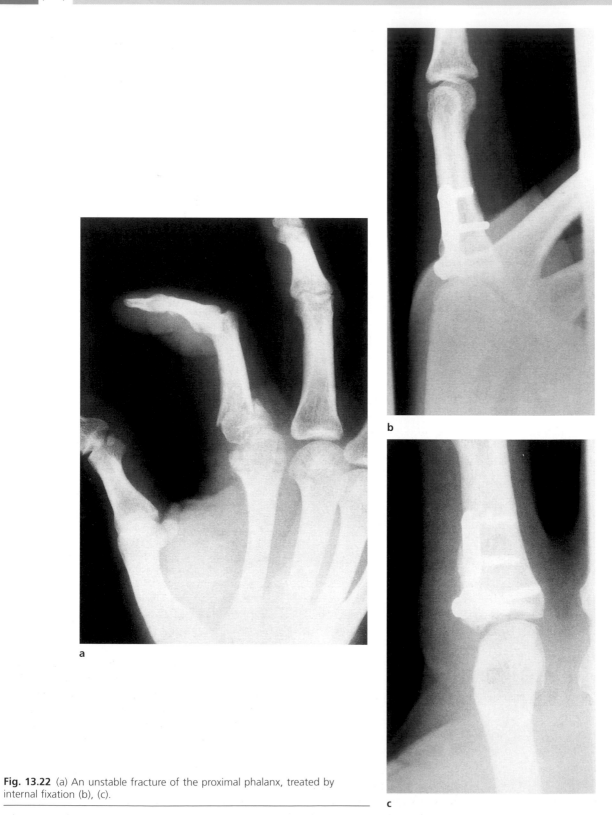

Fig. 13.22 (a) An unstable fracture of the proximal phalanx, treated by internal fixation (b), (c).

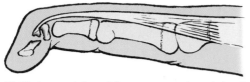

Fig. 13.23 Juxta-epiphyseal fracture separation of the distal phalanx.

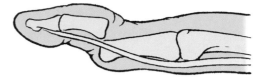

Fig. 13.25 Dislocation of the p.i.p. joint with dislocation of the head of the proximal phalanx between the superficialis tendons.

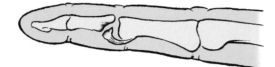

Fig. 13.24 Intra-articular fracture of the p.i.p. joint with avulsed volar plate.

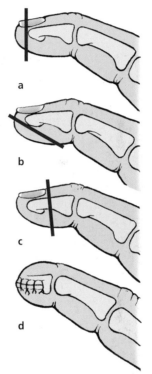

a

b

c

d

Fig. 13.26 Fingertip amputations: (a) amputation through the nail; (b) amputation through the pulp; (c) amputation through the nail and distal phalanx. (d) A skin flap brought up to cover the end of the amputated phalanx.

will not be used and it is far better to take more off the finger if this will leave a better stump. For this reason, it is not always helpful to reattach amputated fingers, however cleanly they may have been amputated.

Treatment

Treatment depends on the level of amputation, of which there are three (Fig. 13.26).

Vertical through the nail. These are treated by a local flap of skin to cover the defect, or by a split skin graft. The defect becomes smaller as the graft contracts to leave a small scar protected by the nail. A split skin graft is easier to apply but the result is not as good as that which follows a successful whole thickness local flap.

Oblique through the pulp. These are closed with a local flap or full thickness graft.

Vertical through the nail and distal phalanx. These are treated by nibbling the end of the phalanx and primary closure, bringing sensitive pulp skin over the tip.

Fingers

Many amputations are clean transverse cuts made with a clean blade. Others are contaminated crushing injuries.

Treatment

Management is directed to producing the most useful stump possible, which may mean shortening it further. It is better to have a finger that ends in the proximal half of the phalanx rather than at an interphalangeal joint and, whenever possible, to leave the flexor and extensor tendon insertions intact.

Sensibility is important. A flap of healthy and innervated skin from the volar aspect can be used to cover the fingertip. If this is not possible, a graft can be stitched over the cut end of the finger to achieve primary closure. If the resulting function is unsatisfactory, the stump can be shortened later.

In some patients, a neuroma forms on the cut end of the digital nerve and produces an exquisitely tender spot that prevents the patient using the finger at all. A protective finger-stall or glove may be helpful but resection of the digital nerve may be needed to place the end of the nerve in a less vulnerable position. Percussion of the neuroma is painful and ineffective but is still recommended in some centres.

Crushing amputations are treated by debridement, elevation and definitive amputation when the swelling has subsided.

Thumb

Traumatic amputation of the thumb is a serious and disabling injury – worse than losing several fingers. If you do not believe this, tuck your thumb into the palm and see how much you can do with just the fingers.

Treatment

Only the thumb can be opposed to the other fingers. If lost, it may be necessary to create a new one by 'pollicizing' the index finger. Even if the resulting 'thumb' is insensitive and stiff, it can still serve as an opposition post for the other digits.

Rehabilitation

Rehabilitation of the hand involves:

- Bones.
- Tendons.
- Joints.
- The whole patient!

Bones

The hand depends for its function upon the movement of its constituent parts over each other. Most fracture management is centred upon encouraging bones to unite soundly in the correct position, even if this means immobilizing soft tissues, but the aim in treating fractures of the hand is to keep the soft tissues moving while the fracture is uniting.

Tendons

Each finger has seven tendons (extensor digitorum, two interossei and one lumbrical, two slips of flexor digitorum superficialis and one flexor digitorum longus). If any of these tendons stick to bone or to another tendon, movement of the finger will be restricted.

Joints

Interphalangeal joints

Joint stiffness is a special problem. The interphalangeal joints become stiff if immobilized in flexion because the volar plate sticks to the front of the phalanx.

Once stuck, the volar plate cannot be mobilized, the collateral ligaments contract and the fingers will never straighten again. The fingers must therefore be immobilized in full extension.

Metacarpophalangeal joints

The metacarpophalangeal joints become stiff in extension because the capsule and collateral ligament are lax in this position and contract.

The metacarpophalangeal joint must therefore be immobilized in flexion to keep the collateral ligaments and the capsule stretched.

Position for splinting

If the hand is immobilized with the metacarpophalangeal joints flexed and the fingers straight (Fig. 13.27) the joints can be made to move again, but if immobilized in the opposite position they will become stiff and normal movement will not return.

In any hand injury it is important to maintain mobility of the fingers and minimize swelling. If

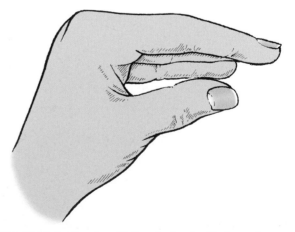

Fig. 13.27 Position for splinting the hand with the metacarpophalangeal joints flexed and the interphalangeal joints extended.

there is abnormal swelling of the hand, the patient should be admitted to hospital and the arm elevated before definitive treatment is begun.

Functions of the hand

The hand can hold things in many ways and it is useful to consider the different grips when reconstructing an injured hand (Fig. 13.28).

Power grip

The power grip is used for holding hammers, tennis racquets and golf clubs. A full range of flexion of the fingers is essential. The little, ring and middle fingers are more important than the thumb and index, which are used primarily for precision work.

In right-handed patients, the power grip in the left hand may be more important than the right because it is the left hand that holds the objects being worked upon by the right hand.

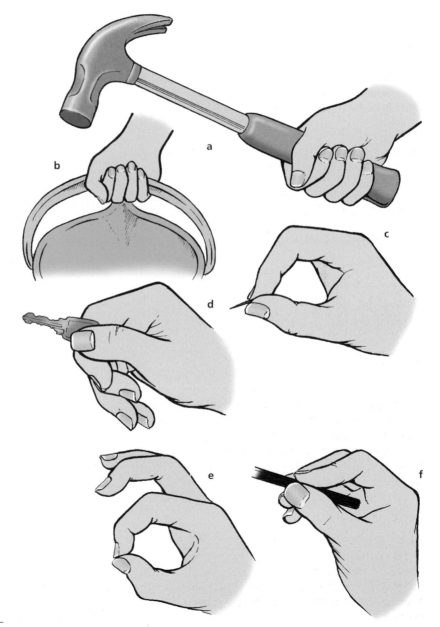

Fig. 13.28 Different functions of the hand: (a) power grip; (b) hook grip; (c) pinch grip; (d) key grip; (e) precision pinch; (f) chuck grip.

Hook grip

The curled fingers can be used as a hook for carrying baskets and swinging from branches. This is one of the few functions still possible if the metacarpophalangeal joints become stiff in extension.

Precision grips

Pinch grip

A pinch grip between the pulps of the thumb and index finger is essential for fine work. If the index is lost, the middle or ring finger can be used almost as well. In some circumstances, the pinch between the middle finger and thumb is so much better than that between the thumb and a stiff insensitive index that the index actually gets in the way and has to be amputated to improve the function of the hand.

Precision pinch

For extra precision the tips of the thumb and index are opposed to meet end to end, reducing the contact area to a minimum. Full flexion of the interphalangeal joints is needed for this function.

Key grip

A pinch grip between the thumb and the side of the flexed index is useful for holding keys and is also useful if the end of the index is lost.

Chuck grip

The fingers of the hand can be used like a drill chuck, grasping an object on all sides.

Other functions

Paperweight

Insensitive hands without motor control are useful as paperweights but little else. Nevertheless, this function is valued by patients to hold down objects being worked upon with the other hand.

Combined functions

These basic functions can be combined or modified for other purposes, e.g. holding a pen or a knife, but the basic concept of giving the patient a power grip to hold objects firmly, and a pinch grip for fine work, should be considered when planning treatment.

Chapter | 14 |

Injuries to the lower limb

By the end of this chapter you should be able to understand and differentiate:

- Femoral neck fractures in the young and the elderly, and appreciate the various treatment options based on age, site of fracture, healing potential.
- High energy injuries to the femoral and tibial shafts, the association with soft tissue injuries and the treatment options in open and closed fractures.
- The severity of intra-articular fractures of the knee and ankle and the poor long term results unless accurate reduction and rehabilitation are undertaken.
- The complexity of ankle fractures, the different mechanisms of injury and the fracture patterns and subsequent treatment.

Fractures at the upper end of the femur: general considerations

Fractures at the upper end of the femur are seen in young patients and high energy injuries or in elderly patients with bones weakened by osteoporosis. Because they live longer than men and the hormonal changes of the menopause make them more subject to osteoporosis, these fractures are commoner in women. The fractures are becoming more and more frequent as the average age of the population increases and in many areas they are the commonest fractures admitted to hospital.

Fractures at the upper end of the femur create clinical, social and economic problems.

Clinical problems

Because the fractures occur in elderly patients, medical problems are seen that are not encountered

in fit young adults with broken bones or in older patients undergoing reconstructive surgery. Assessment therefore requires special attention to the general medical condition, drugs that the patient is taking and the social history.

Bronchopneumonia and cerebral confusion are particular problems and the prognosis for an elderly patient with a fracture at the upper end of the femur is poor.

Approximately 10% of patients die within 6 weeks of this injury and 30% within 1 year.

Of the remaining 70% who survive, one-third are unable to return to their former level of independence or physical activity as the result of the fracture.

Social problems

The fractures are important from the social standpoint because they often connote the end of independent existence, particularly if the patient has unsuitable accommodation and was unfit to live alone even before the fracture. Admission to hospital – a strange and frightening place for an elderly patient at the best of times – always causes anxiety which, when coupled with the upset of operation, may be so great that the patient is quite unable to cope with the problems of rehabilitation.

If return home is impossible and alternative accommodation has to be found, close liaison with the social services, family practitioner and health visitor is mandatory (p. 88). The mental adjustment asked of the patient will be even greater and this must be taken into consideration.

Economic problems

These fractures consume a large part of health service resources in terms of beds, nurses and support outside hospital. As the fractures become more common, pressure on resources becomes greater but there is seldom any increase in the provision of services to match the increased demand.

The result is more pressure on less urgent services, which in practice means that patients with non-urgent conditions cannot be treated and must wait longer for admission to hospital. The level of provision for fractured necks of femur is largely responsible for long orthopaedic waiting lists.

Fractures of the femoral neck

Fractures of the acetabulum are dealt with on pages 178–180.

Clinical features

Fractures of the femoral neck occur after a trivial injury or even without any injury at all; the bone may be so brittle that it snaps as the patient gets out of a chair.

On examination, the affected leg will be short and externally rotated because the fracture allows the shaft of the femur to move independently of the hip joint, which means that the iliopsoas and gravity will rotate the femur externally instead of rotating the hip internally (Fig. 14.1).

Types of fracture

Intracapsular fractures result from a high transcervical fracture and interrupt the blood supply to the

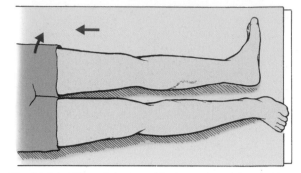

Fig. 14.1 Position of the leg with shortening and external rotation, seen with a displaced fracture at the upper end of the femur.

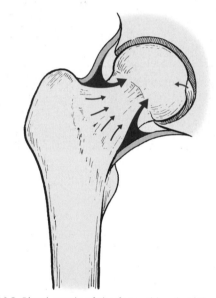

Fig. 14.2 Blood supply of the femoral head via the capsule, intramedullary vessels and ligamentum teres.

femoral head. This is derived from three sources (Fig. 14.2).

Blood supply to the femoral head

1. Synovium and joint capsule.
2. The medullary cavity.
3. A tiny proportion from the ligamentum teres.

An intracapsular fracture can cut off the blood supply to the femoral head completely, leading to aseptic necrosis, non-union, or both. Because the fracture line is inside the capsule, blood is contained within it. This raises the intracapsular pressure and

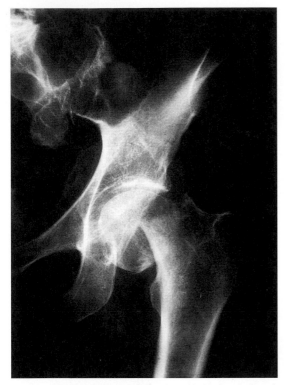

Fig. 14.3 Displaced subcapital fracture of the femoral neck. The femoral shaft has moved proximally.

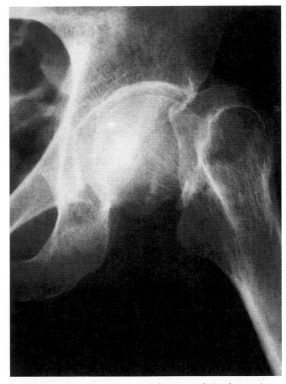

Fig. 14.4 Displaced transcervical fracture of the femoral neck. The femoral head maintains its correct relationship to the pelvis but the femur is rotated.

damages the femoral head still further. It also prevents visible bruising because blood cannot reach the subcutaneous tissues.

To add to these problems, an intracapsular fracture leaves the femoral head very mobile inside the capsule (Figs 14.3, 14.4), particularly if the fracture is just below the head (subcapital). This makes accurate reduction almost impossible. The posterior cortex may also be crushed.

All these factors predispose to non-union and aseptic necrosis (Fig. 14.5), and intracapsular fractures are notorious for their high complication rate.

Extracapsular and basal fractures are less difficult for three reasons (Fig. 14.6):

1. The blood supply is not interrupted so seriously.
2. The surface area of the fracture available for union is larger and consists of good cancellous bone.
3. The femoral head is less mobile.

Nevertheless, non-union and avascular necrosis can occur, and extracapsular fractures must be treated with great respect.

Undisplaced and impacted fractures of the femoral neck present other problems (Figs 14.7–14.9). Because the bones are jammed tightly together the fracture appears stable and the patient may even be able to bear weight on the leg (Fig. 14.10). Many impacted fractures probably pass undiagnosed and do very well without medical attention, but in some patients the fracture becomes displaced days or even weeks after the injury. An impacted fracture must therefore be carefully observed to be certain that it remains stable, and should be protected until the bones are united.

Treatment (intracapsular)

The choice of treatment for femoral neck fractures depends upon three factors:

1. The age and fitness of the patient.
2. The type of fracture.
3. The degree of displacement.

241

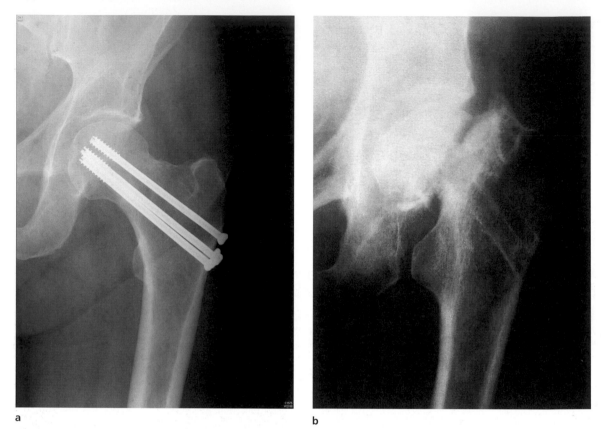

a   b

Fig. 14.5 (a) Internal fixation of a femoral neck fracture with screws. (b) Non-union of a femoral neck fracture with aseptic necrosis of the femoral head. Note how the head has become smaller and denser.

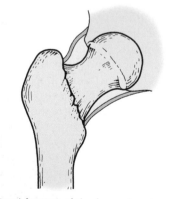

Fig. 14.6 Basal fracture of the femoral neck.

Undisplaced fractures are treated by protected weight-bearing until union occurs or by internal fixation in situ to prevent displacement. If it is decided not to operate, regular radiographs are needed to be sure that the position does not change.

Displaced fractures can be treated by internal fixation or prosthetic replacement.

Internal fixation. The fracture can be held with several fine pins, a pair of crossed nails, cannulated screws or a dynamic compression screw and plate. All of these are inserted under image intensifier control (Fig. 14.11).

The fracture must be protected from full weight-bearing after fixation, which is difficult in the elderly patient, who may not be able to use crutches easily.

If successful, internal fixation of the fracture produces an almost perfect hip, but if the fracture is complicated by aseptic necrosis or non-union, a second operation will be required to replace the head with a prosthesis (Table 14.1). The femoral head may also collapse onto the pins, damaging the acetabulum.

Prosthetic replacement. Immediate replacement of the head with a hemiarthroplasty (e.g. Thompson or Austin Moore prosthesis; Fig. 14.12) avoids the

Table 14.1 Internal fixation versus prosthetic replacement

Indications

Internal fixation: fit; young, little displacement

Prosthesis: unfit, old, displaced fractures

Results

Internal fixation: better long-term result. More complications. May need second operation. Slow rehabilitation

Prosthesis: early mobilization. Long-term complications are rarer but more serious. A good guideline is to fix the fractures of fit patients under 65 and replace the rest

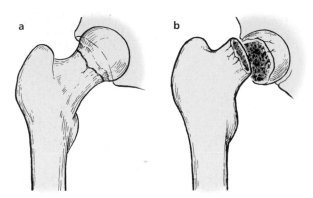

Fig. 14.9 (a) Undisplaced fracture of the femoral neck; (b) displaced fracture of the femoral neck.

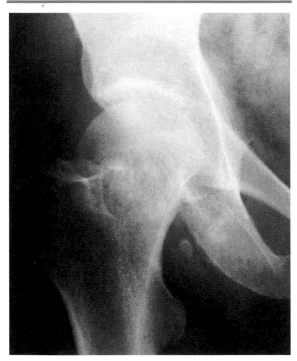

Fig. 14.7 Impacted fracture of the femoral neck with the head in valgus.

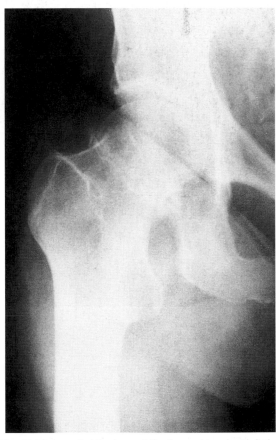

Fig. 14.10 Impacted fracture of the femoral head with little valgus deformity. The patient had walked on this fracture.

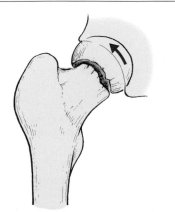

Fig. 14.8 Impacted fracture of the femoral neck. The head rolls into valgus and there is double density of the bone at the site of impaction.

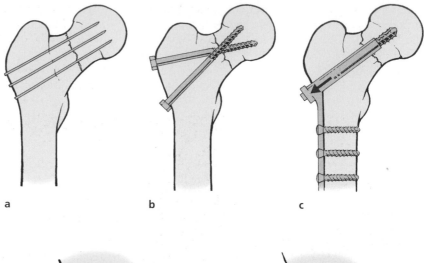

Fig. 14.11 Methods of internal fixation of femoral neck fractures: (a) multiple pins; (b) crossed screw-nails; (c) compression with dynamic screw and plate.

a   b   c

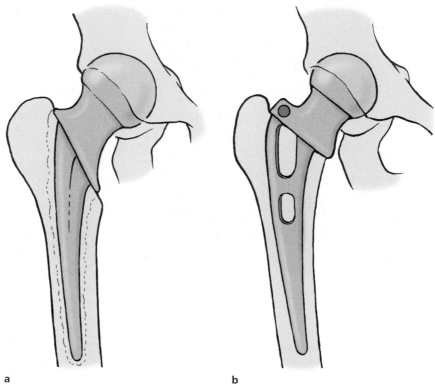

Fig. 14.12 Hip prosthesis for fracture of the femoral neck: (a) Thompson prosthesis secured with cement; (b) Austin Moore prosthesis with no cement.

a   b

complications of non-union and aseptic necrosis and allows immediate full weight-bearing (Fig. 14.13).

Early mobilization has many advantages, but the prosthesis may loosen or the femoral head may erode the floor of the acetabulum. If either complication occurs, a total hip replacement will be needed. The wound may also become infected, making excision arthroplasty necessary.

As always with prosthetic replacement, the results are better than other techniques when they are successful but far worse when they are not.

Bipolar prostheses. 'Bipolar prostheses' are useful in younger patients. A bipolar prosthesis includes a ball and socket bearing within the space occupied by the femoral head. Thus, the outside diameter of the prosthesis replaces the femoral head and fills the acetabulum. Within this sphere there is a second bearing, usually about 22 mm in diameter. Ball and socket movement can therefore occur at two joints, the interface between the acetabulum and the outer circumference of the prosthesis and the smaller bearing within.

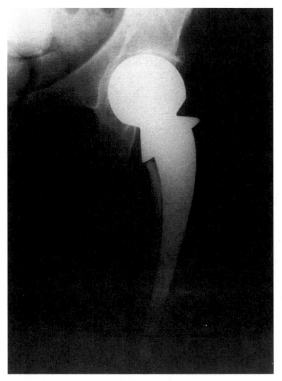

Fig. 14.13 A Thompson prosthesis in position.

These prostheses are more expensive than simple femoral prostheses but they reduce the forces imposed on the interface between the outer circumference and the acetabulum. They are particularly suitable for younger patients with femoral neck fractures not suitable for internal fixation.

Trochanteric fractures

There are four types of trochanteric fracture (Fig. 14.14):

1. Pertrochanteric – through both trochanters.
2. Intertrochanteric – between the trochanters.
3. Subtrochanteric – below the trochanters.
4. Avulsion of the trochanters.

Pertrochanteric and intertrochanteric fractures

Clinical features

In contrast to fractures through the femoral neck, which occur with little or no trauma, these fractures are caused by a sharp twisting injury, and a history of trauma is usual (Fig 14.15). A further point of difference is that fractures of the femoral neck do not occur in joints affected by osteoarthritis because osteoarthritic bone is denser than normal and the femoral neck is not the weakest point.

Fractures through or between the trochanters present different problems from those of the femoral

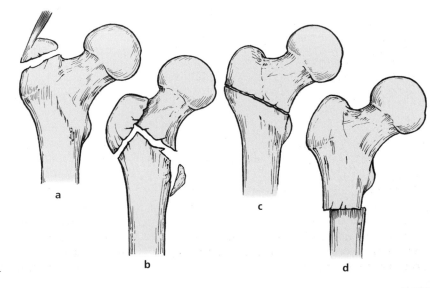

Fig. 14.14 Types of trochanteric fracture: (a) avulsion of the greater tuberosity; (b) pertrochanteric fracture; (c) intertrochanteric fracture between the trochanters; (d) subtrochanteric fracture.

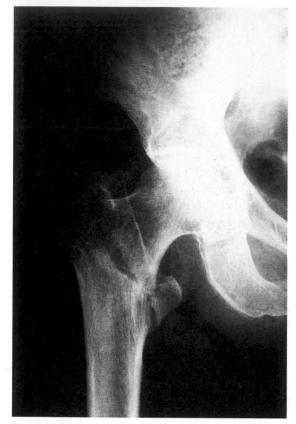

Fig. 14.15 Pertrochanteric fracture of the femur following a fall.

neck. Because the fractures occur through cancellous bone and are surrounded by muscle, they almost always unite but are very unstable and malunion is almost inevitable unless they are fixed internally.

Treatment

Pertrochanteric or intertrochanteric fractures must be held in good position, preferably with a dynamic hip screw or intramedullary hip screw, until united (Fig. 14.16). These implants are not strong enough to take over the mechanical functions of the femur and allow the patient to put all his or her weight through the limb, but they will hold the bones together for the 8 weeks or so needed for union to occur.

Subtrochanteric fractures

Subtrochanteric fractures are rarer than fractures of the neck or pertrochanteric fractures and are often pathological, occurring through areas of Paget's disease or metastases (Fig. 14.17a).

Treatment

Subtrochanteric fractures usually require internal fixation using a nail-plate with a long femoral plate or an intramedullary implant (Fig. 14.17b). If the fracture is pathological, the underlying disorder will also need attention.

Avulsion of the greater trochanter

The greater trochanter can be avulsed by a violent adduction strain.

Clinical presentation

The patient experiences severe pain over the trochanter, abduction is painful and the Trendelenburg sign (p. 25) is positive because the abductor muscles are separated from their bony attachment.

Treatment

Large fragments with much displacement should be reattached if the patient is fit enough but many patients achieve a good result without internal fixation. Non-union is common and causes marked weakness of the abductors, with a Trendelenburg gait.

Fractures at the upper end of the femur in children

Slipped upper femoral epiphysis

In children, the anatomical equivalent of an intracapsular fracture of the femoral neck is a slipped upper femoral epiphysis (Fig. 14.18). The condition occurs most often during the adolescent growth spurt, is commoner in boys than girls, and consists of a medial and backward displacement of the epiphysis, which rolls the limb into external rotation. The slip is either as a result of a Salter I fracture due to trauma or as an insidious gradual event. The slip is probably the result of weakening of the epiphyseal plate and soft tissues by the hormones of adolescence and this may explain why plump gynaecoid boys are most often affected.

Clinical features

A slipped upper femoral epiphysis often causes referred pain to the knee and the diagnosis should

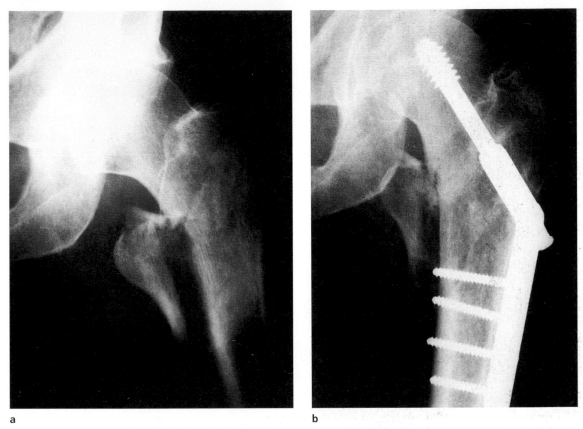

a b

Fig. 14.16 (a), (b) Pertrochanteric fracture fixed with compression screw and nail-plate.

be suspected in any adolescent with aching around the knee but no abnormality at the knee on clinical examination.

On examination, the appearance is very like that of a femoral neck fracture, the leg lying shortened and externally rotated. The condition is bilateral in 40% of cases and the opposite hip should therefore be checked.

Complications

A slipped upper femoral epiphysis can be followed by avascular necrosis of the epiphysis and early osteoarthritis, or by necrosis of the articular cartilage, which also leads to a stiff and painful hip.

Treatment

Slight or moderate displacement should be treated by fixation with pins to prevent further slip.

Manipulation or traction, however gentle, may cause aseptic necrosis of the epiphysis and should

not be attempted. *Do not manipulate a slipped upper femoral epiphysis.* Although this was once standard practice it is now thought to cause further damage to the epiphysis and its blood supply.

Gross displacement may be irreducible, particularly if there is a long history. In these patients it may be better to accept the deformity and correct it by osteotomy when growth is complete, although there is a high incidence of aseptic necrosis of the head.

Femoral neck fractures

Fractures at the upper end of the femur are essentially an injury of the elderly but they are seen very occasionally in children, when they behave very differently. The fractures are usually basal and the prognosis is worse than in adults.

Although rare, these fractures are serious when they occur and the entire femoral head and neck may undergo aseptic necrosis.

247

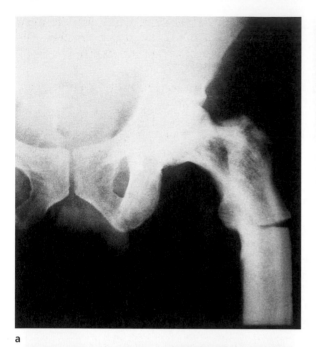

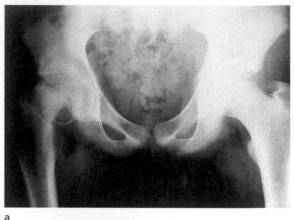

a

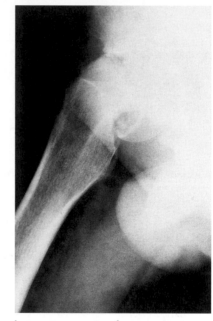

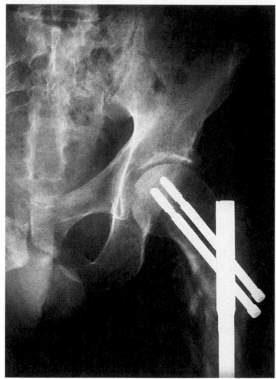

b

Fig. 14.18 Slipped upper femoral epiphysis: (a) anteroposterior view; (b) lateral view.

b

Fig. 14.17 (a) Subtrochanteric fracture through an area of Paget's disease. (b) Subtrochanteric fracture with intramedullary nail.

Treatment

Treatment is by careful reduction and internal fixation.

Fractures of the femoral shaft

The femoral shaft can be fractured by direct trauma, twisting or a blow to the front of the flexed knee in a road traffic accident. This injury can also produce a fracture of the patella, ruptured posterior cruciate ligament and posterior dislocation of the hip.

Clinical features

A broken thigh is shorter and fatter than normal and lies with the distal fragment in external rotation and adduction for four reasons (Fig. 14.19):

1. Without the longitudinal stability of the femur, the muscles attached to the upper and lower ends contract and the thigh shortens, which makes it look swollen (Fig. 14.20).

2. The adductors are attached to the distal fragment and the abductors to the upper fragment. The fracture separates the two groups, which then act unopposed (p. 39).

3. The weight of the foot rolls the distal fragment into external rotation.

4. The femur is surrounded by muscle which is lacerated by the sharp ends of the fractured bone and the thigh fills with blood. The bone also bleeds.

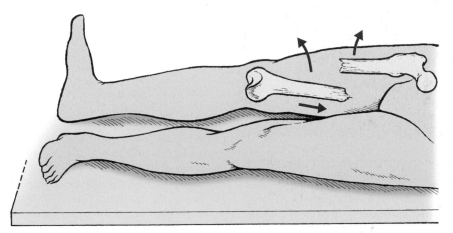

Fig. 14.19 Position of the fragments after a fracture of the femoral shaft. The upper fragment swings upwards and outwards, the distal fragment is adducted and the foot is externally rotated.

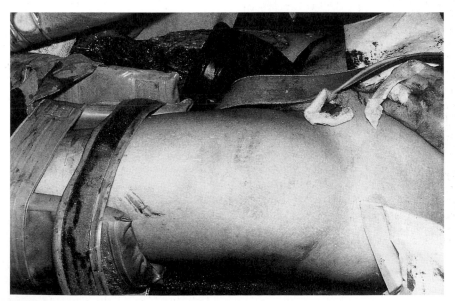

Fig. 14.20 Swelling of the thigh in a patient with a fracture of the femur. An inflatable air splint has been applied for a fracture of the tibial shaft.

Complications

- *Haemorrhage*, which can lead to cardiovascular collapse. This can be corrected by adequate transfusion.
- *Infection*, particularly if a wound is contaminated and wound debridement has been inadequate.
- *Non-union*, which is common in midshaft fractures, high speed trauma and fractures with soft tissues interposed between the fragments. Non-united fractures need bone grafting and internal fixation.
- *Malunion*, caused by abductors and adductors acting unopposed on the proximal and distal fragments, respectively. A varus deformity results from this combination of forces.
- *Arterial and nerve injury* is uncommon but does occur. The neurological and vascular state of the foot should always be checked and recorded.

Treatment

Immediate care

The blood loss from a fractured femur, whether open or closed, is between 2 and 4 units (1–2 litres). An intravenous line should therefore be set up and blood sent to the laboratory for haemoglobin estimation and cross-matching. If there are no other fractures, it may be possible to avoid transfusion, but if any other injuries are present, 2 units of blood should be given as soon as it is available.

Open fractures are usually open from within out, with a wound on the lateral side or the front of the thigh. The wound should be debrided meticulously in the operating theatre and all foreign material removed. It is usually wise to pack the wound and treat it by delayed primary suture (p. 139). Only in very exceptional circumstances can a wound be made clean enough to close immediately. Antibiotics and antitetanus treatment should be given, as for any open fracture.

Treatment of the fracture

When the patient's condition is stable and the wound has been dealt with, the fracture can be immobilized in one of four ways:

1. Traction.
2. Internal fixation.
3. External fixation.
4. Cast bracing.

Traction. Traction used to be the mainstay of treatment of these fractures in the past. Patients were in bed for up to 3 months at times. Traction is now rarely used and is only advocated when surgery is contraindicated or in children. A single, balanced, skeletal traction apparatus is shown applied via a femoral pin in Figure 14.21.

Adequate longitudinal traction is needed for the first 24 h to overcome muscle spasm and prevent shortening and the fragments must be supported posteriorly to prevent sagging. Six kilograms (13lb) is usually enough, but heavy patients need more and light patients less. Check radiographs after 24 h will show if the weight is correct; if there is overdistraction, the weight should be reduced. If there is overlap, it should be increased.

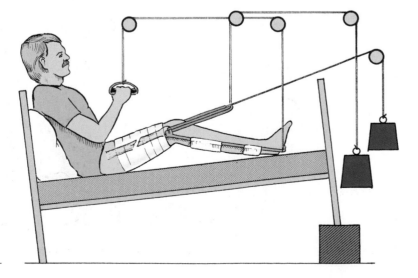

Fig. 14.21 Conservative treatment of a femoral shaft fracture with balanced sliding traction and a knee flexion piece.

Check radiographs are then needed twice weekly for the first 2 weeks and weekly thereafter to ensure that the position is maintained. If this is not done, the fracture may slip gradually and unite in poor position.

Internal fixation. An intramedullary nail is ideal for most fractures (Fig. 14.22). Fractures can be held straight and out to length by a nail, but the fixation may not be firm enough to control rotation. The advent of locking nails – where screws are inserted through the bone and nail – can now control rotation. Open reduction and fixation with a plate is not often performed owing to the extensive soft tissue exposure needed, the devitalization of the bone, and the mechanical failure of the plates.

The advantages of intramedullary nailing are that it provides longitudinal stability as well as alignment and enables the patient to be mobilized rapidly enough to leave hospital within days of fracture. Disadvantages include the anaesthetic, additional surgical trauma and the risk of infection.

Intramedullary nails are inserted through the proximal or distal femur. They can be 'reamed' or 'unreamed'. This simply means that the medullary cavity of the bone is enlarged to allow the nail to fit into the bone. The theoretical advantage of unreamed nails is that there is no excessive damage to the endosteal blood supply, which may further weaken the bone. By reaming the intramedullary canal, the intact endosteal blood supply is damaged throughout the length of the reamed segment and this, in conjunction with the damage to the periosteal layer, may delay healing.

Intramedullary nails can be used for comminuted fractures with shortening, provided the bone can be pulled out to length and held there. Locking nails which maintain length and rotation (p. 135) are required for such fractures.

External fixation. External fixation is used for contaminated and unstable open fractures or in the emergency situation.

Cast bracing. When a fracture treated on traction is stable and a mass of callus is visible radiologically, usually at about 6 weeks, a cast brace can be applied. Fractures in which fixation is less than 100% secure are also suitable.

The cast brace (p. 131) will enable the patient to leave hospital and begin rehabilitation more rapidly.

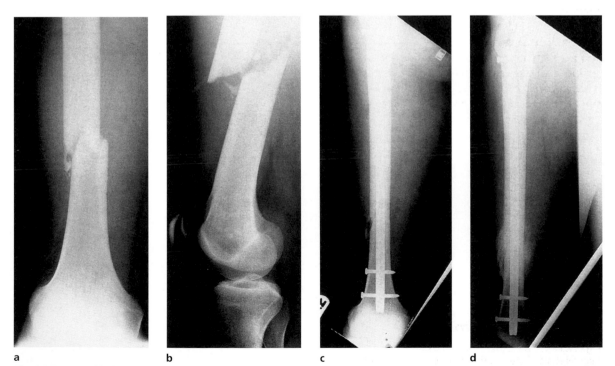

a   b   c   d

Fig. 14.22 Unstable fracture of the femur: (a), (b) before operation; (c) after fixation with a locking nail; (d) united with callus.

Fractures of the lower end of the femur

Supracondylar fractures

Supracondylar fractures are commonest in older patients with soft porotic bone (Fig. 14.23). The fractures are caused by either forced flexion or hyper-extension and are unstable. Gastrocnemius flexes the distal fragment and increases the deformity (Fig. 14.24).

Treatment

These fractures are difficult to control conservatively because of the mobility of the distal fragment. Inter-

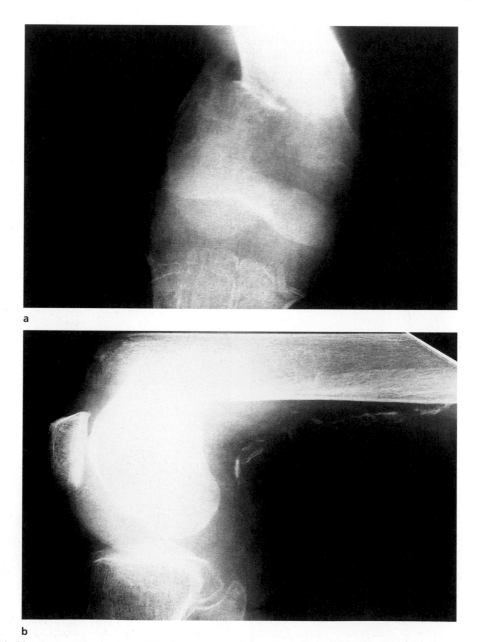

a

b

Fig. 14.23 (a), (b) Supracondylar fracture of the femur in an elderly patient. Note the calcification in the femoral vessels and the extreme flexion of the distal fragment.

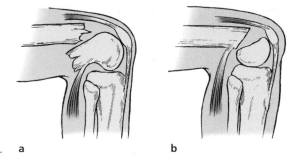

Fig. 14.24 Injuries of the lower end of the femur: (a) the mechanism of flexion of the distal fragment in a supracondylar fracture; (b) slipped lower femoral epiphysis.

nal fixation is the method of choice. A blade or dynamic compression screw can be used and the newer locking plates may be of value in the porotic bone. An intramedullary implant, when inserted through the intercondylar notch of the femur, will hold the bone out to length and in the reduced position. This can be supplemented with additional screws to hold fragments together.

Slipped lower femoral epiphysis

In children, the equivalent of a supracondylar fracture is a slipped lower femoral epiphysis caused by a sharp flexion injury. Surgeons of the 19th century recorded that the fracture occurred in boys who fell backward while sitting on railings or whose feet became caught in the spokes of the wheel while riding on the back of a horse-drawn cart. Today, these injuries are less common.

Treatment

Reduction is usually easy but accuracy is important because angular deformities occur if the reduction is not perfect or the epiphysis is damaged.

Comminuted fractures

Violent trauma, particularly from motor cycle accidents, produces a very nasty comminuted fracture just above the condyle, often accompanied by a condylar fracture. The comminution is usually so great that the bone fragments cannot be reassembled and bone length is lost.

Treatment

Traction or external fixation may hold the bone out to its correct length but grafting may be required to fill the defect. Circular frames with wire fixation

may hold the fragments. Again, locking plates may be of use.

Condylar fractures

Fractures entering the intercondylar notch can break one or both condyles away from the femoral shaft, or follow an oblique line (Fig. 14.25). The relation-

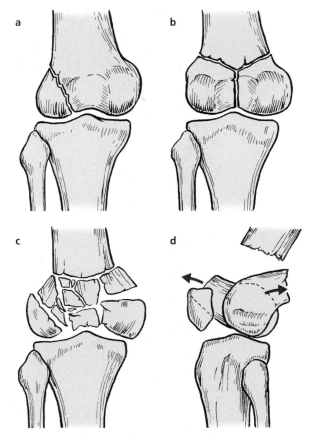

Fig. 14.25 Fractures of the femoral condyles: (a) oblique fracture of the lateral condyle; (b) Y-shaped fracture into the notch; (c) comminuted fracture with (d) rotation of the condyles.

ship of the two condyles is essential for normal knee function and accurate reduction is important; even a millimetre of proximal displacement leaves a valgus or varus deformity and rotation of one condyle relative to the other interferes with flexion.

Treatment

Treatment depends on the degree of displacement.

Undisplaced fractures and those with negligible displacement can be treated by aspiration of the joint to remove blood, followed by rest on traction for at least 4 weeks until the fracture is sufficiently united to be safe in a cast.

Displaced fractures must be accurately reduced to avoid degenerative changes, which usually means open reduction and internal fixation.

If one condyle is involved it can be fixed onto the femur with screws. If both condyles are separated they can be fixed together, converting the lesion into a supracondylar fracture.

Oblique fractures are managed in the same way, with conservative treatment for slight displacement and internal fixation for the rest. Elderly or infirm patients can be managed conservatively.

Complications

The fragments often lose their blood supply at the time of injury or at operation. This can lead to aseptic necrosis, collapse and a gross deformity.

If the fragments are not repositioned exactly there will be a valgus or varus deformity, which may lead to osteoarthritis.

Fractures of the patella

Comminuted fractures

The patella is easily fractured by a blow to the flexed knee, often in a road traffic accident (Fig. 14.26).

Treatment

The shear stresses on the back of the patella are enormous and any irregularity of its surface will cause osteoarthritis in later life.

Unless the fragments can be accurately reassembled, which is usually impossible, it is best to remove the patella and encourage early movement.

Stellate fractures

A blow to the patella may crack it without displacing the fragments, like a boiled sweet broken inside its wrapper (Fig. 14.27).

Treatment

Stellate fractures can be managed conservatively by aspirating blood from the knee and supporting it in a long leg cast for 3 weeks, when mobilization is begun.

Transverse fractures

The patella can be split transversely by indirect violence, e.g. a forced flexion injury caused by falling with the flexed knee under the body or stepping onto a non-existent step. These injuries split not

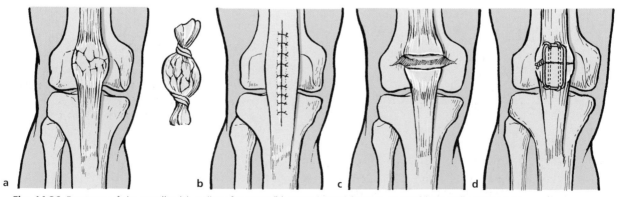

Fig. 14.26 Fractures of the patella: (a) stellate fracture; (b) comminuted fracture treated by patellectomy; (c) transverse fracture; (d) transverse fracture treated by tension band wiring.

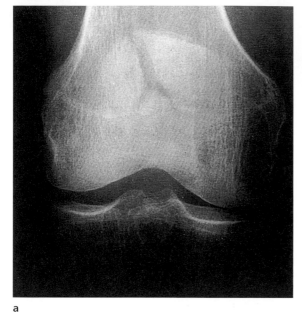

a

Fig. 14.27 (a), (b) Stellate fracture of the patella with little displacement.

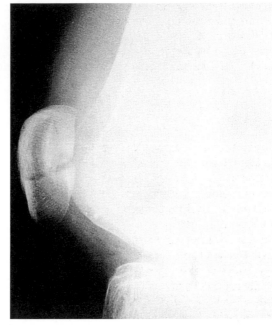

b

only the patella but also the quadriceps expansions on either side.

Left untreated, the fragments separate widely and quadriceps function is lost (Fig. 14.28).

Treatment

Internal fixation is required. A tension band wire is usually adequate.

Injuries of the extensor mechanism

Rupture of the rectus femoris

Sudden violent contraction of the quadriceps is enough to tear rectus femoris transversely in its mid portion (Fig. 14.29). The patient feels sudden severe pain and a defect can be felt in the muscle.

Treatment

None is effective apart from the application of ice wrapped in a towel, elevation, analgesics and mobilization within the limits of comfort. The defect in the muscle remains but the functional deficit is negligible.

Ruptured quadriceps tendon

The same forces that cause transverse fractures of the patella also rupture the quadriceps tendon above the patella.

Treatment

Ruptured quadriceps tendons must be repaired surgically or the defect will widen and quadriceps power will be lost.

Ruptured patellar tendon

The patellar tendon may also be ruptured by a forced flexion injury and this, like the quadriceps tendon, must be repaired. Very rarely, the tendon may pull a fragment of bone from the lower pole of the patella.

Treatment

The defect must be repaired if a serious weakness and extensor lag are to be avoided.

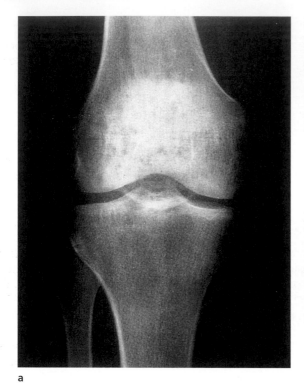

a

Fig. 14.28 (a), (b) Non-union of a transverse fracture of the patella. Note the disuse osteoporosis in the patella and underlying femur.

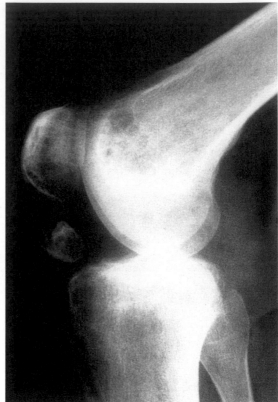

b

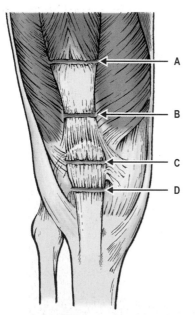

Fig. 14.29 Sites of rupture of the extensor mechanism: (*A*) rectus femoris; (*B*) quadriceps tendon; (*C*) patella; (*D*) patellar tendon.

Dislocation of the patella

The patella can be dislocated by a sharp twisting movement of the knee in very slight flexion (Fig. 14.30) and is common in adolescents, particularly girls with loose ligaments. The dislocation often used to occur on the dance floor during the Charleston, the twist and their successors. The patella sometimes reduces itself at once, but if it remains dislocated, the patient will remember seeing the kneecap lying on the outer side of the knee and may report that the 'knee dislocated' (Fig. 14.31).

On examination soon after a dislocation, the knee will be swollen because of the haemarthrosis and there will be tenderness on the medial side of the patella because the medial structures are torn (medial patella femoral ligament).

Radiographs will show a haemarthrosis, perhaps with a fat–fluid level (see Fig. 5.1) and sometimes an osteochondral fracture. This fracture can be an avulsion fracture from the medial side of the patella or from the lateral femoral condyle.

In over 70% of cases an underlying abnormality is found. These include joint hypermobility, patella alta, patella maltracking and axial malalignments.

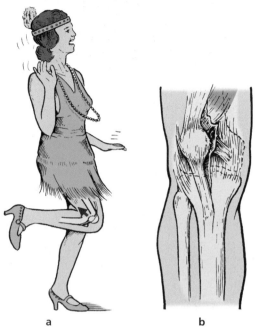

Fig. 14.30 Dislocation of the patella: (a) the patella can be dislocated by sharp twisting movements; (b) dislocation accompanied by a tear in the medial capsule.

Complications

In some patients the patella continues to dislocate with progressively less trauma. Recurrent dislocation of the patella is described on page 426.

If the articular surface is disrupted, patellofemoral osteoarthrosis is likely.

Treatment

All blood should be aspirated to help reduce pain. Immobilization of the knee will weaken the quadriceps further and early active rehabilitation is preferable.

If an osteochondral fracture is present, the fragment must be dealt with. Large fragments in the weight-bearing area should be fixed back into their bed and small ones removed. If there is any doubt about the diagnosis or the size of the fragment, the joint should be examined arthroscopically. Fat within the aspirate should alert one to the osteochondral injury.

If the patella has dislocated more than three times a stabilizing operation will probably be required (p. 426).

Fractures within the knee

Osteochondral fractures

Slivers of bone can be sheared off the articular surfaces by twisting stresses under load, or chipped off

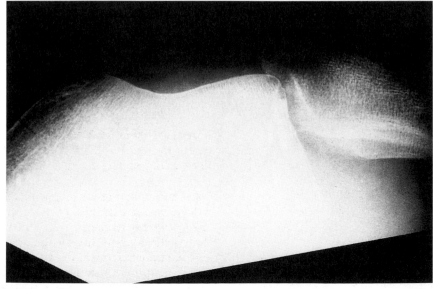

Fig. 14.31 A dislocated patella.

by direct trauma. Indirect violence is commoner in adolescents, and direct violence in young adults. Both are accompanied by haemarthrosis, and fat from the cancellous bone forms a fat–fluid level on the lateral radiograph.

The diagnosis is often missed because the loose body and the defect on the articular surface may be small and escape detection. If left untreated, the fragment will present later as a loose body.

Treatment

Large fragments should be reattached and small ones removed.

Fractures of the tibial plateau

If the knee is struck violently on the lateral side, one of two things can happen:

1. The medial ligament tears.
2. The lateral tibial plateau fractures.

If the bone fractures, four patterns of fracture can occur (Fig. 14.32):

1. The lateral condyle acts like a blunt chisel and splits the lateral tibial plateau vertically (Fig. 14.33).
2. Part of the tibial plateau may be thrust downwards into the tibia producing a depressed plateau fracture (Fig. 14.34).
3. Both of these can occur together.
4. The whole tibial plateau may be depressed (Fig. 14.35).

The full extent of the fracture may not be apparent on a plain radiograph, and CT or MRI scanning may be needed to define the anatomy of the fracture.

Treatment

If a large fragment is split off the tibia it must be screwed back to restore the contour of the tibia. Large depressed fragments can be elevated to reconstitute the bone surface but a cavity will remain at the site of the fragment because the bone was crushed. The chondral surface should be reconstructed and the underlying cavity must be filled with a cancellous bone graft as support.

If there is only a slight depression in the plateau, the fracture can be managed conservatively with early mobilization. The defect will fill in with fibrocartilage and the patient will probably achieve good function despite a slight valgus deformity. This is adequate for an infirm patient with few physical demands on the limb but those younger, requiring a more physical lifestyle, may need reconstruction.

Ligament injuries at the knee

The knee depends heavily on its ligaments for stability. The hip and the shoulder move freely in any direction, the range being limited by the shape of the bones as much as the ligament. The knee has a very restricted range of movement from 0 to 150° in one plane only, and it is the ligaments which prevent unwanted movement.

Because ligaments never heal soundly or regain their normal strength, as bone does, ligament injuries of the knee have more serious long-term implications for the patient than a fracture of the tibia or femur.

Ligaments do not show on radiographs and patients with serious injuries are sometimes sent home from the accident department with the good news that 'no bones are broken'. *If the*

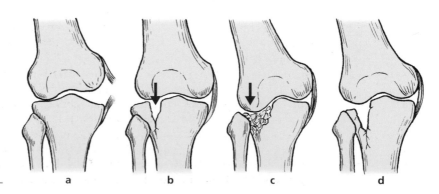

Fig. 14.32 Injuries from a force to the lateral side of the knee: (a) medial ligament rupture; (b) vertical split in the lateral plateau; (c) crush fracture of the lateral plateau; (d) crush and split of the lateral plateau.

a   b   c   d

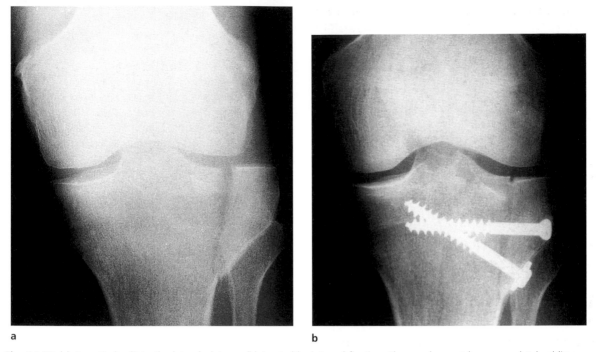

a   b

Fig. 14.33 (a) A vertical split in the lateral plateau; (b) treated by internal fixation. The gap has not been completely obliterated and the depressed fragment has not been elevated. This unsatisfactory result illustrates the difficulties caused by this fracture.

patient felt something break in the leg but the bones are intact, there is a major ligament injury until proved otherwise.

Anterior cruciate rupture

The anterior cruciate limits forward movement of the tibia on the femur and is often ruptured in sporting activities by a sharp twisting movement, or by a tackle which pushes the upper part of the tibia forwards (Fig. 14.36).

Acute anterior cruciate rupture is a common injury. About 80% of acute haemarthroses are caused by this lesion, and about 60% of these patients will have other associated injuries.

The patient often feels something 'go' in the knee at the moment of injury and may think a bone has broken, particularly as breaking a cruciate makes a snapping sound that is audible to those nearby. The patient is unable to carry on and feels the knee is very weak. The event is so dramatic that patients can remember the incident with great clarity many years later.

The instability is easy to assess immediately after injury, before bleeding has occurred and the tissues have swollen. Within 15 minutes the instability is difficult to assess because of swelling and protective muscle spasm.

Natural history

There are three possible outcomes of anterior cruciate ligament rupture. Roughly one-third of patients with anterior cruciate rupture achieve a good result without operation and lead a normal life, including sport, without any difficulties.

In another third, the knee becomes so unstable that it gives way even when walking over level ground. The instability may be so great that the patient is even afraid of crossing a road in case they fall. These patients need reconstruction of the ligament (p. 420).

The remaining third experience symptoms of instability which interfere with life to a variable degree. Some are happy to give up sport or simply to avoid those activities that cause symptoms. Others prefer a reconstruction.

There is no way of knowing for certain what the long-term outcome will be in any one patient on the day of injury. Solidly built rugby players with

259

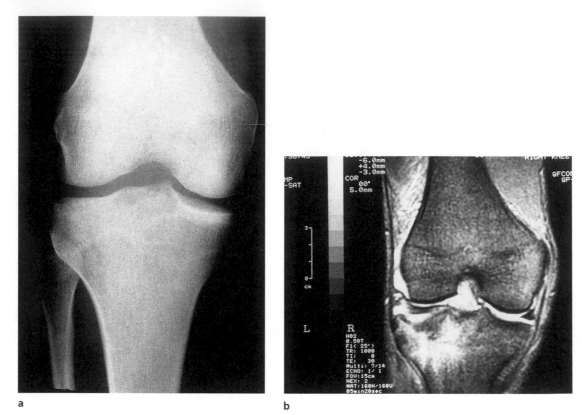

Fig. 14.34 (a) Anteroposterior radiograph of a depressed plateau fracture. The fracture is hard to see. (b) MRI scan of the same fracture showing the full extent of the damage.

big bones are likely to have fewer symptoms of instability than lightly built female netball players with slim bones and generalized ligamentous laxity, but apart from these groups it is hard to give a prognosis.

Because the outcome cannot be accurately predicted, it is better to opt for conservative treatment in most patients and to defer reconstruction until the outcome is known.

Treatment

Conservative. This consists of removing blood from the knee by thorough aspiration or arthroscopy. Arthroscopy is hazardous in patients with ligamentous and possible capsular injury and should only be undertaken by an experienced arthroscopist. It may nevertheless be needed both to remove blood and to assess the condition of the intra-articular structures.

Once blood has been removed, physiotherapy can be instituted to build up all muscle groups, espe-

cially the hamstrings. The hamstrings prevent excessive forward movement of the tibia and are therefore more important than the quadriceps, which work in the opposite direction (exacerbating the anterior draw).

There is no need to apply a cast to a patient with an isolated rupture of the anterior cruciate ligament, provided the diagnosis is certain. In some circumstances a cast may be appropriate as a pain-relieving measure, particularly if the patient has to travel a long distance after injury.

Operative. Effective repair of the anterior cruciate ligament is impossible and has largely been abandoned. The ligament crosses the synovial cavity of the knee, and its torn ends, which look like pieces of soggy string, are devitalized at the moment of injury and retract very rapidly. Apposing two such structures with inert non-absorbable suture material does not produce a functioning anterior cruciate ligament.

If operation is to be undertaken it should be a full reconstruction, of the type described on page 421.

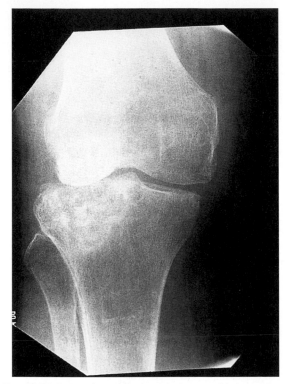

Fig. 14.35 Depression of the lateral plateau with impaction.

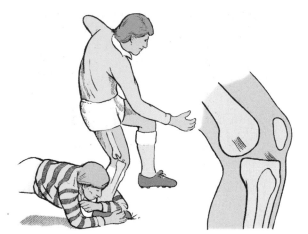

Fig. 14.36 Mechanism of injury of the anterior cruciate ligament.

This should only be advised immediately after injury if the patient needs to return to top class sport without delay, e.g. a professional footballer, or for a patient with gross instability.

Avulsion of the anterior cruciate

In young patients the tibial insertion of the anterior cruciate may be avulsed instead of the ligament tearing (Fig. 14.37).

Treatment

The fragment should be accurately replaced by manipulation, or by reduction and fixation under arthroscopic control, and immobilized for 6 weeks. The results are unpredictable because the avulsed ligament is often devitalized.

Medial collateral ligament

Complete tears of the medial collateral ligament are usually associated with a tear of the anterior cruciate ligament. Isolated tears of the medial collateral are caused by a pure valgus strain. In the UK, blows to the side of the knee from impetuous Labradors and other large dogs are a frequent cause.

Isolated lesions of the medial collateral usually heal well without operation. Lesions near the femoral attachment can heal with the formation of a flake of new bone, which can be seen radiographically, but the site of injury may remain tender for many years. Tenderness associated with the radiological signs of an old medial ligament injury is known as 'Pellegrini–Stieda disease' but it is not a disease in the accepted sense.

Treatment

Although isolated partial medial collateral ligament tears probably heal well whatever is done, it is prudent to apply a long leg cast brace from groin to ankle for about 6 weeks. This brace should allow a degree of knee flexion as this aids ligamentous healing. This brace can be modified to a removable brace to aid with physiotherapy.

Tears of the medial collateral ligament (MCL) and anterior cruciate ligament (ACL) together should be immobilized in a cast for 6 weeks, as above, unless it is decided to proceed to immediate anterior cruciate reconstruction, which may be combined with repair of the medial collateral ligament. It is often better to allow the MCL to heal first and then come back and do an ACL reconstruction, if indicated, in the future.

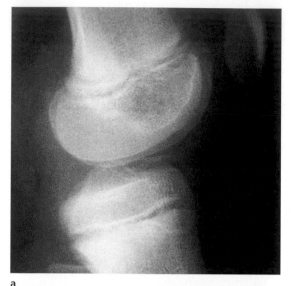

a

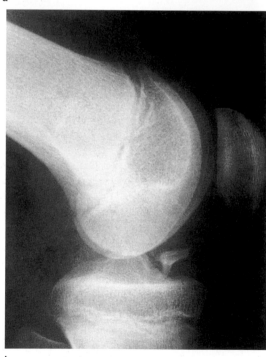

b

Fig. 14.37 (a) Avulsion of the anterior cruciate attachment of the tibia; (b) the fragment has not united in its bed.

Posterior cruciate ligament

The posterior cruciate ligament can be torn in three ways:

1. A blow to the upper end of the tibia when the knee is flexed, as when seated on a motorcycle or in the front seat of a car involved in a head-on collision (Fig. 14.38).

2. By hyperextension.

3. In combination with other ligament injuries (dislocations).

On examination soon after injury, there will be a haemarthrosis and a backward sag of the tibia relative to the femur. This is not disguised by muscle spasm.

Natural history

Most patients make an excellent recovery from an isolated posterior cruciate ligament rupture without treatment and there are many international athletes competing at their former level with posterior cruciate insufficiency.

A few patients, usually those with an associated posterior capsular rupture or damage to the posterior lateral ligamentous structures, do very badly but there is no way of knowing on the day of injury which patients will fall into this category.

Treatment

Conservative. Conservative treatment consists of removing blood from the joint by careful aspiration or arthroscopy and then immobilizing the knee in extension. Following removal of the plaster, a vigorous quadriceps exercises regimen is begun. These should be continued until the quadriceps is more powerful on the side of the injured limb than on the side of the uninjured opposite limb.

Operative. Operation should only be considered if there is considerable instability, associated damage to other ligamentous structures, or when the tibial insertion of the posterior cruciate has been avulsed with a block of bone. If such a block of bone is present it can be reattached with a screw using the posterior approach to the knee.

Most patients manage well without a posterior cruciate ligament and it is usually best to treat the lesion conservatively and perform a late reconstruction if necessary.

Lateral collateral ligament

The lateral collateral ligament is seldom injured on its own, except in lacerations. The ligament joins the femur to the fibula, not the tibia, and it is not as important as the other ligaments. When

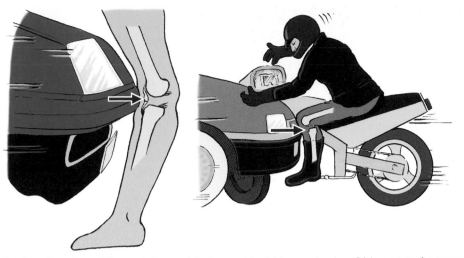

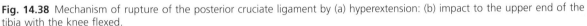

Fig. 14.38 Mechanism of rupture of the posterior cruciate ligament by (a) hyperextension: (b) impact to the upper end of the tibia with the knee flexed.

injured, there is, however, a high incidence of damage to the common peroneal nerve (30%). It is often injured together with the other lateral stabilizers of the joint (popliteus, arcuate, capsule, hamstrings).

Treatment

Early operative repair is preferable as conservative management is often unsatisfactory.

Dislocation of the knee

Complete separation of the tibia from the femur requires enough trauma to tear at least two of the four major ligaments. Trauma as great as this is enough to damage the popliteal vessels and nerves. Both vascular and neurological functions must be assessed carefully and recorded so that any deterioration will be noticed. Damage to the popliteal vessels occurs in 50% of cases and an angiogram is mandatory if there is doubt about the peripheral vascularity. Exploration of the popliteal artery and repair should be performed as an emergency as there is a high chance of an amputation if this is delayed more than 6 hours from the time of the injury.

Treatment

Management consists of attention to the nerves and vessels and watching for compartment syndromes.

Accurate reconstruction of a dislocated knee is difficult. Reattachment of avulsed ligaments is often possible but reconstructing both the cruciates is very difficult. Conservative treatment involves immobilizing the knee for 6 weeks in a plaster cast. Care is taken to ensure there is no displacement of the joint while it is in plaster. Reconstruction may be required later.

Conservative treatment of the ligaments is indicated if damage to the vessels or nerves is suspected but definite damage to the vessels and nerves is an indication for immediate repair of those structures.

Meniscal injuries

Meniscal injuries are described on page 413.

Haemarthrosis of the knee

Management

Bleeding into the knee always indicates a serious injury. Roughly 80% of patients with a haemarthrosis have a major ligament injury, usually the anterior cruciate ligament; 15% are as a result of a patella dislocation and 5% from other causes including osteochondral fractures and peripheral third meniscal tears. The principles of managing a haemarthrosis are twofold:

1. To remove blood from the knee.

2. To make a diagnosis.

Blood in the knee acts like superglue. If not removed, it will clot inside the joint and cause intra-articular adhesions that limit mobility. Even if it does not clot, blood is an irritant and causes an intense synovitis that takes many weeks to resolve. For both these reasons, rehabilitation is much more rapid if the joint is free of blood.

Treatment

Because a haemarthrosis always indicates a serious injury, a diagnosis must be made and treatment begun as soon as possible. Arthroscopy may be needed to remove blood and confirm the diagnosis but this is difficult.

If arthroscopy is not available, blood should be aspirated from the joint as thoroughly as possible and the aspirate examined for fat globules. Fat can only enter the knee from a fracture site or a contused area of subcutaneous fat communicating with the knee. The presence of fat in the aspirate indicates a serious injury. A fat–fluid level may also be visible on a lateral radiograph (see Fig. 5.1).

If the diagnosis remains unclear the knee should be examined by MRI or CT. It is not acceptable to immobilize the knee in a cast or firm supporting bandage and refer the patient to the fracture clinic 2 weeks later. This allows adhesions to form within the joint, the muscles waste and definitive treatment such as replacement of osteochondral fragments is delayed.

Fracture of the tibia and fibula

Fracture of the fibula alone

The fibula can be fractured alone in three ways (Fig. 14.39):

1. Direct trauma to the outer side of the leg, which produces a transverse or a comminuted fracture.

2. Twisting injuries, which produce a spiral fracture. Beware of an isolated spiral fracture at the upper end of the fibula: it may be associated with a fracture of the tibia at the ankle. This combination is a Maisonneuve fracture and will do badly with conservative treatment. The ankle must be examined radiologically in every patient with an apparently isolated fracture of the fibula, so that

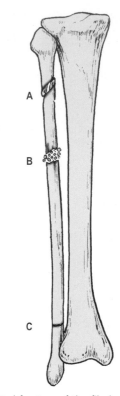

Fig. 14.39 Isolated fracture of the fibula: (A) spiral fracture; (B) comminuted fracture from direct trauma; (C) fatigue fracture.

a tibial fracture is not missed (Fig. 14.40). Maisonneuve, Monteggia and Galeazzi fractures have much in common.

3. Repeated stress in long-distance runners can cause a fatigue fracture, usually just above the inferior tibiofibular ligament (see Fig. 15.2).

On examination, the fracture site will be tender, and perhaps bruised. Dorsiflexion of the ankle may be painful because the fibula takes part in the ankle joint and movement of the ankle causes movement of the fracture site. As long as the tibia remains intact the patient can bear weight through the limb, but will avoid the heel-strike phase of gait if possible.

Treatment

If the fracture is undisplaced and the tibia is intact, no immobilization is required unless movement is painful. A cast may then be required to immobilize the ankle.

Fatigue fractures need immobilization.

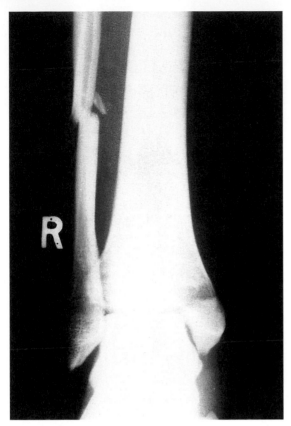

Fig. 14.40 A fracture of the fibula associated with a medial malleolar fracture. This was caused by a pronation injury of the foot.

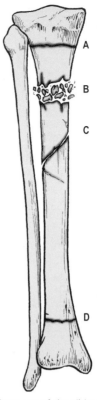

Fig. 14.41 Isolated fractures of the tibia: (*A*) fatigue fracture at the upper end; (*B*) comminuted fracture; (*C*) spiral fracture; (*D*) 'boot top' fracture.

Fracture of the tibia alone

The tibia can be broken, leaving the fibula intact, in three ways (Fig. 14.41):

1. Direct trauma.
2. Very rarely by twisting injuries.
3. Repeated stress can cause a fatigue fracture at the junction of the middle and upper thirds. The lesion is commonly seen in long-distance road runners, hurdlers, and male ballet dancers who jump to excess.

Note: Congenital pseudarthrosis of the tibia is not a true fracture; it is dealt with on page 364.

Treatment

The fracture is treated in the same way as a fracture of both bones. It might seem helpful to have the fibula intact, but this is not so because the intact fibula holds the ends of the tibia apart (Figs 14.42,

14.43) and it may be necessary to cut the fibula in order to achieve satisfactory alignment of the tibia.

Fractures of both tibia and fibula

Fracture of both the tibia and fibula is a common injury and occupies much orthopaedic time. Road traffic accidents and twisting injuries on the sports field are the commonest causes.

Complications (Fig. 14.44)

- Non-union.
- Delayed union.
- Malunion.
- Vascular damage.
- Soft tissue damage.
- Skin loss.
- Compartment syndrome.

265

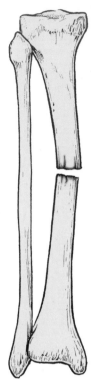

Fig. 14.42 Isolated fracture of the tibia. If the tibia alone is fractured, the intact fibula can hold the ends apart.

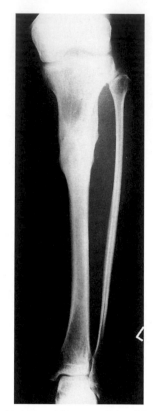

Fig. 14.43 In this isolated fracture of the tibia, the fracture has united with loss of length. The fibula is thus relatively long, causing dislocation of the head of the fibula.

Non-union is common in fractures at the middle of the tibia, particularly if the fracture is open, contaminated, and the result of high speed trauma, with extensive soft tissue damage. It is uncommon in closed fractures resulting from low speed trauma. The problem is therefore much more common following road traffic accidents than injuries on the sports field.

If non-union occurs, plating and grafting will be required.

Delayed union is common in the same group of patients who develop non-union.

Malunion is also common and causes increased wear on the knee and ankle, which in turn causes osteoarthritis.

Vascular damage may lead to gangrene of the foot and ankle. The circulation must always be observed carefully if it is likely that the vessels are seriously stretched or contused at the moment of impact, and the findings recorded. Neurological damage often accompanies vascular injury.

Soft tissue damage around a fractured tibia and fibula interferes with the final function of the leg; management of the soft tissues is often more difficult than treating the fracture.

Skin loss over the subcutaneous surface of the tibia presents a particular problem. Exposed bone does not heal well and it is often necessary to seek the help of a plastic surgeon to achieve skin cover. Any skin cover is better than none, but a free flap transferred with its own blood supply by microvascular surgery may be the most satisfactory solution. A cross-leg flap is an alternative.

Compartment syndromes. Closed fractures cause bleeding and oedema in the closed fascial spaces and a compartment syndrome with ischaemic fibrosis of the muscles if untreated. If a patient develops a tense calf with loss of passive extension and diminished sensibility following a fracture of the tibia, decompression of all four compartments of

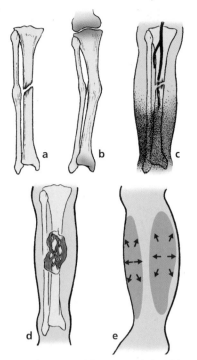

Fig. 14.44 Complications of fractures of the tibia and fibula: (a) non-union of the tibia with union of the fibula: (b) malunion with osteoarthrosis of knee and ankle; (c) ischaemia of the foot due to vascular damage; (d) skin necrosis over the fracture; (e) compartment syndrome.

the leg is required. This can conveniently be done by excising a 5 cm segment of the fibula with its periosteum, but a wide fasciotomy through a long skin incision is equally effective.

Treatment

Treatment begins at the scene of the accident.

Immediate care. The wounds of an open fracture should be covered with the cleanest material available. For transport to hospital the injured limb can be supported by bandaging it to the other leg but air splints are better and readily available in most ambulances. The blood loss from a fractured tibia is between 1 and 3 units and transfusion is not required unless there is haemorrhage from elsewhere.

Definitive treatment. The fragments must be held in the reduced position for 10–16 weeks by one of the following techniques:

1. Cast immobilization.
2. Internal fixation.
3. External fixation.

> **Very basic summary of choice of management in fractures of the tibia and fibula:**
>
> - Stable – cast immobilization.
> - Unstable – internal fixation.
> - Contaminated and unstable – external fixation.

Cast immobilization. The fracture is reduced under general anaesthesia and a cast applied from groin to toe (Fig. 14.45). Until skilled in plastering, apply the cast in stages, beginning with a gaiter round the shin and extending this above and below to include the knee and foot separately. The circulation in the foot must be carefully observed for the first 24 h.

The fracture should be examined radiologically immediately after the reduction, 24 h later and at 1 week, 2 weeks and then monthly after injury. A walking heel can be applied and weight-bearing permitted after a month if the fracture is stable and the position satisfactory.

Internal fixation is indicated for unstable fractures and patients with multiple fractures (p. 132). Plates and screws, screws alone, wires or intramedullary nails can all be used; the choice of technique depends upon the pattern of the fracture (Fig. 14.46). Although rigid anatomical fixation is attractive, the operation is a second injury to the limb and may be followed by infection.

External fixation is needed if there is a dirty wound or extensive skin loss. The fixation is not as rigid as a plate or intramedullary nail but will maintain reduction and length until the soft tissues have healed. Although the fixation apparatus looks gruesome it is well tolerated by patients.

Choice of treatment depends on the shape of the bone ends and the state of the soft tissues.

Transverse fractures of the tibia are stable if the ends can be hitched. Provided that the fracture is truly stable on longitudinal pressure, full weight-bearing can be permitted in a long leg cast as soon as the patient can tolerate it. The cast can be changed to a patellar tendon-bearing or below-knee cast as soon as callus is visible and the fracture appears firm, usually about 8 weeks from injury. The cast can be discarded altogether after about 12 weeks.

Spiral fractures are caused by twisting injuries and are always unstable (Fig. 14.47). The instability is worse if one of the bone ends is broken off as a 'butterfly' fragment. Internal fixation by plating or

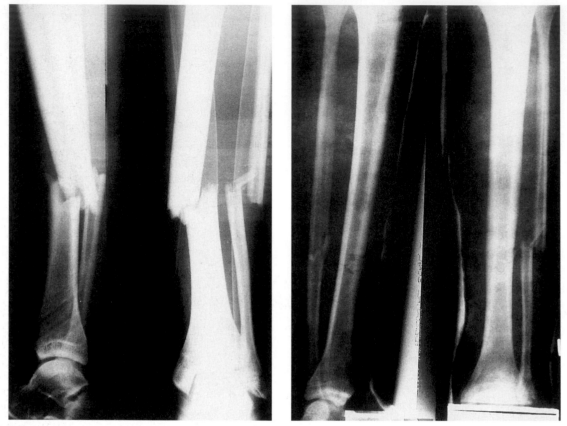

Fig. 14.45 (a) Transverse fracture of the tibia and fibula treated by (b) closed reduction and plaster immobilization.

intramedullary nailing is usually needed for these fractures.

Segmental fractures, in which the tibia and fibula are fractured in two places, with a mobile central fragment, are very unstable and best treated by a locking intramedullary nail.

Boot-top fractures. A ski boot immobilizes the ankle so firmly that rapid deceleration breaks the leg at the top of the boot. These fractures are unstable and usually need internal fixation.

Contaminated fractures are frequently seen after road traffic accidents and are usually comminuted and unstable.

The wound must be meticulously cleaned of all foreign material and dead tissue *under general anaesthesia*.

External fixation is ideal for contaminated fractures, provided that the proximal and distal fragments are large enough to hold the pins needed for sound fixation. Locked reamed or unreamed intra-medullary nails are used frequently with excellent results. If neither of these two methods is possible, skeletal traction can be applied by a calcaneal pin. When the wounds are healed the patient can either be discharged with the external fixation device still in position or after the fractures have been stabilized.

Internal fixation with a plate and screws is very occasionally advised for contaminated wounds on the basis that infection is less likely to persist in a stable skeleton than an unstable fracture. This is an interesting but very controversial subject. It is much safer, especially in examinations, to remember that internal fixation should only be used on clean and healthy tissues.

'*Technically compound*' fractures, in which the skin is punctured from inside, must be cleaned and debrided meticulously because dirt and clothing can be drawn into the wound at the moment of injury. They are just as dangerous as any other open fractures.

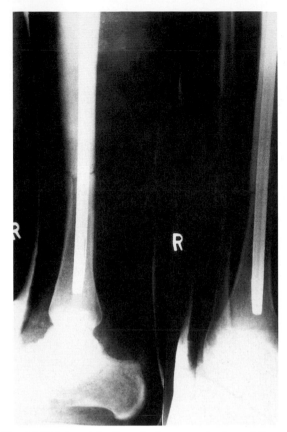

Fig. 14.46 Internal fixation of a transverse fracture of the tibia with an intramedullary nail. The nail is too small to hold rotation but alignment is maintained. A locking nail would have been more secure.

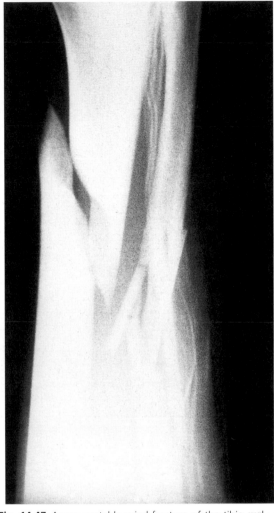

Fig. 14.47 A very unstable spiral fracture of the tibia and fibula.

Injuries of the ankle

In 1769 Sir Percival Pott of St Bartholomew's Hospital described a fracture of the lower end of the fibula with lateral displacement of the talus. 'Pott's fracture' is still often applied loosely to any fracture dislocation of the ankle. This is confusing because the type that Pott described is quite rare. There are many different types of fracture caused by a variety of mechanisms, and each needs to be treated differently.

Bones may be broken in the ankle at three points:

1. The medial malleolus of the tibia.
2. The lower end of the fibula, including the lateral malleolus.

3. The 'posterior malleolus', or posterior margin of the tibia.

Three ligaments may be torn (Fig. 14.48):

1. The inferior tibiofibular ligament.
2. The medial ligament.
3. The lateral collateral ligament.

Four forces may contribute to the injury (Fig. 14.49):

1. Abduction.
2. Adduction.
3. External rotation.
4. Vertical compression.

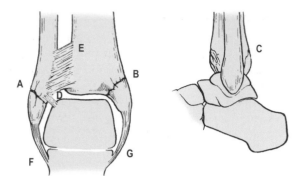

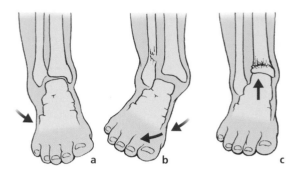

Fig. 14.48 Structures that may be injured at the ankle: (*A*) lateral malleolus; (*B*) medial malleolus; (*C*) posterior malleolus; (*D*) anterior inferior talofibular ligament; (*E*) inferior tibiofibular syndesmosis; (*F*) lateral ligament; (*G*) medial ligament.

Fig. 14.49 Forces that may injure the ankle: (a) adduction; (b) abduction; (c) upward compression.

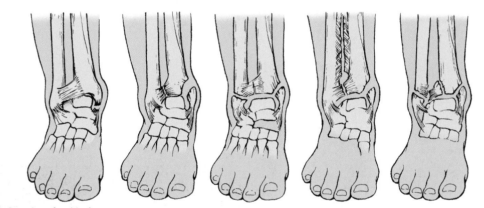

Fig. 14.50 Severity of ankle fracture. Ligaments may be ruptured and bones broken around the ankle in many different combinations.

Five grades of severity are seen (Fig. 14.50):
1. Ligament injury alone.
2. Ligament injury plus one malleolus.
3. Ligament injury plus two malleoli.
4. Ligament injury plus all three malleoli.
5. Ligament injury plus diastasis of the inferior tibiofibular joint plus fracture.

Management

Treatment can be conservative or operative. Both methods consist of reversing the movement that caused the fracture and holding the foot reduced. In some patients a good position will be achieved by manipulation alone but internal fixation is needed if the fractures are unstable or the joint surface of the ankle is disturbed.

The choice between internal fixation and conservative treatment is often difficult and depends on the type of the fracture, its stability and the patient's age.

Conservative treatment

Fractures treated conservatively should be re-examined radiologically at 10 days to be sure that the position has not slipped, and the plaster retained for at least 8 weeks. If the fracture is stable, weight-bearing can be permitted at about 4 weeks. Physiotherapy after the plaster is removed will help to restore ankle movement.

Internal fixation

There are two principal objectives:

1. To reconstitute the joint surface.
2. To create a stable joint.

If these two aims can be achieved, the ankle can be left free and early movement commenced. If not, a cast is needed.

Complications

The main complications of fracture dislocation of the ankle are malunion and secondary osteoarthritis. Because the ankle is at the lowest point of the body it takes all the body's weight and even a slight imperfection of the joint causes degenerative change. Nevertheless, if alignment is good (Fig. 14.51), function may be surprisingly good.

Abduction injuries

Violent abduction of the ankle can tear the deltoid ligament or pull the medial malleolus away from the rest of the tibia. The abduction force also knocks the lower end of the fibula off at the level of the joint surface, but leaves the inferior tibiofibular ligaments intact. The damage on the medial side causes much soft tissue swelling.

Treatment

These fractures are difficult to hold in a cast. The initial position may be satisfactory but as the swelling subsides the cast becomes loose and the fragments can slip. Internal fixation is more reliable and allows earlier mobilization.

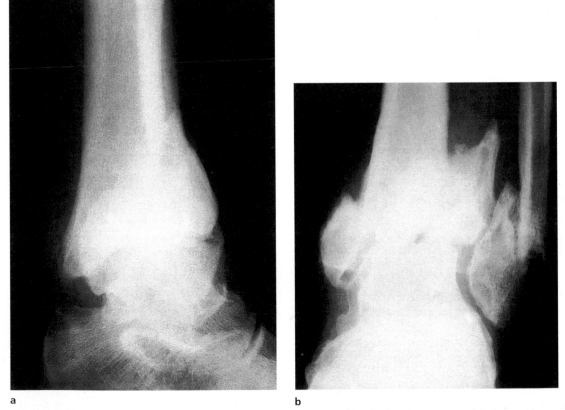

a   b

Fig. 14.51 (a), (b) Malunion following a severe fracture dislocation of the ankle. The function was surprisingly good because the foot was correctly aligned on the tibia in the anterior posterior view.

Adduction injuries

Pure adduction injuries are rare because there is usually an element of rotation if the deforming force is strongly applied.

Sprained ankle

The commonest ankle injury of all, a sprained ankle, is a partial tear of the anterior inferior talofibular ligament caused by sudden adduction of the foot when the ankle is plantar-flexed. The patient is aware of pain at the time of injury, and on clinical examination there is tenderness over the ligament. There may be a haemarthrosis as well.

Treatment. A firm elastic support is usually sufficient to relieve the pain but some patients need a below-knee cast.

The pain settles substantially after 10 days, but it will be uncomfortable for 8–12 weeks. The ankle may be painful if it is twisted accidentally for up to 2 years afterwards.

Lateral collateral ligament rupture

Lateral collateral ligament rupture can occur without a fracture. The radiograph is normal but the diagnosis can be made by the history, clinical examination and a stress radiograph to demonstrate abnormal mobility.

Treatment. Protected mobilization is required for 4–6 weeks.

Complications. Recurrent instability of the ankle can follow rupture of the lateral collateral ligament and may require a reconstructive procedure later (p. 431).

Avulsion of the lateral malleolus

The lateral collateral ligament of the ankle is strong enough to avulse a fragment of the lateral malleolus.

Treatment. The injury can be regarded as a severe sprain rather than a fracture of the fibula but pain can be so severe that a below-knee cast is needed. If the fragment is more than 1 cm wide or displaced, it should be replaced and fixed.

Fracture of the malleoli

In adduction injuries the medial malleolus is pushed away from the rest of the tibia and may break off.

The lateral malleolus may be avulsed and the fragment is sometimes substantial.

Treatment. Fractures with no displacement can be treated conservatively in a below-knee cast. Displaced or unstable fragments will need internal fixation.

External rotation injuries

External rotation of the foot pushes the talus against the lateral malleolus (Fig. 14.52). The deltoid ligament may be torn or the medial malleolus avulsed, but the lateral side is more severely damaged. The fibula may be broken at the level of the inferior tibiofibular ligament and the back of the tibia, or 'posterior malleolus', may also be broken. The fracture of the fibula is sometimes well above the ankle.

Treatment. These fractures are very unstable and internal fixation is usually needed to restore the inferior tibiofibular joint and the surface of the ankle joint (Fig. 14.53). If the posterior malleolus involves more than one-quarter of the joint surface, it will also need to be reduced and fixed.

Diastasis

In very severe external rotation injuries the inferior tibiofibular joint may be completely disrupted with diastasis and a fracture higher up the fibular shaft (Fig. 14.54).

Treatment. The diastasis should be closed with a transverse screw after fixation of the fibular shaft fracture (Fig. 14.55). This screw must be removed after about 8 weeks, when the ligament has healed. There is a little movement between the tibia and fibula in the normal leg, which is not possible with a screw across the syndesmosis. If the screw is not removed, either it will break through fatigue or the ankle will be stiff.

Vertical compression injuries

Vertical compression or hyperextension of the ankle can cause a comminuted crush fracture of the anterior cortex of the tibia. The fracture is often caused by a sharp upward movement of the foot when it catches on a protruding object as the patient is falling from a height.

Treatment. Because the joint surface of the tibia is crushed and the fracture is unstable, it must be held with a plate and, if necessary, a bone graft to fill the

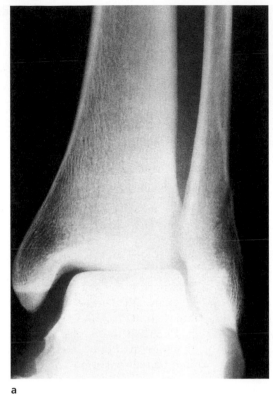

a

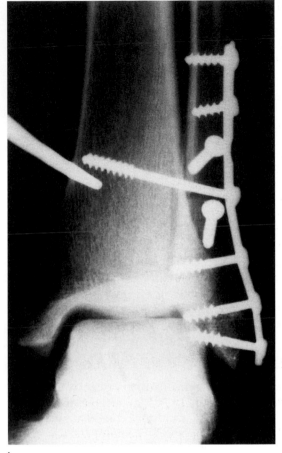

Fig. 14.52 Anteroposterior view of external rotation injury of ankle before (a) and after fixation (b). The talus and lateral malleolus are shifted laterally. *Note*: The diastasis screw was unnecessary once the fibula had been held reduced.

b

defect. The aim is to produce a joint surface in the normal relationship to the talus. An articulated external fixator can be used to hold the bone out to length at the same time as allowing the ankle to move.

Achilles tendon rupture

The Achilles tendon can be torn by a forward lunge on the sports field or squash court. These are the same movements that tear the head of the gastrocnemius (p. 286). The patient will feel as though somebody has kicked him on the Achilles tendon and there are legendary stories of the victim feeling a kick, turning round and punching the person behind – usually a policeman – in retribution.

On examination, there is swelling around the tendon but a defect will be felt in the tendon. The

'squeeze' test will be positive because the fascial sheath is ruptured (Fig. 14.56).

Treatment

Treatment can be conservative or operative but both methods rely on holding the torn ends of the tendon together until healed, and this can be done in a below-knee cast with the ankle in full flexion. Operation is difficult because the ends are not cut cleanly across and at operation look like two untidy shaving brushes, but it is generally preferred, especially for athletes.

Cast immobilization is required for both conservative and operative treatment. A below-knee cast in full ankle flexion is maintained for 4 weeks and then changed to bring the foot halfway up to neutral for a further 2 weeks, when the cast is removed. A

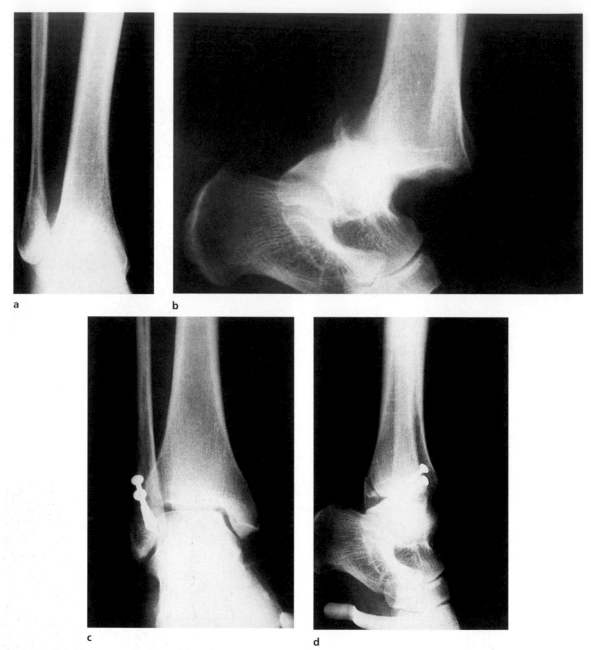

Fig. 14.53 (a), (b) Anteroposterior and lateral views of an external rotation fracture dislocation of the ankle with a small fracture of the posterior malleolus. (c), (d) The same fracture after open reduction and internal fixation of the lateral malleolus.

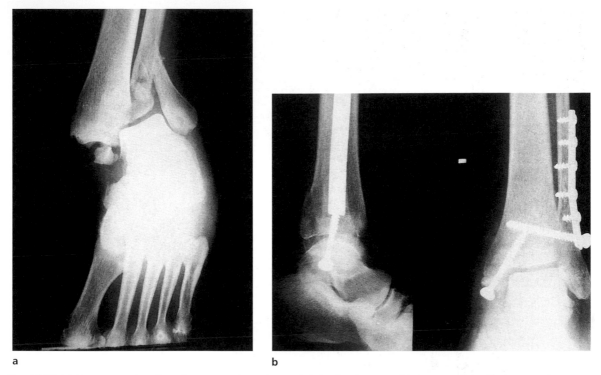

a   b

Fig. 14.54 (a) Anteroposterior view of an external rotation and abduction fracture with fracture of the fibula, posterior malleolus and medial malleolus. (b) The result of open reduction and internal fixation of the fracture in (a).

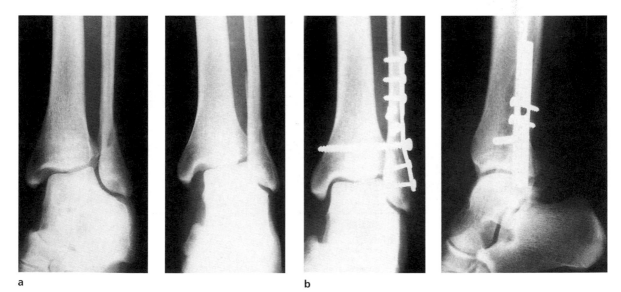

a   b

Fig. 14.55 (a) External rotation and abduction fracture of the fibula, with diastasis treated by internal fixation (b).

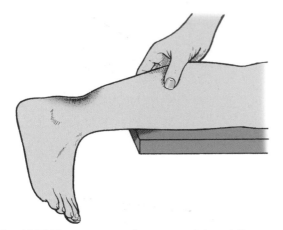

Fig. 14.56 The squeeze test for rupture of the Achilles tendon. If the tendon is ruptured, the foot does not move when the calf is squeezed.

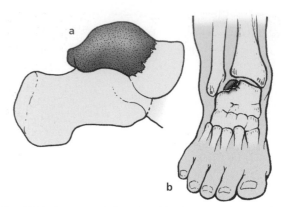

Fig. 14.57 Fractures of the talus: (a) a fracture of the neck may cause aseptic necrosis of the body; (b) osteochondral fracture of the talus.

further walking cast is used for 2 weeks and then the patient starts on an intensive physiotherapy regimen. Recently a removable brace has been used which holds the foot in the desired position but allows physiotherapy to start sooner.

Ultrasound to reduce the swelling and physiotherapy to restore movement can be started when the cast is removed, but no vigorous activity or sport should be permitted until a full range of movement has been restored. This is likely to be at least 16 weeks from injury and usually longer.

Fractures of the talus and hindfoot

Fractures of the talus

The talus can be fractured by twisting injuries to the foot, violent dorsiflexion or impact from below.

The talus takes part in the ankle, subtalar and midtarsal joints. The function of all these joints is affected if the talus is fractured.

There are three types of fracture of the talus (Fig. 14.57):
1. Fractures of the body of the talus.
2. Fractures through the neck of the talus.
3. Osteochondral fractures.

Complications

Fractures of the neck of the talus are serious and often followed by complications:

1. Skin necrosis if the talus is extruded subcutaneously, when it stretches the skin severely.
2. Non-union.
3. Aseptic necrosis because the blood supply of the body of the talus is interrupted by a fracture through its neck.
4. Late osteoarthrosis of the subtalar and talonavicular joints.
5. Unrecognized osteochondral fragments may need to be removed later as loose bodies.

Treatment

Fractures of the neck should be reduced in good position, by open reduction and internal fixation if necessary, and protected from stress until united.

Fractures of the body cannot be reduced accurately and may be treated by early mobilization within the limits of pain.

Fractures of the calcaneum

The calcaneum is broken by a blow to the heel, most often caused by landing from a height. Because the calcaneum is made of cancellous bone, it is crushed at the moment of impact and restoration of the anatomy is difficult (Fig. 14.58). If the cortical fragments are placed in their correct position, a cavity remains and must be filled with a bone graft.

Recognition

Many different patterns of fracture occur, and many escape recognition in the accident department. To

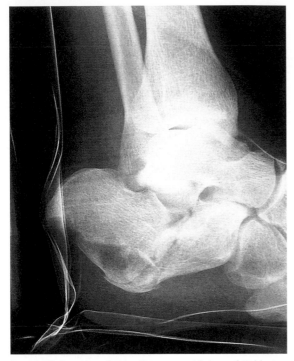

Fig. 14.58 Fracture of the calcaneum with loss of Bohler's angle.

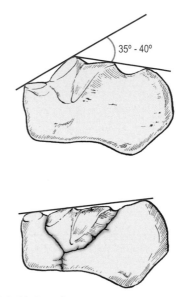

Fig. 14.59 Bohler's angle.

assess the calcaneum radiologically, look for three things:

1. Loss of 'Bohler's angle' (Fig. 14.59).
2. Widening or disruption of the body on an axial view (Fig. 14.60).
3. Separation of the 'beak' at the back of the bone (see Fig. 14.58).

The fracture is very painful and stops the patient from putting the foot to the ground. After a day, bruising begins to appear in a horseshoe around the heel (Fig. 14.61). If this pattern of bruising is present and no fracture has been seen, look again at the radiographs.

Complications

Undisplaced fractures of the calcaneum are unimportant but major fractures destroy the subtalar joint and cause stiffness of the subtalar and midtarsal joints. This leads to disabling pain when walking on rough surfaces. These symptoms go on improving for 2 years but seldom resolve completely.

Treatment

Treatment can be conservative or operative.

Conservative treatment consists of rest and protection from weight-bearing for 6 weeks or until the patient can bear weight on the foot in comfort.

Operative treatment consists of open reduction and bone grafting of the bony defect. Operation is most often advised for severe crushing injuries in young adults. The results are reasonable and perhaps better than the results of conservative management in severe injuries.

Fractures of the tarsus

The tarsal bones are hard, solid bones resistant to fracture but they have flat surfaces and dislocations or fracture dislocations occur at two points (Fig. 14.62): (1) the midtarsal joint and (2) the tarsometatarsal joint (Fig. 14.63).

The injuries are caused by apparently trivial twisting injuries of the forefoot and can easily escape detection both clinically and radiologically. These fractures are a pitfall for the unwary.

Treatment

If not correctly diagnosed and accurately reduced, the dislocation becomes permanent and a disabling deformity results. Open reduction and internal fixation is often needed.

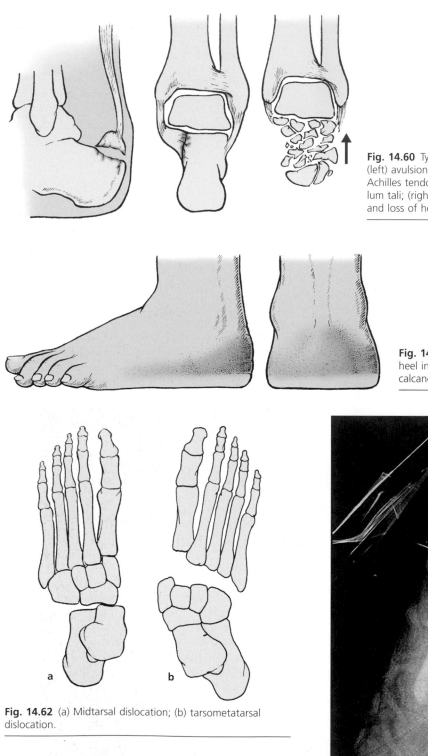

Fig. 14.60 Types of fracture of the calcaneum: (left) avulsion of posterior segment by the Achilles tendon; (middle) fracture of sustentaculum tali; (right) burst fracture with compression and loss of height.

Fig. 14.61 Horseshoe bruise around the heel in the presence of a fracture of the calcaneum.

Fig. 14.62 (a) Midtarsal dislocation; (b) tarsometatarsal dislocation.

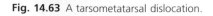

Fig. 14.63 A tarsometatarsal dislocation.

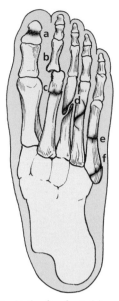

Fig. 14.64 Fractures in the forefoot: (a) crush fracture of the phalanx; (b) dislocation of the metatarsophalangeal joint; (c) fatigue fracture; (d) spiral fracture of the metatarsals; (e) transverse fracture of the fifth metatarsal; (f) fracture of the styloid process of the fifth metatarsal.

Fractures of the forefoot (Fig. 14.64)

Fifth metatarsal

The styloid process of the fifth metatarsal can be avulsed by trivial twisting injuries of the forefoot. Left untreated, the fracture usually joins soundly with bone or fibrous tissue and little long-term disability follows. The shaft may also be fractured (Fig. 14.65).

Treatment

There is considerable pain and tenderness of the fracture site immediately after the injury and a below-knee cast may be needed to relieve pain. Some patients can manage well with just a firm crêpe bandage.

Multiple spiral fractures

Twisting injuries of the forefoot may cause spiral fractures of several metatarsals, sometimes accompanied by dislocation of the tarsometatarsal joints (Fig. 14.66).

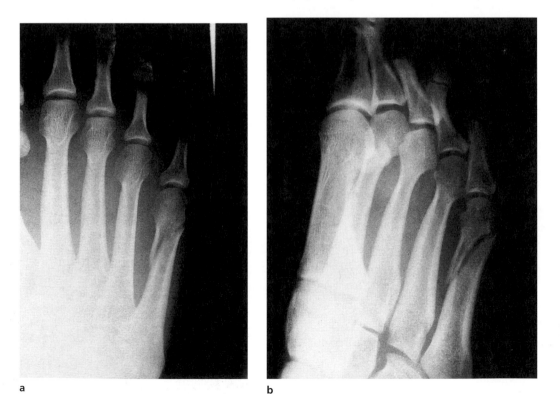

a   b

Fig. 14.65 (a), (b) Spiral fracture of the fifth metatarsal.

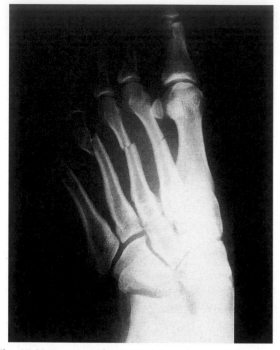

Fig. 14.66 Transverse fractures of the second, third and fourth metatarsals with a spiral fracture of the neck of the third metatarsal.

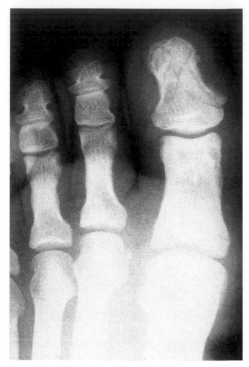

Fig. 14.67 Crush fracture of the distal phalanx of the great toe.

Treatment

The normal relationship of the metatarsal heads must be restored so that the area of contact with the ground remains flat and excessive loading of any single metatarsal head is avoided. Immobilization of the fractures with percutaneous pins may be necessary.

Fatigue fractures

Fatigue fractures are described on pages 100 and 286.

Fractures of the phalanges

The phalanges are in a vulnerable position and easily broken by falling objects (Fig. 14.67). These fractures are common industrial injuries and can be avoided by wearing shoes with protective toecaps.

Treatment

Crush injuries of the distal phalanges should be treated as severe soft tissue injuries without regard to bony continuity. The foot should be elevated until swelling has subsided and adequate pain relief has been given. Elevation for several days may be required.

Fractures of the proximal phalanx seldom require treatment but rotational deformities should be reduced and held in position by securing the toe lightly to its neighbour with strapping, as for the comparable fracture of the fingers (pp. 232–233).

Crushed foot

Crushing injuries of the foot, like crushing injuries of the hand, cause persistent stiffness.

Treatment

The foot should be elevated with the patient in bed until the swelling has settled. This may take 2 weeks. Walking can then be allowed, with a supporting bandage to reduce swelling.

Case reports

These three case studies represent the different management of femoral neck fractures.

Patient A

A 78-year-old lady tripped over the carpet at home, sustaining a heavy fall on to her right hip. She was unable to weight bear, but was fortunate that she had an 'alert' button close to hand and was able to summon help to her home. She had recently been experiencing many falls and her son had insisted that she wear a call button to alert her neighbours should she fall.

Her general practitioner arranged for the ambulance to transfer her to hospital where it was clear that she had no other injuries, but had sustained an intracapsular fracture of the right neck of femur.

She was treated the following day in theatre and had a cemented hemiarthroplasty performed. This allowed her to mobilize slowly over the next few days and she was discharged from hospital after 10 days back to her own home. Home care was arranged. Both occupational and physiotherapy services helped her to rehabilitate in the short term and regain her mobility and independence in the long term.

Patient B

A 10-year-old, slightly overweight boy was playing football and noticed an aching discomfort in his right hip, which failed to settle. There was no specific history of trauma and it was initially felt that he had sprained his hip.

The symptoms failed to settle and, indeed, worsened over the next few days. He was taken to the general practitioner where it was noted that he had a limitation of movement of the hip, but no sign suggestive of infection. A subsequent radiograph confirmed a potential slipped femoral epiphysis and an urgent orthopaedic review was requested. The diagnosis was confirmed and the epiphysis was fixed using a single screw to ensure that there was no further slippage.

After appropriate discussion with the patient's parents the opposite hip was also fixed to avoid potential risks of this physis slipping at a later date (up to 50% chance).

Patient C

A 67-year-old lady sustained a fall while walking to the local shops. She fell on to the pavement sustaining an injury to her right hip. She was unable to mobilize and was taken by the ambulance crew to the local hospital where it was clear that she had sustained a fracture of the right proximal femur.

Radiographs confirmed a transverse subtrochanteric fracture. She was referred to the orthopaedic team and after careful review of the radiographs there was suspicion about not only the position of the fracture, but also the quality of the bone around the proximal femur. A skeletal review was requested and further lytic areas in the skeleton noted.

This lady had had a breast carcinoma 2 years previously and it had been thought at her last follow-up that she was all clear, but there were now multiple bony metastases. The fracture was fixed using an intramedullary hip screw and the oncologists continued with her future management.

Summary

Femoral neck fractures are exceedingly common in the elderly. A small percentage of these are pathological, especially those in the subtrochanteric region.

In benign, innocent, fractures it is important to stabilize the fracture or replace the femoral head early to allow early mobility and rehabilitation.

Fractures of the femoral neck in younger patients are rare. These are either associated with significant high energy trauma (road traffic accidents) or in those patients with a slipped upper femoral epiphysis. In these cases there is a high chance of a contralateral side slipping and it is common practice in some units to prophylactically pin that side at the same time.

Chapter |15|

Sports injuries

By the end of this chapter you should be able to:

- Appreciate the importance of the medical management of the injured athlete.
- Recognize and treat appropriately overuse and fatigue injuries.
- Be aware of the importance of avoidance of these injuries by using the correct equipment and training methods.

Sports medicine is essentially a type of occupational health medicine and this should not be forgotten just because many of the patients are well-known public figures.

No injury is unique to athletes and the conditions described in this chapter could equally well be described elsewhere. The chapter deals with the particular problems of the sporting world and describes lesions that occur more often in sporting activities than everyday life.

Psychology and the athlete

Many sports injuries are treated by orthopaedic surgeons because of their involvement with trauma, but sports medicine is very different from the rest of orthopaedic surgery. For one thing, an athlete who is 100% fit will be unhappy – an athlete needs to be not less than 110% fit, at least in his or her own estimation, and will strive for 120%. This belief, coupled with the athlete's drive to achieve goals beyond the scope of ordinary people, may loosen their hold on reality and prevent them understanding that their body is made of the same stuff as ordinary mortals.

A further problem is that many athletes have a compulsive–obsessional approach to their sport. A cyclist or a runner who does not put in the allotted number of miles per week will feel uneasy and fear their performance will be permanently impaired. In this regard the behaviour of some athletes is similar to that of other compulsive neuroses such as alcoholism, compulsive gambling and anorexia nervosa. Fortunately, most sportsmen and women have a healthy approach to their sport, but compulsive individuals do exist and must be recognized at an early stage.

For many well-balanced athletes fitness is an integral part of their way of life and self-image. Occasional recreational athletes may feel that their sporting activities distinguish them from their more everyday contemporaries. To find that their sporting prowess has been taken away can make both groups clinically depressed and produce a similar reaction to bereavement or the loss of a limb.

Reasons for athletes to seek treatment:

1. Poor performance, which may be due to:
   - lack of ability
   - unfitness
   - age
   - poor mental approach.
2. Injury.
3. A disease that affects performance, e.g.:
   - glandular fever
   - leukaemia
   - osteogenic sarcoma.

Ageing

Athletes have great difficulty in accepting the ageing process. Ageing athletes – over 30 years of age – may be so convinced of their own eternal youth that they will seek medical advice to find out why they cannot run as fast or jump as high as they did 10 years earlier. The simple explanation that they are 'growing old' will not be believed.

Other patients may, unconsciously, be a little more subtle in their approach to advancing age and look to injury as an excuse for graceful retirement or a gradual descent to a lower level of performance. Neither of these conditions can be treated by operation.

The ageing process cannot be denied. However rigorous the training programme and however assiduously it may be pursued, hair still goes grey, skin wrinkles, articular surfaces become less resilient and more fragile, muscles waste, tendons weaken and soft tissue degenerates. These are biological facts that cannot be altered by training or 'dedication'.

For these reasons the approach to the athlete cannot be based on organic features of the injury alone. Many athletes may have a perfectly straightforward organic injury but to treat that without understanding the feeling of the athlete towards his or her own physical fitness will lead to disillusionment on both sides.

Practical and professional considerations

Sports medicine presents practical and ethical problems. In other specialties doctors are in no doubt that they are the patient's medical attendant, but in the field of sports medicine there may be more concern for the success of the player's club than for the long-term future of the player.

The welfare of any patient has to be considered not only from the short-term point of view but also from the long-term. Considerable pressure is sometimes applied to the doctor by the team manager or club, as well as by the player, to achieve a good short-term result without regard for the long-term.

Enabling a player to take part in an important match soon after a serious injury or operation, for example, could have harmful long-term effects. To complicate matters, the players themselves are not always in a position to disagree with their club official and may enthusiastically embrace the prospect of osteoarthritis in middle age if only they can play on Saturday.

The need for rapid results and the fast return to sport after injury also means that athletes demand priority over other patients. If health service resources are in short supply, it is hard to justify treating a recreational athlete in preference to a wage-earner who cannot work. Injured sportsmen are seldom ill or disabled in the common sense of the word, yet their powerful motivation will often find a way through the normal channels to be treated in preference to patients with genuine organic illness. This can lead to ill-feeling when resources are scarce.

To avoid this problem, sports clinics treating athletes only are often set up outside hospitals and orthopaedic departments, but this leads to the paradox that in some places the only way to receive prompt treatment for a musculoskeletal disorder is to declare that it was the result of a sporting injury rather than an accident at work.

These observations do not detract from the need for a specialized service for sportsmen or deny the existence of injuries specific to individual sports. Provided that the doctor can come to terms with the psychological aspects of sportsmen and women and the practical problems of establishing a clinic for sports injuries, sports medicine is a rewarding and fascinating specialty.

The conditions described below are commonly seen in athletes but are not unique to them.

Injuries to muscles

Musculotendinous injuries

- Ruptures of the muscle belly.
- Haematoma in the muscle belly.
- Rupture of the musculotendinous junction.
- Rupture of the tendon.
- Tendinitis.
- Tears at the muscle insertion.

Ruptures of the muscle belly

Clinical features

Rupture of a muscle is felt as a tearing sensation. Swelling and tenderness at the site of the rupture follow within hours, and bruising about 24 h later. The bruising is caused by bleeding from the ends of the ruptured muscle and can be quite dramatic, even alarming.

On examination a defect can be felt in the muscle belly and the belly becomes prominent as the muscle contracts. The swelling can occasionally be mistaken for a soft tissue mass. The rectus femoris and hamstrings are the muscles most often affected.

Haematoma

A haematoma in a muscle is a serious lesion, sometimes called a 'Charley horse' for no obvious reason. The lesion usually follows direct trauma or, more rarely, a tear of the central fibres of the muscle. The quadriceps is most commonly affected.

As the blood in the haematoma becomes organized it interferes with normal muscle function and in some patients the haematoma becomes ossified, which restricts muscle movement severely. The mass of bone usually resolves within 2 years of injury but may have to be excised.

Ossification can occur in any haematoma, but is said to be more common if the muscle is mobilized too rapidly after the injury.

Treatment

The immediate treatment for a ruptured muscle, as for other soft tissue injuries, is to cool the limb with ice wrapped in a towel to prevent cold injury, elevate the limb, apply gentle compression and avoid contracting the torn muscle.

Ruptures of a muscle belly cannot be repaired successfully. The tears take at least 6 weeks to heal with sound fibrous tissue and the healing process cannot be accelerated artificially. Operation causes more soft tissue destruction, sutures will not hold in the torn muscle ends, and rehabilitation is delayed. Ultrasound reduces localized swelling and passive joint movement maintains joint mobility.

Active contraction of the ruptured muscle is harmful during the first 6 weeks, but physiotherapy can then be started to increase muscle power gradually while maintaining joint mobility. When normal power and mobility have been obtained, a gradual return to full sporting activities is permitted. If this regimen is not followed, a re-rupture of the muscle is likely.

Musculotendinous ruptures

Like ruptures of the muscle belly, rupture of the musculotendinous junction is felt as a tearing sensation followed by pain and bruising (Fig. 15.1). The commonest site is the medial belly of the gastrocnemius, which can be torn by a sharp dorsiflexion of the ankle, often during a game of squash or tennis. The area of tenderness is localized and a defect can be felt in the muscle belly.

Treatment

Treatment is the same as for other soft tissue injuries; i.e. ice, elevation and compression. Ultrasound will reduce swelling, and joint movement should be maintained. Pain after this injury lasts for a predictable 8 weeks and complete recovery is the rule.

Emergency treatment of soft tissue injuries:

Rest
Ice (wrapped in a towel if from the deepfreeze)
Compression
Elevation.

Injuries to muscle insertions

Tennis elbow, golfer's elbow and *jumper's knee* are described on pages 371, 372 and 424.

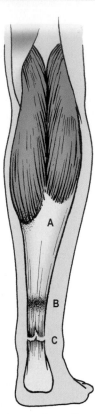

Fig. 15.1 Sites of damage to the calf and Achilles tendon: (*A*) partial rupture of the medial belly of the gastrocnemius; (*B*) paratenonitis; (*C*) rupture of the Achilles tendon.

Tendons

Tendons, like muscles, can be ruptured by sudden violent contraction. The commonest tendon to rupture is the Achilles tendon, but the tendons to the long head of biceps and supraspinatus may also rupture.

Achilles tendon rupture is described on page 273.

Paratenonitis

The paratenon becomes inflamed by repeated friction. The paratenon of the Achilles tendon and extensor muscles of the wrist are commonly affected, and this may be due to poor technique such as holding a racquet wrongly.

Treatment

Paratenonitis at the heel is made worse by running on hard surfaces and wearing shoes with a worn heel. Proper footwear or a soft heel-pad may resolve the problem.

At the wrist, if attention to racquet technique is ineffective, rest in a splint is usually helpful, but unacceptable to athletes.

Injection of a steroid preparation into the paratenon – but not the tendon – is also effective. In persistent cases the paratenon must be explored and adhesions between it and the underlying tendon divided.

Tendinitis

The patellar tendon can be irritated or its central fibres torn by repeated jumping, particularly in high jump training and basketball, to produce a condition similar to jumper's knee. The patient will experience pain in the patellar tendon, worse on quadriceps contraction, but without localized tenderness. Steroid injection around, but not into, the tendon may be helpful.

Treatment

Treatment is by rest and anti-inflammatory drugs. Do not inject steroids into the tendon or it may rupture. Eccentric exercises are beneficial.

Bones and joints

Fatigue fractures

Fatigue fractures in the metatarsals follow overuse and repeated loading. March fracture of the second metatarsal is the best known (p. 100) but fatigue fractures are also seen in the tibia and fibula of long-distance runners and other athletes in whom repeated stress is placed on the lower leg (Figs 15.2, 15.3). Spondylolisthesis, a fatigue fracture of the pars interarticularis, occurs in athletes who hyperextend their spine, such as fast bowlers in cricket and javelin throwers.

Treatment

Treatment consists of rest until the fracture has united. Brace immobilization may allow the patient to start physiotherapy sooner.

Cruciate ligament injuries

Cruciate ligament injuries are common on the sports field and are dealt with on page 420.

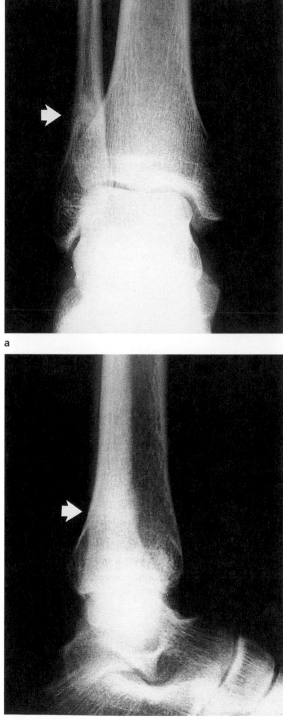

a

b

Fig. 15.2 (a), (b) Fatigue fracture of the lower end of the fibula in a road runner.

Breast-stroke knee

Breast-stroke swimmers adduct the legs forcefully against the resistance of the water (Fig. 15.4). This produces a chronic irritation of the distal insertion of the medial ligament, which becomes tender and painful when a valgus strain is applied.

Treatment

Apart from modifying training there is little to offer for this lesion.

Jogger's knee

Between the ages of 30 and 40 years the articular cartilage begins to lose its resilience and becomes more brittle. Repeated loading of the articular cartilage, as in road running or jogging, can cause pain in the weight-bearing joints, particularly the knee and patellofemoral joint.

Treatment

The symptoms can be relieved by running on soft ground instead of road or by wearing properly designed running shoes with well-padded heels. In persistent cases it may be necessary to advise the patient to stop. Moulded insoles (orthoses) may help by changing the forces on the heel when it strikes the ground.

Other injuries

A full catalogue of the many injuries that can be caused by specific sporting activities would be very long indeed.

Javelin throwers can disrupt the acromioclavicular joint by the violent forward movement of the shoulder (Fig. 15.5). No treatment will restore the joint to complete normality.

Archers develop a similar lesion. On the Tudor warship the *Mary Rose*, many skeletons were found with exaggerated muscle attachments around the right shoulder girdle and disrupted acromioclavicular joints. It is likely that these were archers.

Fast bowlers can rupture their external oblique muscle during delivery. The injury is occasionally seen in other throwing sports.

Footballers may damage the pubic symphysis through kicking the ball at speed while twisting on

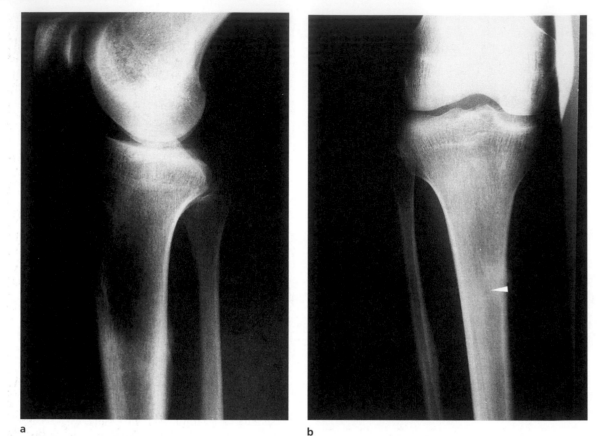

a   b

Fig. 15.3 (a), (b) Fatigue fracture of the tibia in a runner, shown by sclerosis of the tibial cortex.

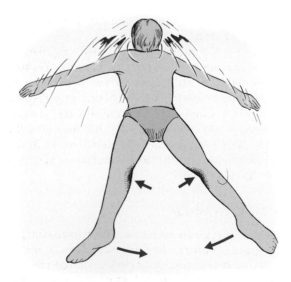

Fig. 15.4 Breast-stroke knee. The breast-stroke action stresses the medial ligaments and may cause pain and tenderness.

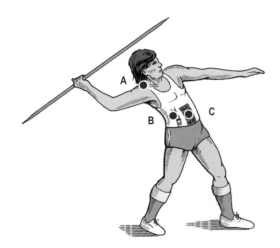

Fig. 15.5 Injuries in javelin throwers: (*A*) subluxation of the acromioclavicular joint; (*B*) hyperextension of the spine, which may cause spondylolysis; (*C*) rupture of the rectus abdominis.

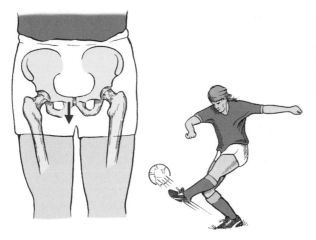

Fig. 15.6 Strain on the pubic symphysis in a footballer.

one leg (Fig. 15.6). This can be resistant to treatment.

Footballers also develop symptoms from small inguinal hernias.

Repetitive stress injuries

Many sports injuries are the result of repeated stress, often from training techniques. This group of injuries includes tenosynovitis, fatigue fractures and a host of other problems caused by repeating the same movement over and over again in an attempt to achieve perfection. Once identified, the problem can usually be corrected by changing the training technique.

Prevention

Prevention of sports injuries

- Adequate 'warm-up'.
- Gradual return after lay-off from injury, off-season, etc.
- Correct footwear and clothing.
- Good protective wear – helmets, etc.

Warming up

Sporting injuries can be minimized by correct training, proper warm-up and using the correct equipment. In particular, muscle and tendon injuries can be reduced by ensuring that players do not go into

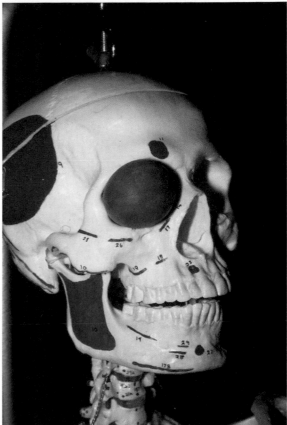

Fig. 15.7 A squash ball fits neatly into the orbit. Protective spectacles should be worn when playing squash.

full athletic activity without stretching the muscles adequately beforehand.

If athletic training is discontinued, suppleness, strength and stamina are lost, in that order. Because suppleness is so important in the prevention of muscle and tendon injuries, and because preseason training is so often neglected, injuries are far more common in the first half of the first match of the season than in any other. An adequate warm-up and muscle stretching routine before a match is essential.

Protective wear

Protective wear is important if patients are engaged in a sport in which they are likely to sustain an impact, such as in boxing or cricket. Correct training shoes help to prevent jogger's knee and plastic spectacles should always be worn when playing squash; the squash ball fits neatly into the orbit and several eyes are lost every year from this injury (Fig. 15.7).

289

Equipment should be of good quality and well maintained. Training shoes with worn heels cause abnormal strains on the foot, and the dangers of defective apparatus such as diving boards and fencing masks are obvious.

Sport, like life, is dangerous!

Case reports

More and more people are playing sport for longer and longer. Unfortunately, as mentioned, a number of injuries can occur. These include not only the acute injuries but also the more chronic injuries that result from overuse, poor technique or bad equipment. The following examples illustrate some of these common chronic injuries.

Patient A

An 18-year-old army recruit suddenly developed right foot pain following prolonged exercise. The pain was worse with activity and relieved slightly by rest.

He was able to walk but found running and marching difficult. He attended the sick bay and was provided with simple analgesics but this failed to settle the pain. He continued with the vigorous army exercises, but was unable to cope and had to stop after the first week.

Clinical examination confirmed pain over the second metatarsal with localized soft tissue swelling but no other abnormality. Radiographs confirmed a periosteal reaction and a possible hairline fracture. This was treated as a stress fracture with rest, avoidance of further injury and a graduated rehabilitation programme.

The patient was able to return to sporting activities and the army regime after 3 months.

Patient B

A keen club runner who frequently ran between 30 and 50 km (20–30 miles) per week noted increasing pain in the calf muscles of the left leg. He noticed that he was able to run a couple of miles before he developed a cramping sensation in the calf, which failed to resolve.

He was forced to rest and the pain did settle slightly, although he was left with a dull aching sensation in the calf. He described the calf as feeling 'woody, hard' when painful. When not running he had no symptoms and was able to continue with his normal lifestyle.

He consulted the local physiotherapists and was informed that he had shin splints and was treated with an orthosis in his shoe. He attempted to continue running, but had a recurrence of the pain after running 2 miles.

When reviewed by the orthopaedic surgeon, intracompartmental pressure studies confirmed an elevation of the compartment pressure with exercise. He subsequently underwent a decompressive fasciotomy which cured the pain and allowed him to continue with his running career.

Patient C

A 45-year-old company director took up competitive tennis after a break of 10 years. Being a highly competitive individual he practised and competed regularly but noted an increasing pain over the lateral aspect of his right elbow with most ground shots.

The local physiotherapist made the diagnosis of a 'tennis elbow' and provided him with an epicondylitis strap. This failed to relieve his pain as he continued to play tennis on a regular basis.

When asked about the equipment that he used it was clear that he continued to use his old racquet, which had a very narrow grip. He had also changed his technique and grip recently. The pain settled in his elbow with the appropriate conservative treatment of physiotherapy, rest and alteration in not only the technique but also the type of racquet that he was using.

Summary

These three cases represent common chronic sporting injuries. With a sudden increase in intensity or duration of activity the bone can fatigue and fracture. This type of stress fracture will only heal when the limb is rested and an appropriate rehabilitation training programme is instituted.

Similarly, overuse injuries are common, especially with runners, and the use of poor equipment or bad technique can result in injury to the joint. Simple treatment of the injury without removing the cause fails to resolve these injuries.

Part | 3 |

Orthopaedics

Chapter |16|

Osteoarthritis

By the end of this chapter you should:

- Be aware of the impact of osteoarthritic conditions on lifestyle.
- Be able to make the correct diagnosis of arthritis on history and clinical findings without the need for expensive investigations.
- Advise on the treatment options and understand the risks (early and late) of joint replacement surgery.

Pathology

Osteoarthritis is a poor name for degenerative joint disease. Articular cartilage is involved more than bone, and inflammation is secondary to the disease and not the cause. 'Osteoarthrosis' is often used as an alternative and 'osteochondrosis' would be more accurate, but 'osteoarthritis' is so well established that it is unlikely to be displaced.

Osteoarthritis is the result of progressive breakdown of the joint surface and can follow any insult to any joint. Infection, direct or indirect trauma to the articular cartilage and joint diseases can all lead to osteoarthritis. The disease involves mainly the large weight-bearing joints. In this respect it differs from rheumatoid arthritis, which involves the synovium of many joints and is commoner in the small joints of the hands and feet (Fig. 16.1).

Primary osteoarthritis includes several different conditions, the commonest of which is generalized nodal osteoarthritis. White women are most often affected, during the fifth and sixth decades, by polyarticular involvement of many joints. The onset can be relatively sudden with hot, inflamed, distal interphalangeal joints.

Hip disease behaves differently. The condition is more common in men, is often unilateral with no other joint involvement and may have no obvious precipitating cause.

Secondary osteoarthritis has many causes, of which the commonest are:

1. Obesity.
2. Abnormal contour of the articular surfaces, particularly malunited fractures.
3. Malalignment of the joints from deformity, fracture or the distortion of the anatomy by previous surgery, particularly meniscectomy at the knee.
4. Joint instability due to trauma or generalized ligamentous laxity.
5. Genetic or developmental abnormalities, such as epiphyseal dysplasia, Perthes disease or slipped epiphysis.
6. Metabolic or endocrine disease, including ochronosis (alkaptonuria), acromegaly and the mucopolysaccharidoses.

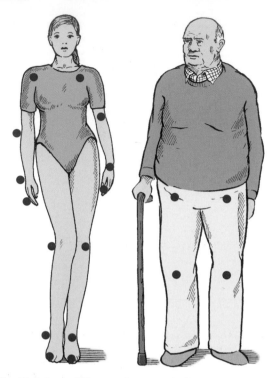

Fig. 16.1 Some differences between rheumatoid arthritis and osteoarthritis. Osteoarthritis mainly affects the weight-bearing joints and is more common in elderly and heavy-weight people. Rheumatoid arthritis affects small joints, is symmetrical and is commonest in young women.

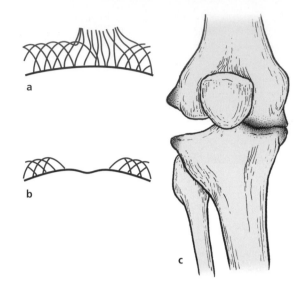

Fig. 16.2 The development of osteoarthritis: (a) breakdown of the articular surface with rupture of the collagen arcades; (b) exposed bone with eburnation; (c) deformity and collapse.

7. Inflammatory diseases such as rheumatoid arthritis, gout and infection.

8. Osteonecrosis.

9. The neuropathies, especially denervated joints and Charcot's disease.

In short, any joint disease can cause osteoarthritis!

The development of osteoarthrosis can be considered in five stages:

1. Breakdown of articular surface.
2. Synovial irritation.
3. Remodelling.
4. Eburnation of bone and cyst formation.
5. Disorganization.

Breakdown of articular surface

Degenerative osteoarthritis begins with failure of the articular surface (Fig. 16.2). The normal smooth surface of articular cartilage is breached, the arcades of collagen fibres break and the surface becomes rough, like a shaggy carpet. Friction against the rough surface generates particles of articular cartilage that are shed into the joint and absorbed by the synovium, where they cause an inflammatory response which the patient feels as stiffness or aching in the joint after exercise rather than at the time of use.

Synovial irritation

The irritation of the synovium is probably due to the release of intracellular enzymes, including lysozymes, which produce hyperaemia and a cellular response in the synovial layers. The synovium can also produce degradative enzymes and mediators such as interleukin-1, which may influence chondrocyte activity. Other potential causes of damage include free radicals and the deposition of immune complexes.

Remodelling

Limited cartilage repair can occur. Superficial lesions of articular cartilage show little healing but deep lesions that penetrate cortical bone allow the influx of marrow cells and the formation of fibrocartilage. Hyaline cartilage, however, is a once-in-a-lifetime tissue and does not regenerate.

The subchondral bone is also abnormally active, with an increase in both the density of the tissue and the number of cells. At the margin of the joint, new bone forms as osteophytes covered by fibrocartilage, perhaps induced by wear particles swept to the edge of the joint by joint movement. There, the osteophytes restrict joint movement.

A line of dense, hard, resilient bone forms just below the cartilage and the joint 'remodels' so that there is a change in shape and congruity. This alters the pattern of weight-bearing, which in turn means that the load is taken by different areas of articular cartilage.

Eburnation of bone and cyst formation

If the joint is rested, the wear particles are gradually absorbed. Fibrous tissue may form in the defect on the joint surface but as time goes by this repair process gradually fails and the articular surface is eroded to expose subchondral bone, which subsequently becomes polished and eburnated.

Raw bone rubbing against raw bone is painful. The eburnated bone is not as slippery as healthy articular cartilage, friction across the joint is increased and weight transmission across the joint becomes uneven. This change overloads some parts of the joint surface and microfractures occur in the trabeculae of the cancellous bone.

The microfractures heal with callus, which increases the rigidity of the bone so that the bone gradually becomes denser, more sclerotic and less resilient. This, in turn, causes more microfractures and the normal architecture of the bone is lost.

At this stage, synovial fluid enters the cancellous bone under pressure through cracks in the articular surface, producing cavities that are seen radiologically as 'cysts'. These cysts fill with fibrous tissue and become lined with a thin shell of cortical bone.

Disorganization

As the disease advances, the joint becomes progressively stiffer and more deformed as the osteophytes enlarge and the bone surfaces are worn away. The ball and socket of the hip is gradually converted into a roller bearing and hinge joints develop a valgus or varus deformity as one side is worn away.

As bone is lost the ligaments become looser, not because they lengthen but because the bones that they support become shorter.

Radiological appearance

The radiological appearance of osteoarthritis reflects these pathological changes (Fig. 16.3). The joint

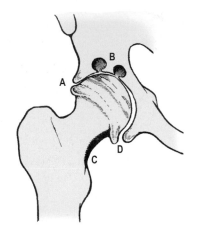

Fig. 16.3 Radiological appearances of osteoarthritis: (A) narrowing of the joint space; (B) cysts; (C) sclerosis; (D) osteophytes.

spaces narrow, the weight-bearing surface becomes sclerotic, osteophytes form around the joint margins and cysts are seen in the subchondral bone. The shape of the bone slowly alters and this deformity can be seen radiologically as well as clinically (Fig. 16.4).

Clinical presentation

The symptoms of osteoarthritis vary from joint to joint but there are three principal features:

1. Pain.
2. Loss of movement.
3. Altered function.

Pain

Pain is worse when the joint is under load and is greatest in the weight-bearing joints of the lower limb. Wear particles cause synovitis after the exercise has ceased. The weekend golfer may experience no pain during the game but will find that the joints are stiff after rest and painful after activity in the early part of the following week.

Loss of movement

Movement is lost as osteophytes form and the joint changes shape. This occurs so slowly that few patients notice any sudden change.

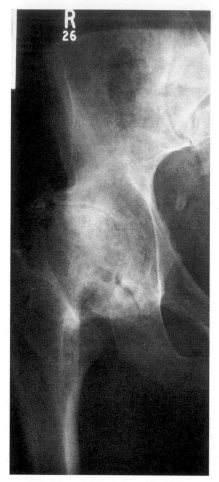

Fig. 16.4 Radiograph of a hip with osteoarthritis.

Altered function

Alterations of joint function occur imperceptibly. Without being aware of it, patients may subconsciously restrict their activities to those that the joints permit. They may choose not to walk as far as they once did, or not to work for as long or as hard without a pause. These limitations gradually increase.

Upper and lower limb osteoarthritis

The progress of osteoarthrosis is different in weight-bearing and non-weight-bearing joints. Weight-bearing joints in the lower limb are subjected to greater load and are more painful than those of the upper limb. Deformities are more apparent and restriction of function is severe.

In contrast, osteoarthritis of the upper limb causes little pain because the joints are seldom under load, but the shape of the joints is unsightly and loss of movement may be disabling.

These differences are important in selecting management. In the lower limb the aim is a joint that will take load without causing pain. Restoration of movement is more important in the upper limbs.

Treatment

Any condition can be treated conservatively or operatively. Osteoarthritis is no exception.

Conservative treatment

Conservative treatment includes the following measures:

1. Explanation of the condition and reassurance.
2. Advice to keep active but modify activities to avoid those things that hurt or aggravate the problem or overload the joint. If it hurts, don't do it.
3. A walking stick and aids in the home.
4. Physiotherapy to maintain muscle bulk and joint movement.
5. Drugs, especially intermittent analgesics and NSAIDs.
6. Very occasional intra-articular steroid injections.

Explanation is important

When patients learn that they have 'arthritis', they see wheelchairs. It is essential to dispel this misconception and adopt a positive approach. Osteoarthritis is not a 'disease' like rheumatoid arthritis; it is simply a patch of fair wear and tear that will probably get very slowly worse over many years and cause some limitation of activity. Widespread and severe osteoarthritis can be disabling but this is fairly uncommon.

Modification of activity

If patients only experience pain during a certain activity they may be able to modify activities to avoid the one that hurts. If a patient with osteoarthritis of the elbow only has pain when clipping the hedge, for example, the simplest solution might be to cut down the hedge or buy an electric hedge-clipper. Similarly, patients with osteoarthritis of the hip who can walk only a few yards are able to cycle for long distances without pain, and a bicycle can solve many of their problems.

These are commonsense solutions that many patients will find without consulting their doctor but they should always be considered before advising operation.

Appliances and aids

Aids such as sticks, elbow crutches or a walking frame are helpful to patients with osteoarthritis of the lower limbs. A tall chair is better for patients who lack full flexion of the hips and the knees, both of which are necessary to sit in a comfortable or 'easy' chair. The same patients are also helped by a high seat when using the lavatory (Fig. 16.5).

Osteoarthritis of the knee or hip can produce real or apparent shortening of the limb. A raise to the heel and sole of the shoe on the shorter side will make good this shortening. Although it will not alter the progress of the disease, the raise will improve the gait and take the strain off other joints and the lumbar spine.

Physiotherapy

Heat treatment by ice, infrared lamps or short-wave diathermy will often produce relief for many months.

Exercises to increase the power of muscles around osteoarthritic joints are of limited value. It is not possible to 'compensate' for worn joints by increasing the strength of the muscles that operate them,

any more than it is possible to improve the body-work of a rusty car by putting in a more powerful engine. It is, however, useful to increase the range of movement in degenerate joints and prevent contractures. Many patients understandably avoid moving their painful joints and function deteriorates; the more painful the joints, the less they are moved, the stiffer they become, the less they are moved, and so on. If the joints are put through their full range of movement every day, function is maintained and stiffness avoided.

Drugs

Both analgesics and anti-inflammatory drugs are available but many drugs act in both ways.

Non-steroidal anti-inflammatory drugs. NSAIDs include fenamate derivatives such as flurbiprofen, ibuprofen, naproxen and mefenamic acid. These drugs are prostaglandin inhibitors and reduce the inflammatory response of the synovium to articular cartilage debris. Aspirin is also a prostaglandin inhibitor as well as an analgesic and should not be underestimated.

These drugs do not abolish pain but they reduce it effectively. They do not affect the articular surfaces but the response of the synovium to wear particles of articular cartilage is reduced. Some patients learn to take their anti-inflammatory drugs before physical activity; the weekend golfer may take tablets on Saturday morning to reduce the inflammatory response that will be felt on Sunday and Monday.

Almost all NSAIDs cause gastrointestinal problems and should be taken either with food or with

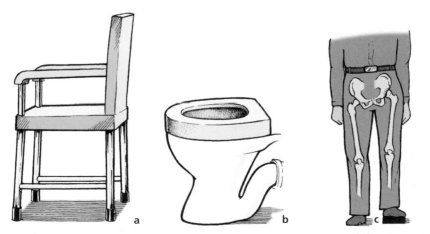

Fig. 16.5 Aids for osteoarthritis of the hip: (a) firm chair with arm supports; (b) a high seat to avoid excessive flexion of the hip; (c) raise the shoe to correct shortening.

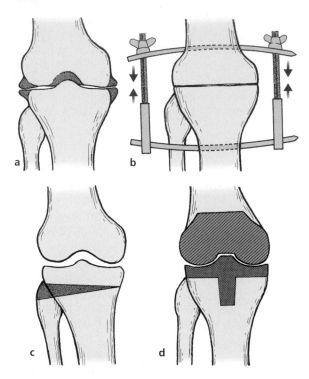

Fig. 16.6 Operations for osteoarthritis: (a) debridement and removal of osteophytes; (b) arthrodesis; (c) osteotomy to correct alignment; (d) total joint replacement.

anti-inflammatory drugs taken at bedtime, perhaps with a mild hypnotic, can be helpful.

Steroid injections are helpful for areas of extra-articular inflammation, particularly along joint margins or over osteophytes, but intra-articular injections are less effective. The steroid can reduce the intra-articular inflammation but the results are transient and leave the underlying pathology unchanged. Intra-articular steroids are given more often by rheumatologists than surgeons.

Operative treatment

Operative treatment should only be considered if conservative measures have failed. The operations can be divided into four groups (Fig. 16.6), described below:

1. Debridement.
2. Arthrodesis.
3. Osteotomy.
4. Arthroplasty.

Debridement

Osteophytes are the most obvious radiological abnormality and it is tempting to remove them in the hope that the radiological appearance, and thus the patient, will be restored to normal. Although the osteophytes can be removed, they quickly recur and the benefit from this procedure is transient.

If the osteophytes seriously obstruct joint movement it is reasonable to excise them. Excision of the osteophytes also improves the appearance, which can be important in the hand where the osteophytes around the distal interphalangeal joints may be very unsightly.

Arthrodesis

Arthrodesis, the fusion of a joint, is one of the oldest operations in orthopaedic surgery and converts a stiff painful joint in bad position into a stiff, painless joint in good position. This is a fair exchange.

Arthrodesis is useful for small joints in the hand, fingers and toes, where the loss of movement in one joint can be disguised by the movement of others. In larger joints the operation has more far-reaching effects. An arthrodesed knee, for example, is good for walking but will not bend when the patient sits down, and creates particular problems when getting out of a car or using a lavatory.

milk and biscuits. This gastrointestinal irritation is partly a systemic phenomenon and cannot be avoided by giving the drug parenterally or by suppository, although this can lessen the problem. In the elderly, NSAIDs may cause confusion.

NSAIDs can depress chondrocyte activity and this may cause the disease to progress more rapidly, especially in weight-bearing joints such as the hip. Because of this, NSAIDs should be given intermittently and cautiously, with courses during exacerbations and at important times for the patient, such as golf tournaments.

Analgesics. Simple analgesics such as paracetamol or dihydrocodeine have an analgesic effect only, but reduce the pain caused by raw bone rubbing on raw bone. They do not reduce the synovitis of osteoarthritis. Comparative studies suggest that NSAIDs are more effective than simple analgesics, but in practice the best results may be achieved by a combination of paracetamol with an NSAID.

In some patients with severe osteoarthritis, pain interferes with sleep and the plight of these patients is made worse by perpetual tiredness. Analgesics or

Arthrodesis should not be performed unless the neighbouring joints are healthy and have a good range of movement. A stiff hip and knee, or two stiff hips, creates great difficulty in walking and getting out of a chair. Abnormal strains are placed on the neighbouring joints in the lumbar spine and the ankle and these joints develop degenerative change.

Accordingly, arthrodesis is best suited to degenerative disease affecting a single joint surrounded by joints that are healthy and likely to stay healthy. It is contraindicated in diseases such as rheumatoid arthritis where many joints are involved.

If arthrodesis is carried out, the joint should be fixed in the position of function; i.e. the most useful position. To be sure that the patient will be pleased with the result it is advisable to apply a cast in the proposed position before operation, so that they can use the limb as if it were arthrodesed and assess the likely benefits for themselves.

Osteotomy

Osteotomy helps osteoarthritic joints in three ways:

1. Correcting the deformity.
2. Altering the architecture at the site of healing.
3. Dividing intraosseous vessels.

Correcting the deformity reduces the abnormal loads across the joints. This is important in the weight-bearing joints of the lower limb, where the hip, knee and ankle should be one above the other in the same vertical line. Correction of the line of weight-bearing does not 'cure' osteoarthritis but can slow the deterioration.

Altering the bone architecture. Cutting across the bone allows some remodelling to occur at the fracture site.

Dividing vessels. Osteotomy divides the medullary cavity of the bone, including the venous channels, and this may have some effect on pain.

Disadvantages of osteotomy. The operation causes considerable discomfort, requires a long period of rehabilitation, and the symptoms can recur. In its favour, the operation does not destroy the joint irreparably, as does an arthrodesis or an arthroplasty, and a second operation is always possible.

Arthroplasty

Arthroplasty means the creation of a joint; several types are available.

Types of arthroplasty

1. Excision arthroplasty.
2. Interposition arthroplasty.
3. Mould arthroplasty.
4. Replacement arthroplasty, including hemiarthroplasty and total replacement.

Excision arthroplasty replaces the normal joint with a fibrous ankylosis with less movement and less stability than a normal joint. Excision arthroplasty is therefore unsuitable for weight-bearing joints, but is effective in those that do not bear weight, e.g. the toe.

Disadvantages are that pain can arise in the new 'joint' from bone-to-bone contact across the pseudarthrosis and the instability can be distressing to the patient. The advantages are that no foreign material is inserted and the complications of infection and loosening are reduced.

Interposition arthroplasty. The formation of a pseudarthrosis can be encouraged by placing something between the bone ends. Skin, fascia and muscle have all been used but the results are little different from a straightforward excision arthroplasty.

An inert spacer, such as Silastic, can also be used as an interposition material. The results are better but the wear particles of the material can be an irritant and the joint is still unstable.

Mould arthroplasty. A hard material, such as metal, placed between the bone ends can act as a mould to shape a new joint. The idea is simple in principle but in practice the joints become stiff and the bone inside the mould can undergo aseptic necrosis. Cup arthroplasty of the hip was a good example but has now been replaced by total hip replacement.

Replacement arthroplasty. If the worn joint surfaces are removed and replaced by a prosthesis, a stable and painless joint resembling the original can be created. Two types of replacement arthroplasty are in current use:

1. *Hemiarthroplasty.* If only one joint surface is replaced the early results are good but the prosthetic material is likely to wear away the opposite joint surface.

   Hemiarthroplasty is useful in femoral neck fractures, which almost invariably occur in patients in whom the joint is healthy. In patients with osteoarthritis and an abnormal acetabulum, hemiarthroplasty has been abandoned.

2. *Total replacement arthroplasty*. If both surfaces are replaced, the result is anatomically better than a hemiarthroplasty and would be the ideal operation if the results were consistently good. This is not so. If the joint becomes infected or the components loosen (p. 398), the results are poor and may be worse than before operation.

Salvage of a loose or infected prosthesis is difficult. Excision arthroplasty is always available but is not ideal in weight-bearing joints because so much bone must be removed that later arthrodesis is impossible. In some circumstances amputation may be necessary as a salvage procedure.

Summary

- Drugs and operation are sometimes needed for patients with osteoarthritis, but not always.
- Management depends on careful assessment of the precise local and general problems for the individual patient.
- Simple non-invasive measures are often the best.
- Much depends on a positive and optimistic approach.
- Polypharmacy and multiple operations should be avoided but the belief that 'nothing can be done' may be just as damaging.

Chapter |17|

Rheumatoid arthritis and other arthropathies

By the end of this chapter you should be able to:

- Distinguish inflammatory arthropathies from those caused by wear and tear.
- Understand the destructive nature of the disease process on the joints and soft tissues.
- Order the correct investigations to make the diagnosis and be aware of the medical and surgical treatment options.

Rheumatoid arthritis

Rheumatoid arthritis is an autoimmune disease that causes chronic inflammation and destruction of synovial joints. It is the commonest chronic inflammatory disease of joints, and affects 3% of women and 1% of men. The inflammation is a result of an abnormality of both cellular and humoral immunity but the cause of the disease itself is still unknown.

Because it is a systemic disease, many different structures all over the body are affected, in contrast to osteoarthritis, which is due to localized mechanical wear. Although rheumatoid arthritis is primarily treated by rheumatologists and described more fully in medical texts, it frequently involves orthopaedic surgeons and the orthopaedic aspects are described here.

Pathology

Rheumatoid arthritis is primarily a disease of the synovium. Affected synovium contains plasma cells and lymphocytes, a reflection of the autoimmune nature of the disease. The aetiology has been thought to be associated with an infectious origin, or possibly genetic (an abnormal HLA-Dw4 focus). Regardless of the exact trigger mechanism, lymphocytes are activated and chemical messengers initiate destructive cascades that may ultimately lead to joint destruction. These chemicals include phospholipase A2, tumor necrosis factor (TNF), plasminogen activators and interleukin-1 (IL1).

Untreated, the synovium swelling and inflammatory reaction gradually affect neighbouring structures. Articular cartilage is damaged and the surrounding ligaments may become lax, and bone destruction makes these even looser.

Ultimately, there is destruction of joint cartilage, capsule and ligaments, which causes instability, mechanical disarray, subluxation and deformity (Figs 17.1, 17.2).

Clinical features

This is often of insidious onset with morning stiffness and polyarthritis. It most commonly affects the

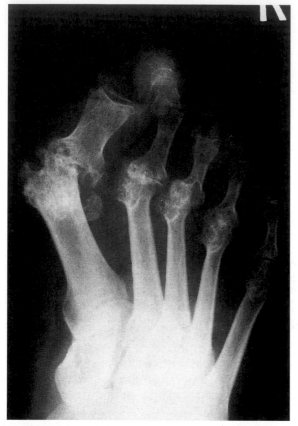

Fig. 17.1 Rheumatoid arthritis of the foot with destruction of the small joints.

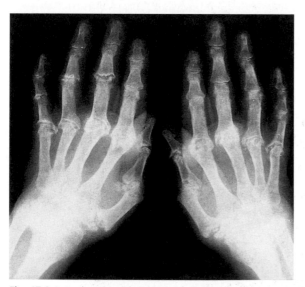

Fig. 17.2 Late rheumatoid arthritis of the hands with destruction of the small joints.

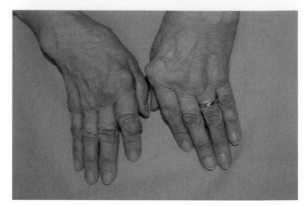

Fig. 17.3 Rheumatoid of the hand and wrist with characteristic deviation and swelling.

small joints of young adults between the ages of 15 and 35. Women are more commonly affected than men.

The disease begins with swelling of the small joints of the hands and feet, and the pannus ingrowth gradually denudes articular cartilage and leads to chondrocyte death. The synovial swelling is best seen in the fingers and the valleys between the metacarpal heads (Fig. 17.3).

Because rheumatoid arthritis is a systemic disease, it also involves extra-articular structures. Rheumatoid nodules form in the subcutaneous tissues and may need to be excised if they rupture or lie on the subcutaneous border of the forearm, where they interfere with the use of crutches (Fig. 17.4). They are, however, prone to recurrence. The skin becomes thin and fragile and this makes wound healing difficult and unpredictable. The sclera of the eye and cardiac muscle can also be affected.

The progress of the disease is variable. Patients experience occasional 'flare-ups' relieved by drugs and rest. A small minority develop the crippling deformities that make rheumatoid arthritis such a disabling disease.

Investigations

The diagnosis of rheumatoid arthritis is essentially clinical. A useful screening tool is the inclusion of one or more of the following:

1. Morning stiffness > 1 h.
2. Swelling (synovitis).
3. Characteristic distribution of joints.
4. ESR 20 mm/h.
5. Nodules.

6. Positive laboratory tests.
7. Radiographic findings – erosions of hands and feet.
8. Non-steroidal anti-inflammatory drugs are beneficial.
9. First degree relative with inflammatory joint disease.

The earliest radiographic changes are seen around the small joints of the hands and feet, where erosions occur at the carpometacarpal and interphalangeal joints (Fig. 17.5). Periarticular erosions and osteopenia are probably the first signs.

Because rheumatoid arthritis is due to an abnormality of the autoimmune system, the ESR and CRP are raised, along with various agglutination tests, such as sheep cell agglutination test (SCAT) and latex tests. Thirty percent of patients test negative despite having the typical clinical appearance of rheumatoid arthritis. Such patients are said to have 'seronegative' rheumatoid arthritis. The rheumatoid factor (antibody test) is positive in 80%.

Recently, anti-cyclic citrullinated peptide (anti-CCP) antibody elevation has been shown to be more sensitive and specific than the rheumatoid factor. These antibodies may be present in 50–60% of patients with early signs of the disease (before rheumatoid factor becomes positive). Their use may help stage the disease and give an accurate prognosis with treatment.

Systemic manifestations include pericarditis and pulmonary disease (pleurisy, nodules and fibrosis). Popliteal cysts in rheumatoids can mimic thrombophlebitis or, when ruptured, a deep vein thrombosis. Felty's syndrome includes an enlargement of the spleen and leucopenia. Still's disease is a rapid onset of rheumatoid arthritis associated with a fever, rash and splenomegaly. When associated with

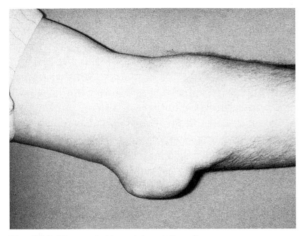

Fig. 17.4 Rheumatoid nodules at the elbow.

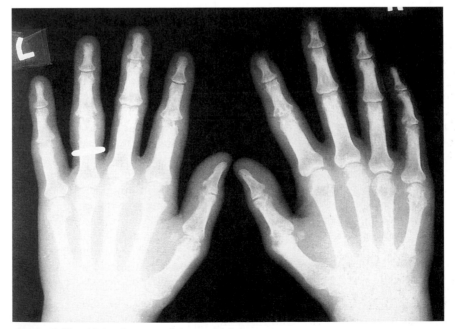

Fig. 17.5 Rheumatoid arthritis with involvement of the small joints.

inflammation of the glands of the eye and mouth giving dryness in these areas it is called Sjögren's syndrome.

Treatment

The aim of treatment is to control synovitis and pain as well as maintaining joint function and the prevention of long-term deformities. A multi-disciplinary approach between rheumatologists, orthopaedic surgeons and physical therapists is often necessary.

Conservative treatment

Conservative treatment of rheumatoid arthritis involves the use of the following:

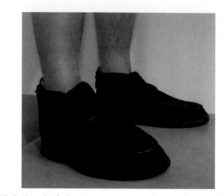

Fig. 17.6 Surgical shoes to accommodate a foot deformity.

> **Conservative measures in rheumatoid arthritis**
>
> 1. Drugs.
> 2. Rest during an attack and mobilization during remission.
> 3. Aids and appliances.

Non-steroidal anti-inflammatory drugs. These are the first line of treatment and include aspirin, ibuprofen, naproxen, etc. Patients may require steroids taken orally, or injected into affected joints in severe cases. These drugs help modify joint pain and inflammation.

Second line drugs or disease-modifying antirheumatic drugs (DMARDS) may help prevent joint destruction and subsequent deformity. These slow-acting drugs may take months to become effective and are often used for long periods of time, sometimes years. If effective, these DMARDS may promote remission, and they are often used in combination and together with first line drugs. Second-line drugs include quinine, sulfasalazine, gold, penicillamine or immunosuppressive therapies such as methotrexate, azathioprine and cyclophosphamide. Newer drugs aim to block the production of the inflammatory mediators such as tumor necrosis factor (antiTNF) and interleukin-1.

Rest and immobilization. Splintage and rest will also reduce the swelling of joints and it can induce remission of the disease in an acute attack. Rest may require admission to hospital. Restoration of joint movement by physiotherapy when the attack has passed is essential.

Aids and appliances. Patients with rheumatoid arthritis need a host of appliances. Sticks, frames and crutches take the weight of lower limbs; splints and braces protect painful joints from unnecessary movement; and soft protective footwear relieves the pressure on vulnerable skin (Fig. 17.6).

Operative treatment

Operative treatment may be required for three reasons, but only if medical treatment has failed.

> **Indications for operations in rheumatoid arthritis**
>
> 1. To remove inflamed synovium by synovectomy.
> 2. To repair damaged soft tissue.
> 3. To salvage destroyed joints.

Synovectomy. If conservative measures do not reduce the synovial swelling, a surgical synovectomy may be required. Unless done arthroscopically this is an extensive operation and requires considerable rehabilitation. Once done, the joint is less liable to flare-ups of the disease in the future and progression of the disease may slow. Synovium can also be removed from around the tendon sheaths, and at the wrist this may reduce the risk of future tendon rupture.

Repair. Ruptured extensor tendons at the wrist need to be repaired and unstable metacarpophalangeal joints stabilized by soft tissue procedures. Rheumatoid nodules and cysts around the joints, such as popliteal cysts at the knee, may need excision.

Salvage. In late rheumatoid arthritis with destroyed joints, salvage operations are necessary. Joint replacement is effective in the weight-bearing joints of the lower limb. Arthrodesis may be the treatment of choice at the wrist and in other joints of the upper limb, although more recently replacement procedures have proved to be effective, in the shoulder and elbow in particular. Spinal fusion is sometimes needed for instability of the cervical spine or segments.

Operating on a patient with widespread joint destruction has far-reaching effects on other joints as well, and the impact of the operation on the patient as a whole must be carefully considered. Surgery should never be undertaken for patients with rheumatoid arthritis without careful assessment. This may not be possible in a single outpatient consultation. Assessment requires many visits to the physiotherapist or occupational therapy department to determine the operation most likely to bring long-standing relief.

Undiagnosed joint pain

Many patients in the second and third decades of life develop symmetrical pains in the small joints of the hands and feet or, less often, the large joints and are referred to a rheumatologist. The majority of these patients, perhaps as many as 80%, yield no abnormality on thorough investigation. Most patients make a complete recovery over a period of months or years and do not have rheumatoid arthritis.

Other arthropathies

Crystal arthropathies

Crystals can be deposited in joints or soft tissue because of a metabolic abnormality. The accumulation of crystals probably begins in infancy but is not usually apparent until the third or fourth decade. Deposits of crystals in and around joints often remain asymptomatic but they can also cause two types of arthritis:

1. Acute self-limiting attacks of inflammation.
2. Chronic destructive joint disease.

Gout

The commonest and best known crystal arthropathy is gout, in which urate crystals are deposited (Fig.

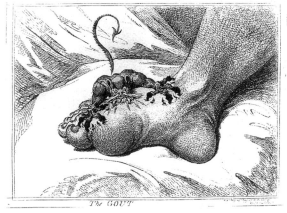

Fig. 17.7 The gout. James Gillray, 1799. By kind permission of the Wellcome Institute Library, London.

17.7). Traditionally, the condition affects the first metatarsophalangeal joint and is precipitated by an excess of red meat or port wine. This bucolic image is incorrect; the condition can occur at any age and diet is only rarely involved. Dehydration following major trauma or operation, soft tissue destruction caused by chemotherapy or radiotherapy for malignant disease, and the use of diuretics in the elderly are more frequent precipitating factors. Alcohol abuse is but one cause of dehydration.

These conditions are most often seen and treated by the rheumatologists but it is important for orthopaedic surgeons to be aware of them because the painful swollen joints can present to an orthopaedic clinic and be mistaken for septic arthritis or an internal mechanical derangement.

Treatment of the acute attack is by anti-inflammatory drugs. Indometacin 50 mg three times daily usually produces dramatic relief but systemic steroids are sometimes required. Aspiration of the knee and irrigation is helpful and allows the joint fluid to be centrifuged and examined for cells and crystals. Polymorphs are usually seen, and birefringent crystals are sometimes identified under polarized light.

If the attacks recur, long-term treatment with allopurinol may be helpful and this is best conducted by a rheumatologist.

Pyrophosphate and hydroxyapatite deposition (pseudogout)

Atypical gout (pseudogout) produces a similar clinical picture to gout but the crystals involved are

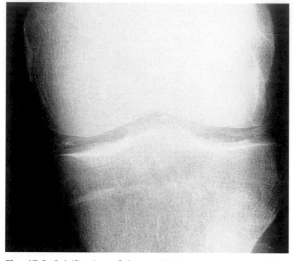

Fig. 17.8 Calcification of the menisci.

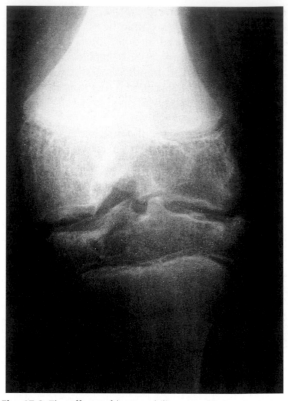

Fig. 17.9 The effects of haemophiliac synovitis.

calcium pyrophosphate. Both pyrophosphate and hydroxyapatite deposition may follow either local or systemic disorders and be associated with acute inflammatory synovitis or chronic joint destruction (Fig. 17.8).

Treatment is similar to that for gout but long-term treatment with allopurinol is not effective.

Psoriatic arthropathy

Psoriatic arthropathy can involve the small joints of the hands and feet but can also cause a large effusion in a single joint. Beware of the patient with psoriasis who has a swollen joint without obvious explanation: operation is unlikely to be helpful.

Treatment is similar to rheumatoid arthritis, but the condition is seldom as severe.

Haemophiliac arthropathy

Bleeding disorders of any type can cause recurrent intra-articular haemorrhage into any joint but the knee is most often affected (Fig. 17.9). The blood causes a synovitis and leads to pigmentation of the synovium. The articular cartilage is also involved and develops craters and pot-holes filled with dark brown synovial fronds. In time the subsynovial layers become fibrotic, the capsule loses its flexibility and the articular surfaces undergo degenerative change.

Diagnosis is usually simple because most haemophiliacs know they have the condition and carry a card with details of the exact diagnosis and the treatment they have received.

Treatment. Most patients nowadays have a supply of cryoprecipitate which they administer themselves at the first sign of bleeding into a joint.

If this is not the case, the first step is to rest the limb and contact the haematologist in charge of treatment. The appropriate clotting factors are then administered and the joint aspirated when it is safe to do so.

If the joint develops a proliferative synovitis that never really settles, recurrent bleeding is likely. In some circumstances it is possible to remove the affected synovium but this is a hazardous undertaking in a haemophiliac unless the synovectomy is done arthroscopically. At the knee, arthroscopic synovectomy yields good results in selected patients.

Remember that many unfortunate haemophiliacs have become infected with the HIV or hepatitis virus through blood products such as cryoprecipitate. Special care must be taken to avoid accidental infection of those caring for these patients.

Pigmented villonodular synovitis (PVNS)

Any chronic synovitis accompanied by recurrent small bleeds stains the synovium dark and causes thickening of the deep layers with patches of proliferative synovial villi. The synovium becomes pigmented, nodular and villous. PVNS is essentially a macroscopic description of the end result of chronic synovitis and recurrent bleeding rather than a separate disease entity.

Treatment. The condition usually settles slowly with time, but recovery can be hastened by excising inflamed areas, if possible by arthroscopy. If the inflammation cannot be controlled, a persistent synovitis a little like haemophilic synovitis will follow.

Synovial chondromatosis

Any joint may be affected by synovial chondromatosis, in which masses of articular cartilage develop either in the synovium or within the synovial cavity. These cartilage masses may become ossified, and appear as multiple loose bodies (Fig. 17.10). If the symptoms are severe, the abnormal tissue must be removed, but recurrence is common.

Bone necrosis

Bone necrosis can occur from the following causes:

1. Corticosteroid administration.
2. Blood dyscrasias (such as sickle cell disease and thalassaemia).
3. Gaucher's disease.
4. Alcoholism.
5. Caisson disease.
6. Spontaneous osteonecrosis.

Steroid necrosis. High doses of corticosteroids are sometimes necessary after transplant surgery or to suppress the immune response for other reasons, and may be accompanied by separation of large fragments of bone (Fig. 17.11). The separated fragments are avascular but the exact pathogenesis is unclear.

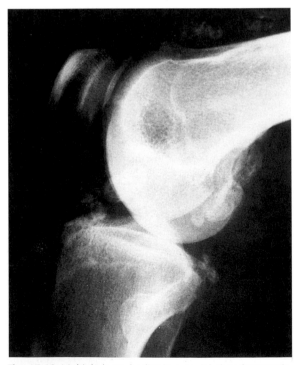

Fig. 17.10 Multiple loose bodies in synovial chondromatosis.

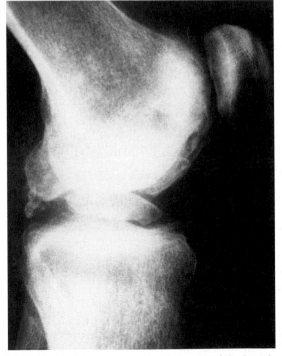

Fig. 17.11 Steroid osteonecrosis. A fragment of the lateral femoral condyle has separated and is lying with the convex femoral surface facing upwards.

The condition causes permanent damage to the joint and replacement may be needed.

Blood dyscrasias. Patients with homozygous sickle cell disease, or occasionally patients with thalassaemia, are susceptible to episodes of spontaneous bone necrosis. This can follow periods of anoxia but can also occur without obvious cause.

Gaucher's disease. This is a rare cause of bone necrosis but should be remembered, if only for examination purposes.

Alcoholism. Alcohol abuse can lead to necrosis of the femoral heads and occasionally the weight-bearing parts of other joints. The diagnosis is often difficult because of the patient's denial of the problem.

Caisson disease. 'Caisson' does not refer to a person and to talk of 'Caisson's' disease is incorrect. A *caisson* is a large metal vessel placed under water and filled with compressed air so that labourers can work within it for tunnelling and bridge-building projects. The workers may develop decompression sickness when they come to the surface, gas bubbles form within the bones and bone necrosis follows. The condition is now more commonly seen in deep-sea divers and may occur even in the presence of strict decompression procedures.

Spontaneous osteonecrosis can occur for no obvious reason, particularly at the knee. The condition is described on page 419.

Neuropathic arthropathy

Joints with deficient sensory innervation develop a rapidly progressive destructive arthropathy. It is suggested that the denervation allows the patient to apply enormous loads to the joint without the protection of normal reflexes, but other factors may be involved.

The condition was described by Charcot in patients with tabes dorsalis, in whom the condition can correctly be called a 'Charcot joint'.

Neuropathic joints can be seen whenever a joint is denervated, but the following are the commonest causes:

1. Diabetes mellitus.
2. Syringomyelia.
3. Late syphilis.
4. Denervated limbs.

A similar appearance is seen in patients taking large doses of analgesic and anti-inflammatory drugs,

perhaps because they also lack the sensory arm of their protective reflexes.

Clinically, the joints are swollen, grossly unstable, inflamed and painless. Radiological examination shows widespread bone destruction and loss of bone architecture.

Treatment. There is no treatment for a neuropathic joint except stabilization in a caliper or orthosis. Operation should not be attempted on a neuropathic joint because arthrodeses do not join and prostheses tear out of the bone.

Reiter's disease

Reiter's disease is acquired through sexual contact or as a sequel to dysentery and includes the following features:

1. Conjunctivitis.
2. Urethritis.
3. Synovitis.

The condition can affect any joint but the small joints of the hands and feet are most often involved. Large joints such as the knee are affected less often. The diagnosis should be considered in any patient, especially men, with these symptoms.

Treatment. The condition usually resolves spontaneously but anti-inflammatory drugs are helpful.

Arthropathies following infection

Brucellosis, typhoid and viral illnesses can all be followed by generalized joint disease resembling rheumatoid arthritis. The orthopaedic surgeon need not become involved in the management of these difficult problems but must always be aware that a single painful joint can be the first manifestation of a generalized joint disorder and should avoid operating without good reason.

Ankylosing spondylitis

Ankylosing spondylitis is essentially a disease of the spine (p. 455) but it also involves the large joints, such as hip, knee and shoulder. The disease is commoner in men than women by 6:1 and usually presents between the ages of 15 and 30 years.

Treatment consists of anti-inflammatory drugs and physiotherapy. Cervical and lumbar osteotomy may be needed for late deformities. Joint replacement is often unsuccessful because the new joints also become ankylosed.

Reflex sympathetic dystrophy

This should be called a complex regional pain syndrome as there were previously a number of terms describing the same process. They included causalgia, Sudek's atrophy (e.g. following a Colles fracture, p. 215), post-traumatic dystrophy, shoulder–hand syndrome, algodystrophy, algoneurodystrophy and reflex sympathetic dystrophy. Regional pain syndrome can be further divided into two types: type 1 with features not associated with a specific nerve injury and type 2 with a specific nerve (more akin to the condition previously described as causalgia). Both types present with an exaggerated pain response, intolerance of temperature and often a blotchy discoloration of the skin. There may also be colour changes on the limb, usually blue or purple patches. The condition can be precipitated by trauma of any kind, including operation.

The syndrome can be made worse by trauma, even by a trivial procedure such as arthroscopy. For this reason, operations should not be undertaken on painful joints that go cold or blue and have no mechanical symptoms.

Investigations are usually unhelpful. A thermogram may show an altered pattern but radiographs are normal except in very late cases when there is osteoporosis.

Treatment

Transcutaneous electric nerve stimulators, beta blockers and guanethidine injections to the affected limb are often helpful and chemical sympathectomy is sometimes required. Calcitonin has been shown to be of value. Physiotherapy and joint mobilization are vital. Prolonged bracing will only lead to stiffness and muscle wasting.

Monarticular synovitis in a large joint

Many patients present with pain and swelling confined to one joint without any history of injury or mechanical symptoms. The common causes are as follows:

1. A mechanical derangement. In the knee, a torn meniscus or defect in the articular cartilage is often responsible.
2. Gout or pseudogout.
3. A disorder of synovium, such as ankylosing spondylitis or rheumatoid arthritis.
4. Psoriatic arthropathy. Always ask a patient with acute monarticular synovitis if they have psoriasis or any other rash.
5. Reiter's disease.
6. Septic arthritis, including gonococcal arthritis.
7. Osteoarthritis. Osteoarthritis is perhaps the commonest cause of pain and swelling in a large joint. Quite severe degenerative changes can be present before any abnormality can be seen on the radiograph.
8. Synovial chondromatosis (p. 307).
9. Spontaneous osteonecrosis (p. 307).

Chapter 18

Bone and joint infections

By the end of this chapter you should be able to:

- Understand the pathology and process of inflammation.
- Understand the severity of the joint destruction caused by infection and therefore appreciate the urgency of making the correct diagnosis and instituting the correct treatment.
- Remember the worldwide problem of tuberculosis.

Acute osteomyelitis

Bone infection usually involves the bone marrow and is therefore called osteomyelitis. The disease can be acute or chronic.

Acute osteomyelitis is seen in both children and adults. In days past it was a common cause of disease and death but in the last 50 years it has become both less common and less serious.

Pathology

The disease begins with an infection in the juxta-epiphyseal region of the bone. The symptoms often begin after minor trauma, perhaps because the trauma creates a small haematoma from rupture of the very profuse blood vessels near the epiphyseal plate. The haematoma provides an ideal breeding ground for bacteria reaching it from the bloodstream.

Clinical features

As the infection proceeds, the patient becomes ill and pyrexial and develops excruciating pain because of the tissue tension within the bone. Untreated, the infection spreads until it erodes the surrounding bone and eventually the cortex, allowing pus to strip the periosteum off the bone, and forms a subperiosteal abscess (Fig. 18.1). The pus will eventually discharge through the skin, leaving a bone abscess discharging through a sinus. At this stage the patient has chronic osteomyelitis.

If the epiphyseal plate lies inside a joint the pus will discharge not through skin but into the joint, causing a septic arthritis. The following joints can become infected in this way (Fig. 18.2):

1. Hip.
2. Knee.
3. Shoulder.
4. Elbow.
5. Wrist.

Treatment

In the first few days of the disease, when there is a hot tender bone and a pyrexia, the child should be admitted to hospital, the limb elevated and blood

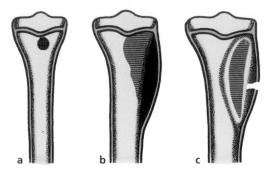

Fig. 18.1 Progress of osteomyelitis: (a) small septic focus next to the epiphyseal plate; (b) collection of pus beneath the periosteum; (c) pus has drained through the skin and an abscess cavity in the bone communicates with skin.

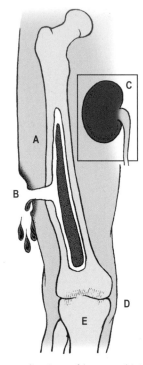

Fig. 18.3 Late complications of bone and joint sepsis: (A) involucrum, sequestrum and sinus; (B) squamous carcinoma at the margin of the sinus; (C) amyloid disease; (D) ankylosed joint following septic arthritis; (E) deformity from growth arrest.

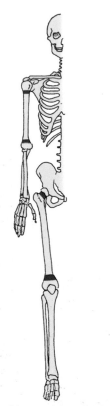

Fig. 18.2 Joints susceptible to septic arthritis.

sent to the laboratory for haemoglobin, ESR, white cell count and blood culture. Only when the blood culture specimens are safely in the laboratory should antibiotic therapy be given.

The antibiotics given should be the 'best guess' based on the prevalent organisms in the hospital and neighbourhood. A good microbiologist will know the most likely organism to cause bone infec-

tion in the area, but *Staphylococcus aureus* and *Haemophilus influenzae* are the usual culprits. A good antibiotic regimen is a combination of ampicillin 500 mg four times daily and flucloxacillin 500 mg four times daily, although 1 g four times daily may be needed.

If the patient is not clinically better after 2 days treatment and the pyrexia remains unchanged, the affected area of bone should be exposed and drilled to release pus.

Almost every patient with acute osteomyelitis can be cured in this way and chronic osteomyelitis has almost become a disease of the past in developed countries.

Brodie's abscess. Not all osteomyelitis behaves in this way. The infection can be partly overcome by natural defences and remain confined in an abscess lined by cortical bone. These lesions, called Brodie's abscesses, are visible radiologically as a small cavity and contain quiescent bacteria.

Chronic osteomyelitis

Chronic osteomyelitis, one of the grand old diseases of orthopaedic surgery a major cause of disability and crippling in the 19th century, is a complication of acute osteomyelitis in which the infection persists.

Pathology

Pus spreads under the periosteum around the cortex, which dies (Fig. 18.3). The periosteum then forms a 'new' bone around the abscess, leaving a mass of dead bone lying in a pocket of pus surrounded by living bone (Fig. 18.4). The dead bone, which is separate from the living and cannot be discharged from the body because it is too large to pass down the sinus, is called a **sequestrum**. The living bone surrounding it is the **involucrum**.

Clinical features

Without treatment, the patient is left with a large bony cavity containing pus and dead bone, communicating with the exterior through a sinus that discharges stinking pus and occasional pieces of dead bone, and requires regular dressing (Fig. 18.5). Apart from the misery of such a condition, there are serious complications:

1. Growth changes follow damage to the epiphyseal growth plates (Fig. 18.6).
2. The chronic infection leads to secondary amyloid disease.
3. The skin margins can undergo malignant change (Marjolin's ulcer).

Treatment

Today, many of the chronic sinuses can be healed by eradication of dead bone and correct antibiotic treatment. This sounds straightforward but, in some patients, to remove all the dead bone means excising a complete segment of bone, bridging the gap with external fixation, and grafting the defect when the infection has been eradicated. This is extensive surgery requiring prolonged admission to hospital

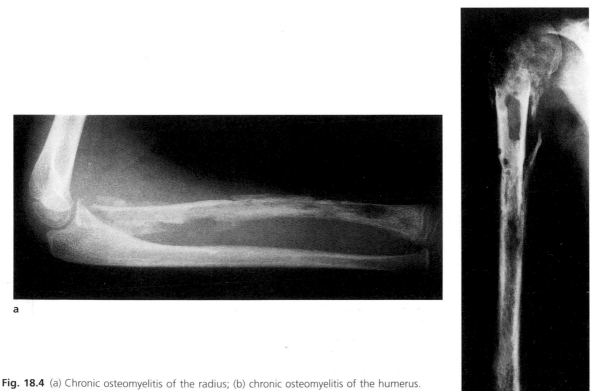

Fig. 18.4 (a) Chronic osteomyelitis of the radius; (b) chronic osteomyelitis of the humerus. The lesion has been drained with drill holes and windowing, but a large sequestrum of dead bone remains in the cavity of the involucrum.

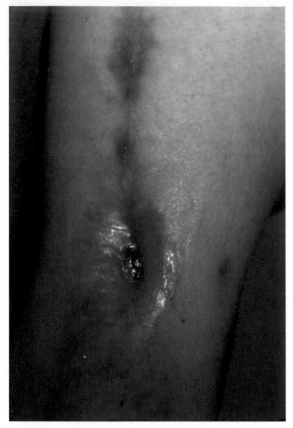

Fig. 18.5 A sinus from osteomyelitis which had been present for more than 20 years.

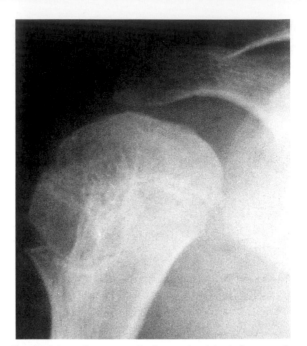

Fig. 18.6 Late damage to the humeral epiphysis from sepsis.

and antibiotics must be given in adequate doses for long periods, sometimes for a year or more.

Septic arthritis

Septic arthritis can arise in three ways:

1. Spread from an infected bone.
2. Direct infection from a penetrating wound.
3. Bacteraemia.

Clinical features

Septic arthritis should be suspected in any hot swollen joint, particularly if there is infection elsewhere or the patient is systemically ill.

Infected joints are extremely painful and the patient is systemically ill unless there is another debilitating condition, such as diabetes. This is an important exception because diabetic patients are particularly susceptible to infection. Any unexplained joint effusion in a diabetic should be aspirated and sent for culture.

Do not forget the gonococcus! The gonococcus has a special affinity for joints, hence its name, and should always be thought of when a young adult presents with septic arthritis.

Untreated, septic arthritis destroys articular cartilage and leads to a bony ankylosis (Fig. 18.7). If the patient is fortunate, the joint becomes ankylosed in the position of function, but more often the patient holds the joint in the position of ease; i.e. the position in which it is least painful because the joint cavity is greatest. The joint then becomes fused in a position that is not ideal for normal use. Occasionally the ankylosis occurs with fibrous tissue instead of bone and an arthrodesis is needed to produce a better result.

Neonatal septicaemia

Neonatal septicaemia causes widespread septic arthritis (Fig. 18.8). Once common, and known as Tom Smith's arthritis, the condition is now rare in developed countries but is sometimes seen after exchange transfusion and invasive procedures on the newborn.

Treatment

Treatment depends on a thorough lavage of the joint and adequate antibiotic treatment. An irrigation–drainage system in which fluid is alternately run into the joint and drained out at hourly or 2-hourly intervals is usually effective if coupled with adequate antibiotic treatment. Thorough irriga-

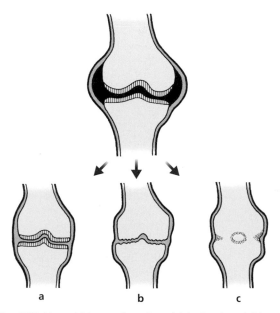

Fig. 18.7 Natural history of septic arthritis. Septic arthritis can lead to: (a) a normal joint; (b) fibrous ankylosis; (c) bony ankylosis.

tion of the joint, if necessary combined with arthroscopy and division of intra-articular adhesions, will usually eradicate septic arthritis.

Tuberculosis

Tuberculosis of bone is still a scourge in undeveloped countries but rare elsewhere (Fig. 18.9). The course of the disease is similar to that of ordinary bone and joint infection, but in slow motion. The illness is chronic, the symptoms develop slowly, the pyrexia is less marked and the abscesses are slow to form. Joint tuberculosis is a disease of synovium and is so similar to rheumatoid arthritis in presentation that it was once thought they were the same condition.

Treatment is similar to that of other infections but taken at a slower pace and with a different drug regimen. A combination of antibiotic drugs such as ethionamide, rifampicin, isoniazid (INH) and ethambutol is usually effective, provided that there is no dead bone within the abscess cavity.

Drugs for tuberculosis
1. Ethionamide.
2. Rifampicin.
3. INH.
4. Ethambutol.

The drugs should be given in combination.

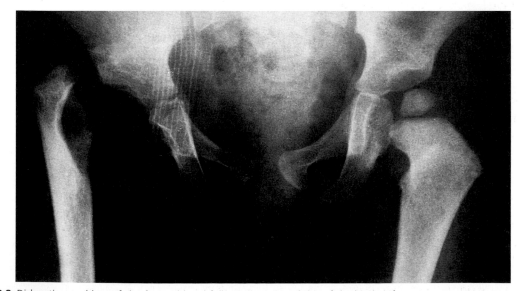

Fig. 18.8 Dislocation and loss of the femoral head following septic arthritis of the hip in infancy.

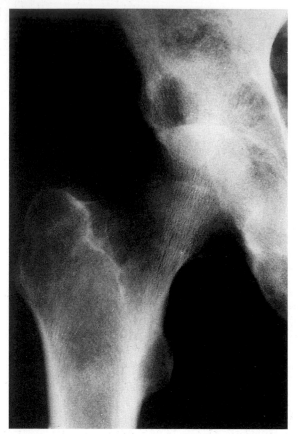

Fig. 18.9 Tuberculosis of the hip with rarefaction and bone destruction.

Spinal tuberculosis (Pott's disease)

See page 463.

Disc infection

The intervertebral discs can become infected with obscure organisms such as brucella, micrococci or fungi, producing severe back pain (p. 463). Providing the infecting organism can be correctly identified, antibiotics are usually effective, but exploration and spinal fusion is sometimes required.

In children, inflammation of the discs can occur in the absence of any detectable infection.

Syphilis

Syphilis of bone is rare in modern days, and the classic sabre tibia caused by syphilitic periostitis is seen more often in museums than orthopaedic clinics.

From an orthopaedic standpoint the most important aspect of syphilis is the Charcot neuropathic joint (p. 308). These joints are grossly unstable, insensitive and often look suitable for joint replacement or arthrodesis. They do badly and the temptation to operate must be resisted.

Chapter |19|

Metabolic disease, dysplasias, osteochondritis and neurological disorders

By the end of this chapter you should be able to:

- Remember the factors affecting bone growth.
- Be aware of the disorders of collagen metabolism and how these affect growth.
- Recall the common sites of the osteochondritic changes in the growing skeleton.

Abnormalities of bone structure

Many disorders of bone occur as a result of the way it is made rather than attack by a disease. These conditions are complex, but learning can be simplified by looking at the different components of bone and the factors that influence their growth.

Bone growth is influenced by the following hormones and vitamins:

Factors affecting bone growth

1. Growth hormone.
2. Sex hormones.
3. Thyroid hormones.
4. Parathyroid hormone.
5. Vitamin C.
6. Vitamin D.
7. Calcitonin.

Growth hormone is responsible for growth until the epiphyses close. Excess secretion after growth is complete causes the thickening of the bones seen in acromegaly; excess secretion before growth is complete causes gigantism.

Sex hormones are involved in the growth spurt of puberty. Release of testosterone causes a rapid increase in growth followed by epiphyseal closure. If testosterone is not released, the epiphyses grow for longer than normal and the patients are tall; hence the legendary giant eunuchs.

Thyroid hormone permits normal growth and deficiency retards it, which is the reason that hypothyroid cretins are small. Thyrotoxicosis does not cause an increase in size but can lead to osteoporosis.

Parathyroid hormone is a polypeptide released when the serum calcium falls. Parathormone acts to increase the serum calcium in two ways:

1. Mobilization of calcium from bone.
2. Increased tubular resorption of calcium.

Vitamin C is necessary for collagen synthesis. Without it, osteoid cannot be properly formed at the epiphyses and children with scurvy have transradiant bands at the epiphyses.

Vitamin D has three actions:

1. It is essential for the absorption of calcium from the gut.

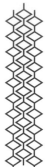

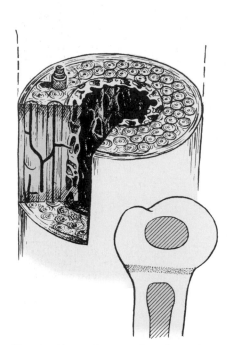

Fig. 19.1 Constituents of bone. Bone consists of crystals arranged along collagen fibres, cartilage, and osteons or haversian systems.

2. It affects the absorption and deposition of calcium in bone.

3. It affects muscle tone; patients with vitamin D deficiency have muscle weakness.

Calcitonin is secreted in the thyroid. Its exact function is unclear but it is secreted if the serum calcium is high and it affects release of calcium from bone.

Bones have four main constituents which can affect growth. Disorders of growth can be considered according to the structure affected (Fig. 19.1).

Constituents of bone

1. Collagen.
2. Crystals of calcium hydroxyapatite arranged in an orderly manner along the collagen fibres. Osteoid is the uncalcified precursor of normal bone.
3. Osteons. Long bones are made up of long tubular units – the haversian systems or osteons. The osteocytes lie in cavities inside dense cortical bone and communicate with other osteocytes by prolongations of the cell body which run through canaliculi. This contact enables the osteocytes to react to abnormal stresses.
4. Cartilage. Growing bones develop from cartilage, which contains proteoglycans.

Abnormalities of collagen

Scurvy

The manifestations of scurvy include abnormal calcification at the epiphyses, and capillary fragility which leads to subperiosteal haemorrhage.

Treatment. Ascorbic acid (vitamin C).

Osteogenesis imperfecta

Osteogenesis imperfecta, or fragilitas ossium, is often sporadic, but can be inherited through either autosomal recessive or autosomal dominant genes (Fig. 19.2). Although the brittleness of bone is the most obvious feature, it is essentially a disorder of type 1 collagen synthesis.

There are four common types:

Type 1. Mildest form with fractures in childhood but less frequent with age. Patients have a slight blue discoloration to the sclera of the eyes. Hearing loss is common in adults.

Type 2. Most severe form with patients having fractures in utero or being stillborn.

Type 3. Severe. Frequent fractures in childhood and adults. Short stature, hearing loss and blue sclera common. Patients will often also have problems with their teeth development.

Type 4. Moderate form with fractures in child and adulthood. Sclera are often white but there is often hearing loss, short stature and possible teeth problems.

The brittleness of the bones is only part of the syndrome (Fig. 19.3). The teeth may also be affected and are often discoloured and abnormally thick – dentogenesis imperfecta. The ground substance in the sclerae of the eye may be abnormal, so that the retinal pigmentation is seen through the sclerae, producing a characteristic bluish discoloration. This is characteristic of the condition but not present in every patient. Mutations in the COL1A1, COL1A2, CRTAP and LEPRE1 genes appear to be the cause.

Bones affected by osteogenesis imperfecta are more plastic than normal and bowing is a recurring problem needing correction by multiple osteotomy and internal fixation.

There are three grades of severity:

1. Some patients are so badly affected that they have multiple fractures in utero and do not survive.

2. Others have multiple fractures during childhood and develop a pigeon chest and scoliosis.

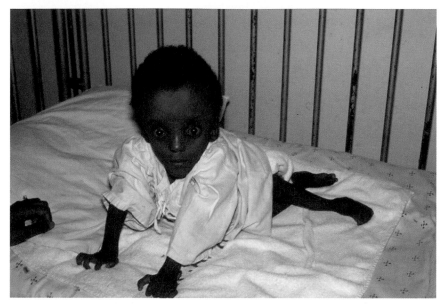

Fig. 19.2 Gross osteogenesis imperfecta.

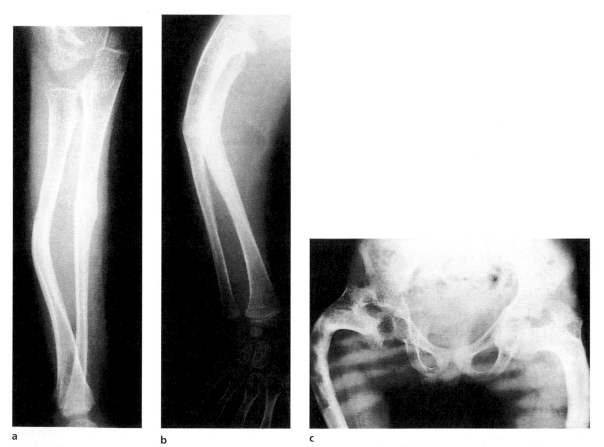

a   b   c

Fig. 19.3 (a), (b) Fractures in osteogenesis imperfecta (note the bowing). (c) Gross bowing of the femora in osteogenesis imperfecta.

3. Some suffer only a few fractures during child-hood, the bones assuming normal strength when skeletal growth is complete.

Although fragilitas ossium does occur, many parents believe that their accident-prone children must have a bony abnormality to account for their fractures and require firm reassurance. In other patients the diagnosis of a non-accidental injury must be considered.

Abnormalities of mineralization

Bone loss

Bone can be lost in three ways:

1. Osteomalacia – decreased mineralization.
2. Osteolysis – increased removal by osteoclasts.
3. Osteopenia – decrease in osteoid tissue. In practice, 'osteopenia' is more often used in the description of radiologically thin bones without implying a specific cause.

These three processes usually occur together in varying degree. The resulting loss of bone is called osteoporosis, of which there are three common types:

1. Idiopathic osteoporosis.
2. Disuse osteoporosis.
3. Steroid osteoporosis.

Idiopathic osteoporosis

Lack of oestrogen causes a reduction in the amount of collagen in the bones of postmenopausal women, which become thin and 'porotic'. Affected bone, particularly cancellous bone, is weaker than normal and susceptible to fractures (Fig. 19.4). Fractures of the femoral neck and crush fractures of the vertebrae are common after trivial injuries in elderly women with senile osteoporosis.

Clinical and radiological features. The patients experience pain in the bones, especially the back. A kyphosis gradually develops. Radiologically, the bones look 'thinner' than normal and pathological fractures may be present.

Treatment. The treatment of osteoporosis is gener-ally unsuccessful because the condition takes so long to appear that, by the time it is recognized, it is too late to treat it. If recognized early, hormonal treat-ment can be instituted, which can, at best, reverse the osteoporosis and restore normal bone texture.

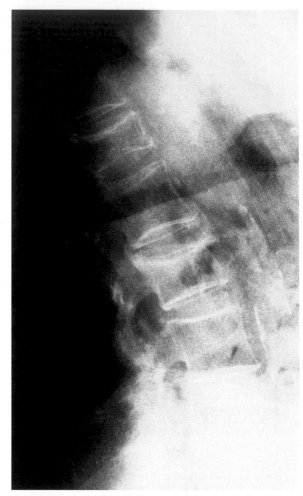

Fig. 19.4 Osteoporosis with crush fractures of the lumbar vertebrae.

The first line of treatment has been hormone replacement therapy (HRT) with special emphasis on oestrogen. The second line is low dose bisphos-phonates (etidronate) given intermittently.

The ideal treatment has yet to be found but there has been a drive to make people and clinicians aware of the problems. Screening programmes have been started and these will hopefully allow earlier detection; this, together with the newer treatments, may help reduce the morbidity suffered by patients.

Disuse osteoporosis

Disuse osteoporosis is seen in bones that are not stressed normally. Patients confined to bed are particularly affected, as are paralysed limbs and

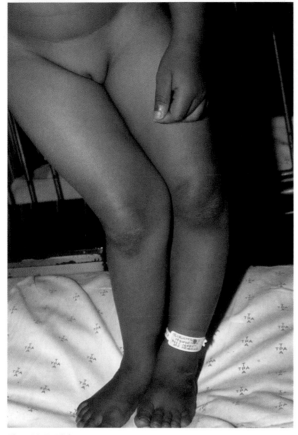

Fig. 19.5 Rickets.

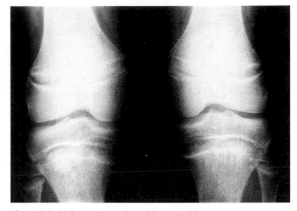

Fig. 19.6 Rickets. Note the wide osteoid seams.

fractures that are treated as non-weight-bearing. Astronauts undergo gross disuse osteoporosis.

Treatment is by mobilization and load-bearing.

Steroid osteoporosis

Steroid osteoporosis is seen in patients receiving large doses of steroids for rheumatoid arthritis or following transplantation, and in Cushing's disease. The consequences include pathological fractures and vertebral collapse.

Treatment is by reducing the dose of steroids or treating the underlying disorder.

Rickets

Rickets is due to deficiency of calcium and phosphate in childhood (Fig. 19.5). Although much less common than in former times, rickets still occurs widely in developing countries. There are four causes:

1. The commonest is vitamin D deficiency due to inadequate diet or lack of natural vitamin D from exposure to sunlight.
2. Malabsorption of calcium due to steatorrhoea.
3. Renal osteodystrophy due to renal abnormality, which affects vitamin D metabolism and causes renal failure.
4. Hypophosphataemia due to a renal tubular abnormality. This condition causes vitamin D-resistant rickets.

Clinical and radiological features. Rickets can be recognized clinically by the curved bones and the prominent epiphyses, which are due to an excess of unmineralized osteoid tissue. Radiologically, the osteoid seams at the epiphyses are widened and there is cupping of the epiphyses (Fig. 19.6).

Investigations. Calcium levels are usually normal, but phosphate levels are low and alkaline phosphatase high.

Treatment. Vitamin D will produce a marked improvement but residual deformities may need correction by osteotomy.

Osteomalacia

Osteomalacia, or softening of the bone, is caused in the adult by vitamin D deficiency. Osteomalacic bone is less rigid than normal bone. The long bones become bowed and small fractures occur on the tension surfaces of these bones.

Clinical and radiological features. The patients are usually malnourished, unwell and complain of bone pain. Crush fractures of the vertebrae may be present. The fractures on the tension surfaces of the bones are visible radiologically as Looser's zones

321

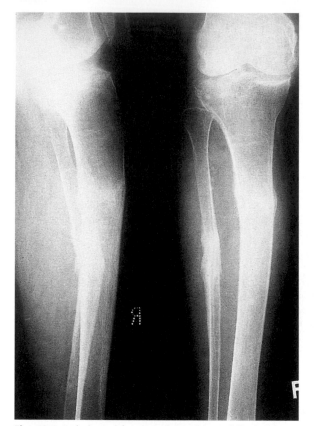

Fig. 19.7 Pathological fracture of the tibia and fibula in osteomalacia. Note the Looser's zone on the front of the tibia.

(Fig. 19.7). The pelvis becomes trefoil in outline as the acetabula and the walls of the pelvis move inwards (Fig. 19.8).

Investigations. Serum calcium and phosphate may be lowered but alkaline phosphatase is raised. Bone biopsy shows wide osteoid seams.

Treatment is by correcting the dietary insufficiency and administering vitamin D.

Hyperparathyroidism

Hyperparathyroidism, also known as von Recklinghausen's disease of bone and osteitis fibrosa cystica, is due to excess production of parathormone (Fig. 19.9). There is excessive resorption of calcium from the skeleton, and cysts full of brownish tissue ('brown tumours') form within the bone in severe disease.

Hyperparathyroidism can be primary, secondary or tertiary:

1. *Primary hyperparathyroidism* is due to excess parathyroid production by a hormone-secreting adenoma.

2. *Secondary hyperparathyroidism* is due to excessive secretion of parathormone in order to mobilize calcium from the bones in response to low calcium levels from renal disease or malabsorption.

3. *Tertiary hyperparathyroidism* occurs when the parathyroid still secretes too much hormone, even when the reason for the excess secretion has been cured. The usual reason is an autonomous nodule of parathyroid tissue which develops while the patient has secondary hyperparathyroidism.

Clinical and radiological features. Classically, the patients have 'moans, sore bones and abdominal groans'. The bone pain is due to softening and resorption of the bones and the moans to personality changes. The cause of abdominal pain is unknown.

Investigations. Serum calcium is high, phosphate low and alkaline phosphatase high in primary hyperparathyroidism. The levels vary in other types according to renal and other pathology.

Treatment. If the excess production of parathormone can be corrected, the bones return to normal. Surgical removal of the parathyroids is usually required.

Disorders of osteon architecture

Paget's disease

Paget's disease, or osteitis deformans, was described by Sir James Paget in 1879 and the cause is still unknown. It is the commonest bone dysplasia.

Bones affected by Paget's disease increase in width, lose their normal architecture and develop an increased blood supply (Fig. 19.10). The increase in size distinguishes the condition from metastases and other disorders which look similar. The increase in blood supply makes the bone warm to touch and in some circumstances can lead to high output cardiac failure. Paget's bone can also become bowed; hence the name, osteitis 'deformans'. The bones can be abnormally soft or excessively hard and break easily.

Paget's disease does not cross joint spaces and is usually confined to individual bones, although many bones may be involved in the same patient.

Clinical and radiological features. The bones are often painful but many patients remain symptom-

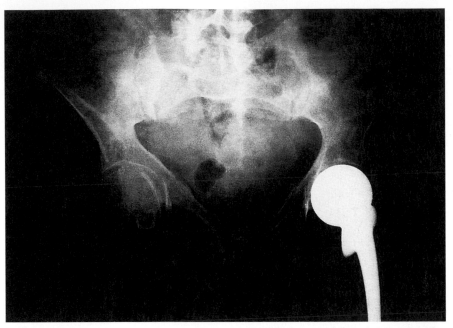

Fig. 19.8 Osteomalacia. Note the trefoil pelvis, fractures of the inferior public rami and right femur and a Thompson prosthesis inserted for a pathological fracture of the neck of the femur.

free, despite gross radiological changes, until they develop osteoarthritis in joints or suffer a pathological fracture. The bones lack the normal arrangement of trabeculae and may be larger than normal. Pseudofractures, like Looser's zones (p. 322), are seen on the tension side of bones.

Investigations. Alkaline phosphatase is high and isotope scans show up affected areas as 'hot'.

Complications. Paget's bone is not as strong as normal bone and pathological fractures occur, but the fractures usually unite as quickly, if not more quickly, than fractures through ordinary bone.

A sinister complication is the development of a particularly malignant tumour, known as Paget's sarcoma, in a small percentage of cases (Fig. 19.11). It is not known why some patients develop this tumour.

Treatment. Simple analgesics are not always effective for the pain. Parenteral calcitonin and oral diphosphonates are effective in 50–70% of patients but this figure is rising as newer biphosphonates are introduced.

Fibrous dysplasia

Fibrous dysplasia causes the formation of fibrous areas within bone (Fig. 19.12). Affected areas are fragile and pathological fractures occur. The cause is not known.

Marble bone disease (Albers–Schönberg disease, osteopetrosis)

The normal tubulation of a long bone may be lost and the bone appears as a solid stick on the radiographs, while the vertebrae have a characteristic striped appearance (Fig. 19.13). The bones look very solid but are in fact very brittle. When they break it is almost impossible to fix the fractures internally because the bone is so hard that it cannot be drilled with ordinary equipment. The condition is usually inherited through an autosomal dominant gene but there is a more severe form inherited through an autosomal recessive gene.

Other dysplasias

There are countless other dysplasias, all interesting and obscure, and many with interesting radiological abnormalities. Striped bones, spotted bones (Fig. 19.14) and candlestick bones (melorheostosis) are all seen.

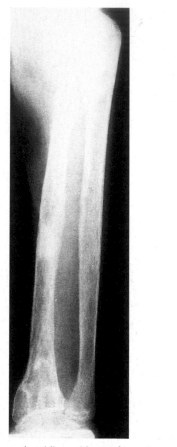

Fig. 19.9 Hyperparathyroidism with cyst formation.

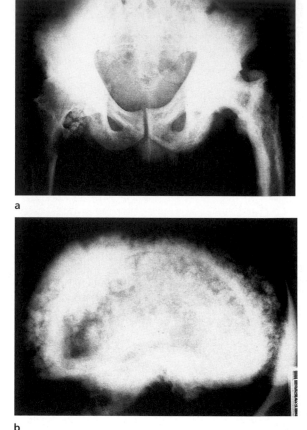

a

b

Fig. 19.10 Paget's disease of: (a) the pelvis and left femur; (b) the skull.

Abnormalities of cartilage

Mucopolysaccharidoses

Mucopolysaccharidoses are due to congenitally determined abnormalities in the composition of cartilage.

Hurler's disease, or 'gargoylism', includes facial deformity, corneal opacities, epiphyseal and vertebral deformity and mental retardation. The disease is inherited through an autosomal recessive gene.

Morquio's disease is similar to Hurler's disease but does not include facial deformity, corneal opacities or mental retardation. The disease is inherited through an autosomal recessive gene.

Achondroplasia

Achondroplasia, or dyschondroplasia, in which the long bones do not grow as much as normal and the patients are very short, is inherited as an autosomal

dominant (Fig. 19.15). The families of dwarves seen in circuses have achondroplasia. Achondroplastic bones are of normal strength and the patients are of normal intelligence. A similar genetic disorder in dogs is responsible for short-legged breeds such as dachshunds, basset hounds and corgis.

Apart from the short stature and the social problems that this can bring, there are other complications of achondroplasia. The pedicles of the vertebrae are shorter than normal and the spinal canal is therefore abnormally narrow, which leads to spinal stenosis (p. 456) and neurological impairment.

Craniocleidodysostosis

This melodiously named condition is the 'opposite' of achondroplasia. Cartilage bones are normal but membrane bones, particularly the skull and clavicle, are imperfectly developed. No treatment is effective.

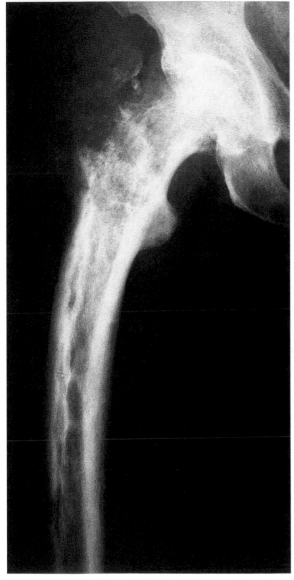

Fig. 19.11 Paget's disease with pseudofractures along the convex side of the bone and sarcoma at the greater trochanter.

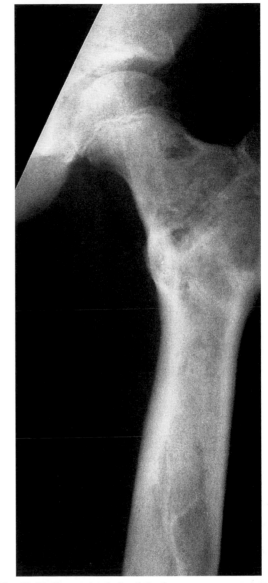

Fig. 19.12 Fibrous dysplasia of the femur.

The disease is inherited through an autosomal dominant gene.

Diaphyseal aclasis

Diaphyseal aclasis is a generalized failure of bone remodelling inherited as an autosomal dominant.

It is easy to understand how a long bone grows from an epiphyseal plate but it is not so easy to understand why the shaft is narrower than the epiphysis. What force makes the bone become narrow? Whatever the mechanism, it sometimes fails and produces the appearance in Figure 19.16.

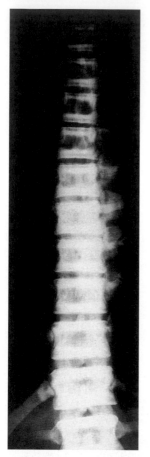

Fig. 19.13 The rugger jersey spine of osteopetrosis (Albers–Schönberg disease).

Dysplasia epiphysealis multiplex

Dysplasia epiphysealis multiplex is an inherited disorder which affects the epiphyseal plates. Growth is irregular and deformities involve many bones (Fig. 19.17).

There are many other rare types of epiphyseal dysplasias affecting the behaviour of the growth plate in different ways.

Osteochondritis

Osteochondritis is a bad term, used to describe conditions which look a little similar but are caused by several different pathological processes:

1. Vascular abnormalities.
2. Damage to apophyses.
3. Conditions of unknown origin.

Vascular abnormalities

Many osteochondritides are caused by a transient disturbance of vascularity (Fig. 19.18). The cause is almost certainly partial venous occlusion, and is quite different from aseptic necrosis.

Perthes' disease

Perthes' disease is an osteochondritis of the upper femoral epiphysis in which the femoral head

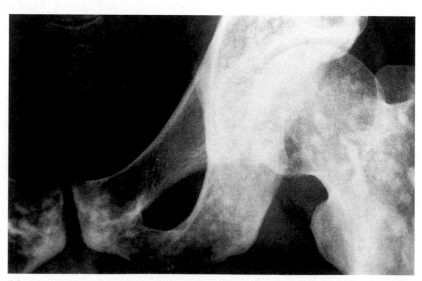

Fig. 19.14 Osteopoikilosis, or 'spotted bones'.

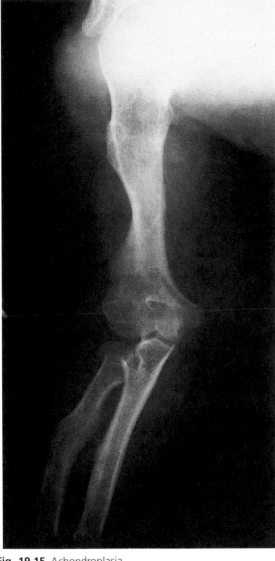

Fig. 19.15 Achondroplasia.

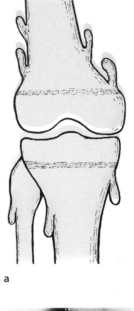

a

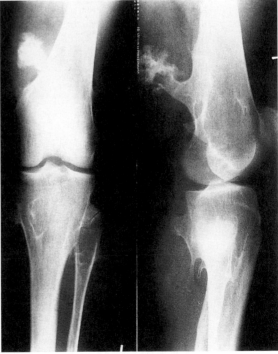

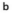
b

Fig. 19.16 (a) Multiple exostoses pointing away from the growth plates in diaphyseal aclasis. (b) Radiograph of diaphyseal aclasis.

becomes soft and then gradually reforms over a period of several years (Fig. 19.19). The condition is seen in children between the ages of 5 and 10 years and is commoner in boys. The primary pathology is an interference with the venous drainage of the femoral head. The reformed head is larger and flatter than the original.

Treatment is directed to containing the femoral head within the acetabulum until it reforms. This can usually be achieved by conservative means, with splints if necessary, but osteotomy is sometimes required.

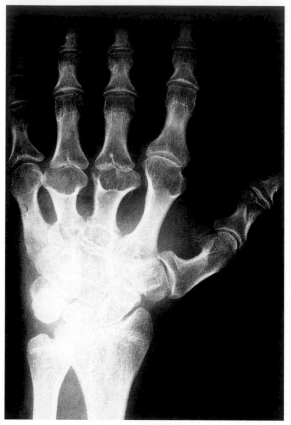

Fig. 19.17 The hand in a patient with multiple epiphyseal dysplasia.

Kienböck's disease

Kienböck's disease is similar to Perthes' disease but affects the lunate, which collapses, becomes dense and gradually reforms (Fig. 19.20). The disease presents with pain on the dorsum of the wrist over the lunate. The pain usually resolves after 1 year, but can recur when the wrist is twisted awkwardly or stressed.

Köhler's disease

Köhler's disease affects the navicular bone in the foot and presents with pain on the dorsum (p. 432).

Other sites

Other epiphyses can be affected by the same cycle of rarefaction, collapse and reformation, including Freiberg's disease of the second and third metatarsal heads.

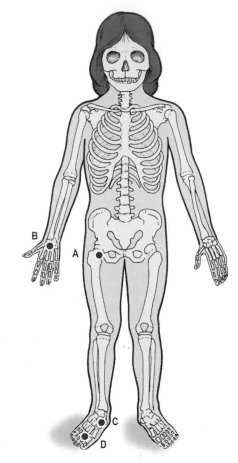

Fig. 19.18 Sites of vascular osteochondritis: (*A*) Perthes' disease at the hip; (*B*) Kienböck's disease of the lunate; (*C*) Köhler's disease of the navicular; (*D*) Freiberg's disease of the metatarsal heads.

Damage to apophyses

Muscles attached to an apophysis can lift all or part of the apophysis away from the bone during the adolescent growth spurt (Fig. 19.21). The bone is painful at first but the pain subsides gradually as the apophysis becomes reattached with growth. In some patients a sliver or spicule of bone remains detached and causes pain, rather like a splinter or foreign body. A better name for these disorders would be 'traction apophysitis'.

Osgood–Schlatter disease

The commonest traction apophysitis is Osgood–Schlatter disease, in which the apophysis of the tibial tubercle is lifted off the tibia. This happens most often in vigorous teenagers at the stage of

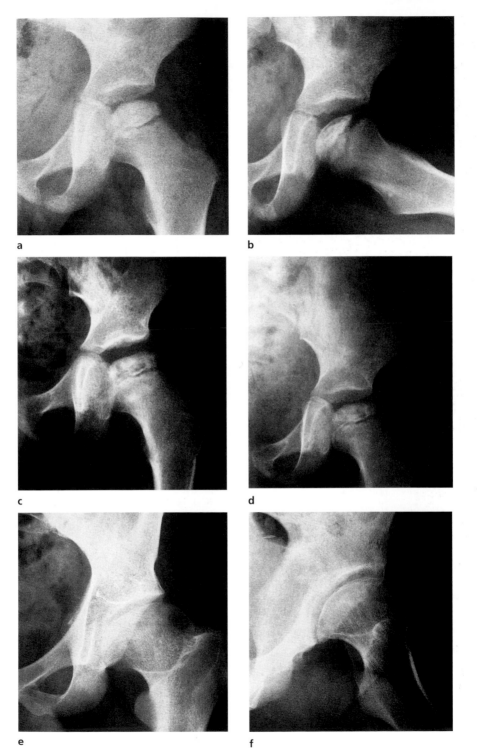

Fig. 19.19 (a), (b) Perthes' disease with increased density of the femoral head and a sequestrum within it; (c) 3 months later the changes have progressed; (d) 12 months later, the same femoral head is beginning to reform. (e), (f) The end result of Perthes' disease, sometimes known as 'coxa plana' or 'coxa magna'.

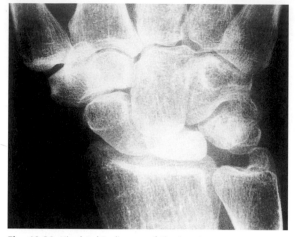

Fig. 19.20 Kienböck's disease of the lunate.

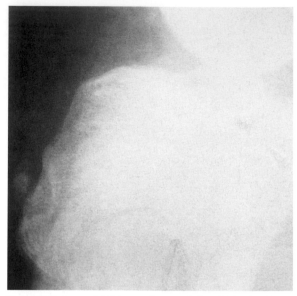

Fig. 19.22 Osgood–Schlatter disease of the tibial tubercle. A fragment of the apophysis has become detached from the tibial tubercle.

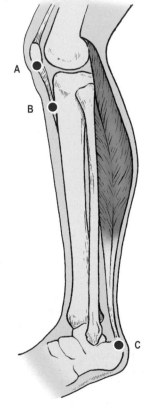

Fig. 19.21 Sites of osteochondritis involving apophyses: (A) Sinding Larsen's disease; (B) Osgood–Schlatter disease; (C) Sever's disease.

growth when the quadriceps has enlarged, but before the apophysis has fused to the tibia – about 12–13 years in boys and a year less in girls.

There was no such person as Osgood–Schlatter. Osgood described the condition in America in 1903, the same year that Schlatter described it in Germany. Confusion about the name of the condition was settled by calling it 'Osgood–Schlatter's disease'. Although this shares the honours evenly, it sounds so serious that parents need reassurance that their child will survive.

Treatment is conservative, by restriction of activities that cause pain. Plaster immobilization is not required. Most lesions heal as growth proceeds, but about 5% have persistent pain from an ununited spicule of bone within the tubercle (Fig. 19.22). Some of these respond to steroid injection, but a few need the spicule excised.

The bump at the tibial tubercle never diminishes in size and persists into adult life. Apart from the appearance, it causes few problems.

Sever's disease

At the heel, pain and tenderness can arise at the upper edge of the calcaneal apophysis from traction apophysitis, which is an injury caused by overuse of the Achilles tendon (p. 433).

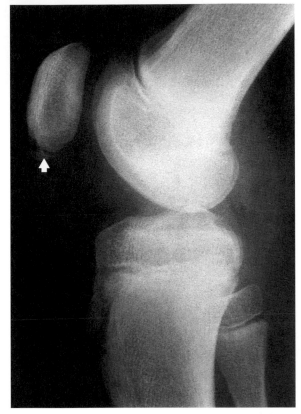

Fig. 19.23 Sinding Larsen's disease. The lower part of the patella shows a separate fragment of apophysis.

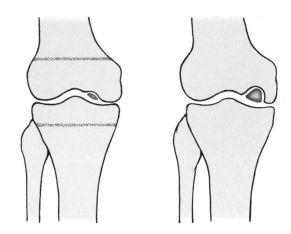

Fig. 19.24 Osteochondritis dissecans. The lesion begins as a small defect on the medial femoral condyle in the growing skeleton and increases in size, sometimes producing a loose body.

Sinding Larsen's disease

Sinding Larsen (one person) described pain at the lower pole of the patella caused by traction of the patellar tendon. The disease is similar to Osgood–Schlatter disease but occurs 1 or 2 years earlier (Fig. 19.23).

Scheuermann's disease

The ring apophyses of the thoracic vertebrae can be damaged at their anterior border, producing pain during the growing period and growth arrest. The cause is unknown but traction is not involved and this separates the condition from the other apophyseal osteochondritides. The condition affects many levels and causes a rounded kyphosis of the thoracic spine (p. 459).

Treatment. No treatment is effective, and there is no disability apart from the shape of the back. Pain ceases when growth is complete. Parents should be told that the child cannot help standing with rounded shoulders and that nagging to 'stand up straight' is unhelpful.

Others

Calvé's disease

A collapse of the vertebral body in children and young adults was formerly described as Calvé's disease but many cases have since been shown to be the result of an eosinophilic granuloma of bone. Calvé's disease does not exist as a separate entity.

Osteochondritis dissecans

Osteochondritis dissecans consists of a gradual dissection (not desiccation) or separation of a block of bone from its bed (Figs 19.24, 19.25). The medial femoral condyle is by far the commonest site. Osteochondritis dissecans of other joints is rare. Progress should be assessed radiologically. The lesions may require reattachment drilling to encourage union, or removal of the affected area if it separates.

Neuromuscular disorders

Although neuromuscular disorders fall within the province of neurologists, many present first to the orthopaedic clinic with abnormal gait. They must not be forgotten just because they are not 'surgical' diseases.

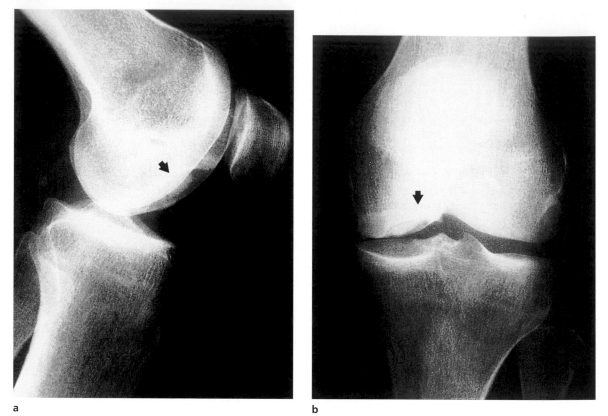

a   b

Fig. 19.25 (a), (b) Osteochondritis dissecans. The end result in an adult, showing a potential loose body lying in a crater beneath intact articular cartilage.

Duchenne muscular dystrophy

Duchenne muscular dystrophy is inherited through an X-linked recessive gene and therefore affects boys almost exclusively. The boy will have passed the early developmental milestones normally but then develops muscular weakness during childhood and presents with a broad-based waddle that can be mistaken for instability of the hips. The diagnosis can be confirmed by high creatinine phosphokinase levels and muscle biopsy.

Apart from splintage to prevent contractures and aids to minimize the impact of the disease, such as an electric wheelchair, there is no treatment to offer for this distressing disease. Progressive and severe scoliosis is common and spinal fusion may be needed to stabilize the spine.

Death from intercurrent infection in early adult life is usual.

Friedreich's ataxia

Friedreich's ataxia often presents with weakness of the ankles and is easily mistaken for a recurrent ankle sprain. The disease is familial and of variable severity.

Peroneal muscular atrophy

This familial condition involves both hands and feet, but principally the feet. There is a high arched foot, absent ankle jerk and an extensor plantar response.

A combination of soft tissue release and arthrodesis is required according to the severity of the disease. Some patients need no treatment.

Acute poliomyelitis

Because poliomyelitis is so rare in the West it is likely to be missed if the patient first presents to an orthopaedic clinic. Think of poliomyelitis if the patient has developed localized muscular weakness after a febrile illness.

Late poliomyelitis

The imbalance of muscle power produces deformity. The treatment of late poliomyelitis consists of balancing the remaining active muscles and splinting joints. Arthrodesis may be required to prevent deformity.

Weakness of the ankle dorsiflexors, for example, can be treated with a toe-raising splint or transfer of a plantarflexor from the calf. The variety of possible problems in poliomyelitis is infinite, and each case must be considered as if it were unique.

Chapter |20|

Granulomatous disorders and tumours

By the end of this chapter you should:
- Appreciate the rarity of primary bone tumours.
- Remember the abnormal presentation of bone pain in the younger patient could represent a tumour.
- Be able to differentiate the radiological signs of benign and malignant cases.
- Be aware of the common classification of different types according to the cell of origin.

Granulomatous conditions

There are three disorders of the reticuloendothelial system that affect bone; all are rare, but they are important because they can be mistaken for tumours:

1. Eosinophilic granuloma.
2. Hand–Schüller–Christian disease.
3. Gaucher's disease.

Eosinophilic granuloma

The lesions of eosinophilic granuloma are 'punched-out' holes in the skull and elsewhere. Radiologically, the lesions resemble metastases or bone cysts (Fig. 20.1). The 'holes' contain a soft brown tissue.

The condition is not fatal and may regress spontaneously.

Hand–Schüller–Christian disease

This condition is similar to eosinophilic granuloma except that the lesions are paler and the brain is often involved, particularly around the pituitary. The condition is slowly progressive and may be fatal.

Gaucher's disease

Gaucher's disease is a systemic disorder in which an abnormal fatty substance (kerasin) is deposited in the liver and other tissues. Bone involved in Gaucher's disease contains irregular cysts and cavities visible radiologically. Affected bones, particularly the femoral head and condyles, may collapse and make joint replacement necessary.

Tumours

Radiological appearance of bone tumours

When looking at bone tumours on a radiograph, ask the following questions:

335

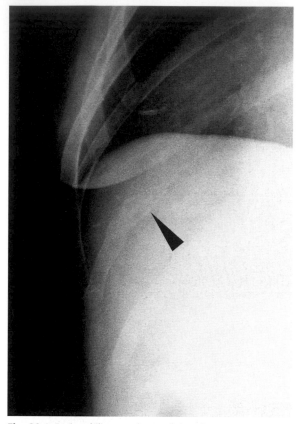

Fig. 20.1 Eosinophilic granuloma of the rib.

Radiological features of bone tumours

1. Is the tumour creating bone or destroying bone?
2. Is the cortex of the bone intact, broken or eroded?
3. If intact, is the cortex thinner than normal and, if so, has it been indented from outside or inside the medullary cavity?
4. Is the medullary cavity wider than normal?
5. Does the shape of the tumour suggest that it is lifting the periosteum off the bone? If it is, there may be a small triangle of bone at the edge of the tumour, known as a Codman's triangle, which is often seen in malignant tumours.
6. If the tumour is fusiform, is there an 'onion skin' appearance? This is often seen in Ewing's tumour and other rapidly growing lesions.
7. Is there any sunray radial calcification? This is often seen in tumours, particularly osteogenic sarcoma.

Table 20.1 A simple classification of benign and malignant bone tumours according to cell of origin

	Benign	Malignant
Fibrogenic	Simple cyst	Malignant fibrous
	Aneurysmal bone cyst	Hystiocytoma
	Fibrous dysplasia	
	Fibrous cortical defect	Fibrosarcoma
Chondrogenic	Enchondroma	Chondrosarcoma
	Periosteal chondroma	
	Osteochondroma	
	Chondromyxoid fibroma	
	Chondroblastoma	
Osteogenic	Osteoid osteoma	Osteosarcoma
	Osteoblastoma	
	Ossifying fibroma	
Unknown origin	Giant cell	Ewing's
		Synovial sarcoma
Bone marrow		Myeloma
		Lymphoma

Classification of bone tumours

The classification of bone tumours should reflect the cell of origin. They can be further subclassified into benign and malignant tumours (Table 20.1).

Simple bone islands (Fig. 20.2) are of no particular significance, although they are often striking on X-ray.

Benign bone tumours

Fibrogenic

Fibrous cortical defect (Fig. 20.3). This most common abnormality has a characteristic oval X-ray appearance with a sharp margin and often multilocular. No specific treatment is required.

Fibrous dysplasia. This can present in mono- or polyostotic forms and is seen more commonly between the second and third decades. The radiographic appearance is of a ground-glass expansile lesion, often with a bowing of the affected bone. A 'shepherd's crook' deformity is seen in the proximal femur as a result of this bowing and possible multiple fractures. The polyostotic form can be associated with hypothyroidism, vitamin D-resistant rickets and the Cushing syndrome. Albright's syndrome includes the polyostotic dysplasia with café-

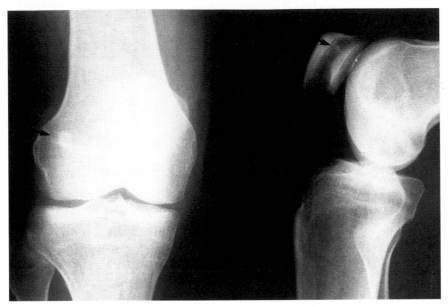

Fig. 20.2 Cortical bone islands.

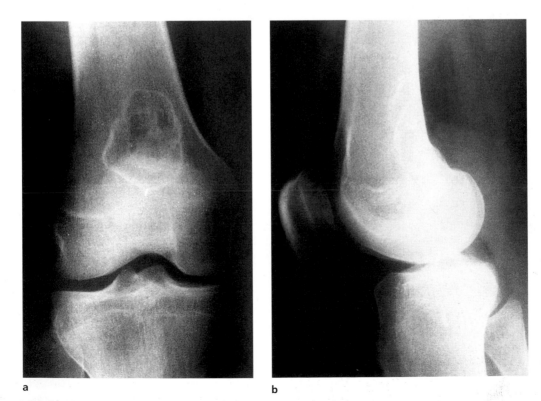

a   b

Fig. 20.3 (a), (b) Fibrous cortical defect at the lower end of femur.

au-lait spots and precocious puberty. The lesions are reasonably characteristic on X-ray but occasionally a biopsy is required. When painful, these are adequately treated with curettage and bone grafting. Occasionally there can be an associated fracture, although this is rare.

Simple bone cyst (Fig. 20.4). These cysts may occur during growth and are commonly located adjacent to the epiphyseal plate. They are usually asymptomatic until pathological fracture occurs. The radiographic appearances show a well defined radiolucent lesion, often with this pathological fracture.

Bone scans confirm a decreased uptake in the area and treatment is unnecessary unless there is a risk of fracture. These cysts can heal spontaneously after a fracture, but when in doubt aspiration and an injection of methylprednisolone acetate has an 80–90% success rate. Curettage and bone grafting is occasionally necessary.

Aneurysmal bone cyst (Fig. 20.5). These cystic cavities contain a thick brown-coloured membrane containing blood. They may occur in any bone, including the vertebrae. Approximately 50% are

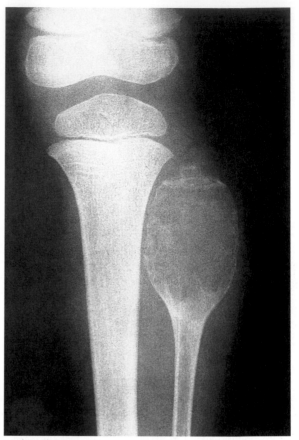

Fig. 20.5 Aneurysmal bone cyst at the upper end of the fibula. It has not crossed the epiphyseal plate.

primary and 50% are the result of a benign lesion such as a chondroblastoma.

Radiographic signs confirm an expansile eccentric lesion and a thin 'eggshell' ring of bone. A CT scan may demonstrate a fluid level within the cyst. Treatment is usually by curettage and bone grafting.

Osteogenic

Osteoid osteoma (Figs 20.6, 20.7). Any bone can be involved but more commonly the femur, tibia and vertebrae. There is a characteristic nidus in the cortical lesions, demonstrated on CT. Patients often have pain, which is particularly worse at night and can be relieved by aspirin. The natural history is thought to be self-limiting and resolution of symptoms has been described. Treatment has traditionally been surgical excision, although it is often difficult to localize the lesion. Guided laser ablation has shown encouraging results.

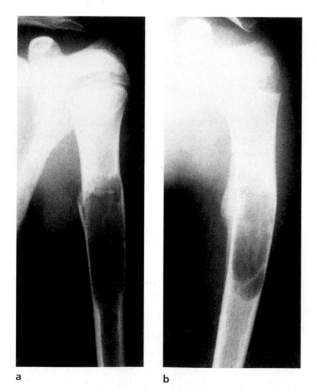

a   b

Fig. 20.4 (a) A pathological fracture through a simple bone cyst of the humerus; (b) the fracture has united and the bone cyst is less obvious.

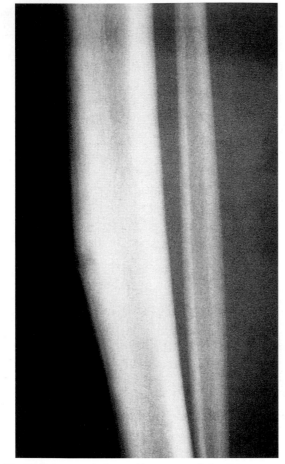

Fig. 20.6 Juxtacortical osteoid osteoma of the tibia.

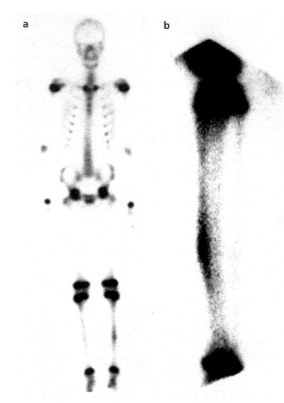

Fig. 20.7 (a) Isotope scan to show an osteoid osteoma in the left tibia of a growing child; (b) lateral view of the left tibia to show the position of the osteoid osteoma on the anterior cortex.

Osteoblastoma. This tumour is characterized by immature osteoid and is more commonly located in the posterior elements of the spine and occasionally the skull. They are larger than the osteoid osteoma (greater than 2 cm). These lesions can be aggressive and have a higher recurrence rate following curettage.

Ossifying fibroma. These are often considered to be a variation of fibrous dysplasia and are located eccentrically, either in the tibia or the fibula in young children. Occasional rapid expansion with or without a fracture is noted, but surgery is rarely indicated.

Chondrogenic

Enchondroma (Fig. 20.8). These benign tumours of mature hyaline cartilage are usually located centrally within the diaphysis of long bones and may represent the remnant of the epiphyseal plate. They can be solitary or multiple (Ollier's disease) or associ-ated with skin haemangiomas (Maffucci syndrome). Less frequently these lesions are located at the periosteum and are either juxtacortical or subperiosteal chondromas. These often involve the small tubular bones of the hand and feet and are noted more commonly in the second, third and fourth decades. Malignant transformation has been reported. Radiographic signs are characteristic, with an expansile nature of the bone, often with punctate calcification within. Treatment by curettage and bone grafting is occasionally required but patients should remain under review, especially with large tumours of the pelvis or spine.

Osteochondroma (Fig. 20.9). These are the most common benign bone tumours and probably represent a disorder of the normal enchondral bone growth. The appearance is either sessile or of a pedunculated lesion arising from the cortex of a long bone, adjacent to the physis (exostosis). Unlike a true neoplasm, the growth normally parallels that of skeletal maturity and is often noted during periods

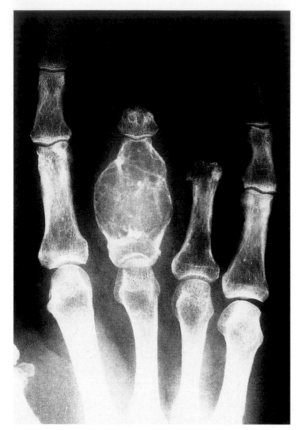

Fig. 20.8 An enchondroma of the proximal phalanx of the middle finger. The distal part of the middle and ring fingers have suffered a previous traumatic amputation.

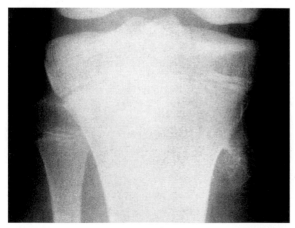

Fig. 20.9 An isolated exostosis of the upper end of the tibia pointing away from the growing epiphysis.

of rapid skeletal growth. Ninety per cent are single, but in 10% multiple osteochondromas occur. Most lesions are asymptomatic but can cause irritation of the surrounding structures (muscle, ligament). The clinical findings are usually of a palpable mass.

A cartilaginous cap of a few millimetres thickness usually covers the lesion. Large lesions can result in growth abnormalities (ulna bowing, etc.). Malignant transformation is possible and may occur in 10–25% of cases, although the exact incidence is unknown.

Chondroblastoma. This rare tumour occurs between 5 and 25 years of age, more commonly in the knee, hip and shoulder area. The tumour usually involves the physis and patients tend to present with pain. The lesion is lytic, with calcification occurring in approximately 50% of cases. Secondary aneurysmal bone cysts may occur. These chondroblastomas are aggressive, benign tumours but metastases can occur. In common with giant cell tumours, they should be regarded as potentially malignant.

Chondromyxoid fibroma. These occur eccentrically in the metaphysis of the proximal tibia commonly. Treatment includes curettage and bone grafting.

Undetermined aetiology

Giant cell tumour (Fig. 20.10). This occurs commonly in the third and fourth decade and more commonly around the knee or distal radius. The radiographic features are of an expansile lesion, which often lies eccentrically. The border is well defined with some sclerosis and is often juxtaposed to the articular cartilage. Pathological fracture is common and treatment includes surgical removal with curettage and bone grafting, with or without phenol ablation, cryosurgery or instillation of methylmethacrylate.

Primary malignant bone tumours

Fibrogenic

Malignant fibrous hystiocytoma (MFH) is a high grade tumour seen in adulthood. It commonly occurs around the metaphysis, in particular of the knee. Radiographs show a 'moth-eaten' osteolytic lesion with extensive cortical disruption but a minimal periosteal reaction and very little, if any, new bone formation. The underlying cell of origin is doubtful and treatment is difficult. The prognosis is unfavourable.

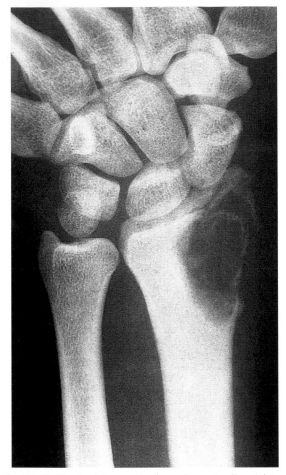

Fig. 20.10 Giant cell tumour in the radius extending right up to the joint margin.

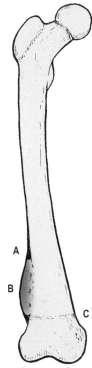

Fig. 20.11 Radiological features of osteogenic sarcoma: (*A*) Codman's triangle at the margins of the tumour; (*B*) 'sunrise' spicules of calcification within the tumour; (*C*) site at growing end of a long bone.

Fibrosarcoma. This rare tumour most probably represents a variation of an MFH but can follow X-ray therapy, Paget's disease, bone infarcts or dedifferentiated chondrosarcomas.

Osteogenic

Osteogenic sarcoma (Figs 20.11, 20.12). These are the most common primary bone tumours and occur more commonly in children and young adults (Fig. 20.11). The tumour often presents as a swelling with a history of minimal trauma. The tumours are classified as primary or secondary (following Paget's disease, X-ray therapy). The primary tumours are further classified according to their position (parosteal, central or multicentric).

Approximately 70% of patients present without a detectable metastasis, but in the 30% that do there is a high percentage of relapse following chemotherapy and local surgery. Limb sparing resection is possible with adjuvant chemotherapy. The prognosis for all types is poor.

Radiographic signs confirm the lytic lesion, elevation of the periosteum and the production of a 'Codman's triangle'.

Chondrogenic

Chondrosarcomas. These may be classified as central or peripheral, or primary versus secondary (secondary to a pre-existing lesion such as an osteochondroma). Patients usually present with a long history of pain, mass or both. These tumours are further differentiated into low, intermediate or high grade lesions. The behaviour of the tumour is related to the aggressive portion of the lesion and the prognosis is poor.

Cells of unknown origin

Ewing's sarcoma (Figs 20.13, 20.14). This rare tumour occurs in the first and second decade of life and the

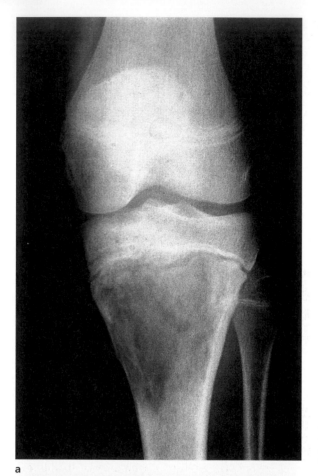

a

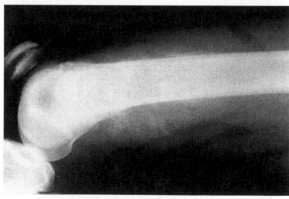

b

Fig. 20.12 (a) Osteogenic sarcoma at the upper end of the tibia in a girl aged 12 years; (b) osteogenic sarcoma at the lower end of the femur showing the classic 'sun ray' cacification.

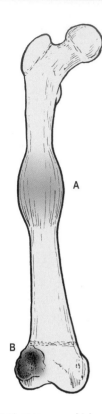

Fig. 20.13 (*A*) Ewing's sarcoma, which may arise anywhere along the shaft of a long bone. (*B*) Giant cell tumour appearing as a multilocular cyst in the epiphysis, but not crossing the line of the epiphysis

small, primitive, round cells have a common karyotypic translocation between chromosome 11 and 22. Previously these were uniformly fatal, but major advances in treatment have been made with the use of chemotherapy and adequate local control. The most important adverse prognostic feature is metastatic disease detectable at the time of diagnosis. The 5-year relapse-free survival rate is 20% for those with metastatic disease, compared with 55% for those without metastases at the time of presentation.

Surgical resection is considered the optimal method of obtaining local control. The radiographic appearances include bone destruction with an 'onion skin' reaction of the periosteum. It may involve large areas of the diathesis and may appear to skip areas of the bone.

Synovial sarcoma. This tumour has histological similarities with the synovium of joint but rarely arises directly from the joint. They are often of a

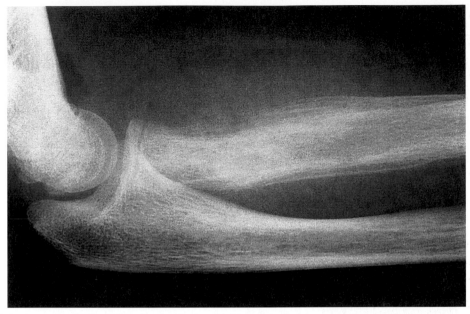

Fig. 20.14 Ewing's sarcoma in the radius showing 'onion skin' layering.

high grade histological appearance but may be well circumscribed or multinodular. Soft tissue calcification occurs in approximately 25% of cases and lymphatic and vascular metastatic spread is common, with a poor long-term prognosis.

Tumours of bone marrow

Myeloma. This is a tumour derived from the plasma cells (highly differentiated B lymphocytes). Presentation includes pain and anaemia in the fifth and sixth decade of life. A monoclonal gammopathy with an elevated M-spike is characteristic. Bence Jones proteins may be demonstrated in the urine. Radiographic changes include multiple 'punched out' lesions of the bones and bone scan appearances may be unusual.

Solitary lesions (plasmocytomas) are seen infrequently and aggressive radiotherapy is the treatment of choice.

Lymphoma of bone. These are usually a sign of disseminated disease and rarely represent a primary tumour. The tumour characteristically presents in the third to fifth decades of life and radiographs may show a 'moth-eaten' appearance. Treatment is by chemotherapy and radiotherapy.

Metastatic bone tumours

The commonest malignant bone tumours are secondary deposits (Fig. 20.15). The tumours that most commonly metastasize to bone (Fig. 20.16) are bronchus, breast, prostate and renal cell carcinomas.

Tumours that metastasize to bone most often (Fig. 20.16)
1. Lung.
2. Breast.
3. Prostate.
4. Renal cell carcinoma.

Treatment

Treatment depends upon the tumour but may involve radiotherapy, chemotherapy or hormone therapy. If pathological fracture occurs, intramedullary nailing is indicated. It is wise to nail the bone prophylactically in those lesions that involve more than 50% of the circumference of the bone to avoid an impending fracture.

An MRI scan of the bone can delineate the extent of the secondary deposit.

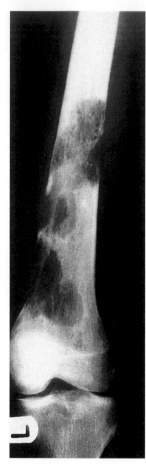

Fig. 20.15 Metastatic deposits in the femur. Note the clear punched-out margins.

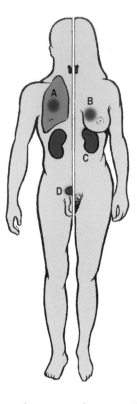

Fig. 20.16 Tumours that commonly metastasize to bone: (*A*) bronchus; (*B*) breast; (*C*) hypernephroma; (*D*) prostate.

Case reports

These three cases represent different presentations of swelling around the knee.

Patient A

An 18-year-old gentleman presented with a painless swelling on the medial side of his right knee. He had noticed a slight increase in size over the last few months, but related the swelling to a minor injury he had while playing football some 3 months previously. The swelling failed to settle and he eventually attended his general practitioner.

A plain radiograph was requested and the radiologist's report suggested an urgent orthopaedic review. The plain radiograph confirmed what appeared to be an osteogenic sarcoma and the patient was subsequently transferred to a bone tumour unit for further management.

Patient B

A 14-year-old boy who was a very keen sportsman noticed a pain on the inner side of his right knee. This pain was associated with a small lump, which he thought was growing in size. He could not remember having injured the knee specifically, but did notice that the pain was getting increasingly severe and was affecting his day-to-day activities.

When reviewed in the orthopaedic department it was noted that he had a small, hard, bony lump on the proximal medial aspect of his right tibia. Plain radiographs confirmed that this was a benign osteochondroma. After careful palpation of the other leg and arms it was clear that this was an isolated osteochondroma. There was no family history to suggest a hereditary link. The patient subsequently underwent an uneventful removal of this bony lump with the cartilagenous cap intact. Histology showed no evidence of malignancy.

Patient C

A 14-year-old boy was admitted with a painful lump over the medial aspect of the proximal tibia. He had noticed this lump increasing in size over the last few weeks. He had been generally unwell and over the last few days had suffered shivers and a fever.

It was thought that he had a recent upper respiratory tract infection, but this had been minor.

On examination he was pyrexial with a tachycardia. The swelling over the proximal tibia was warm and tender. Plain radiographs confirmed a lytic area in the proximal tibia and laboratory investigations confirmed a high ESR and CRP. It was felt that this was an osteomyelitis. The abscess was drained and irrigated thoroughly. Appropriate antibiotics were given and the patient made an uneventful recovery in the long term.

Summary

Swellings around the knee can be simple cysts or benign bony lumps, but it must be remembered that more sinister tumours often present in the younger age group with a slightly tenuous history of previous trauma preceding this. Similarly, infections, although rare in the developed world, are still frequently seen.

Management of malignant tumours should be undertaken in a specialist bone tumour centre where the results of treatment are greatly improved.

Chapter |21|

Deformities in children

By the end of this chapter you should:

- Be able to distinguish normal from abnormal developmental milestones; decide when to investigate and when to reassure.
- Remember the importance of a multidisciplinary team to treat growth disorders.
- Understand developmental hip dysplasia, the importance of early diagnosis and appropriate treatment.
- Recognize common foot abnormalities and know the conservative treatment of club feet.
- Understand the different types of neurological disorder and how the lesser varieties may present with subtle lower limb signs.
- Know the different types of scoliosis and be aware of conservative and operative treatment options.

Crooked children are still referred to orthopaedic surgeons for treatment as they were in Andry's time, but serious deformity is rare today and the majority of children referred to an orthopaedic children's clinic have nothing more than a minor abnormality of the lower limbs requiring firm reassurance. Reassurance is not always easy; well-intentioned advice or a careless remark by a respected relative, usually a grandparent, can cause anxiety that is difficult to eradicate.

Before reassuring the parents that all is well, it is important to confirm that no serious abnormality is present and it is therefore essential to understand what is normal and what is not.

Normal milestones

The milestones of normal development are very variable and accurate assessment may need a child development specialist. From an orthopaedic standpoint the most important milestones are those shown in Figure 21.1.

A paediatric opinion is needed if the child cannot do the following:

1. Sit by the age of 9 months.
2. Pull himself or herself upright by 12 months.
3. Walk by the age of 20 months.

Problems with walking

Not all children learn to walk at the same age and some are not very good at it when they do. Some children walk with an ungainly gait, as do some adults, and some learn to walk by using one leg as a prop at the front while the other pushes forwards from behind. This and other 'trick' gaits look bizarre but should correct spontaneously, although pathological and normal gaits can look very similar.

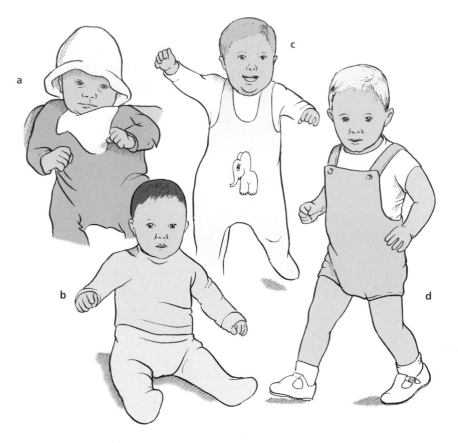

Fig. 21.1 Milestones of development: (a) holds the head up unsupported at 3 months; (b) sits up unaided at 6 months; (c) stands up unaided between 9 and 12 months; (d) walks between 12 and 18 months.

When asked to examine a child or toddler's gait, be sure to watch the child walk into the consulting room. Nobody, child or adult, can walk 'normally' if asked to do so and the entry into the consulting room may be the only chance to observe the gait that is the reason for the consultation.

Remember DDH (p. 354)

Before reassuring a patient that a child's gait is normal, always think of developmental dysplasia of the hip (DDH), particularly if the child is aged between 12 and 18 months (p. 354). If there are any of the following features, assume that the child has a dislocated hip until radiographs prove otherwise:

1. Limbs of unequal length.
2. An asymmetrical range of movement of the hips.
3. Asymmetrical skin creases.
4. A lurching gait.
5. A feeling of instability.

The consequences of missing DDH are very serious and radiographic examination of the pelvis is always justified if there is the slightest doubt about the stability of the hips in a child.

Bow legs and knock knees

Valgus or varus deformities in children are very common but seldom serious. Few children have rickets in this day and age but the herd memory of the disease is still active and bowed legs give very reasonable cause for alarm.

Many babies have varus tibiae at birth, and nappies, which hold the hips in abduction, make the bowing more obvious. The bowing also makes the toes turn slightly inward. If the bowing is very obvious the children are said to have outward-curved tibiae but the borderline between normal and abnormal is very vague.

The varus will usually have corrected itself by the age of 3, when it is replaced by a slight valgus deformity at the knee (Fig. 21.2). The amount of valgus deformity is variable but it is permissible to have

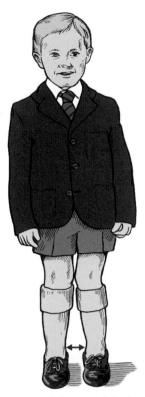

Fig. 21.2 Normal valgus deformity of the leg. Ten centimetres between the medial malleoli at the age of 4 years will correct spontaneously.

10 cm between the ankles at the age of 4 ('4 inches at 4 years') when the deformity is at its greatest. A marked improvement can be expected soon after the child starts school at the age of 4 or 5 years.

Before reassuring the parents, it is important to exclude serious disease, of which the following are the most likely under the age of 5:

1. Vitamin D or C deficiency.
2. Blount's disease, an abnormality of development at the upper end of the tibia which leads to progressive varus deformity.
3. Growth disorders such as epiphyseal injuries and epiphyseal dysplasia.

There are four factors to beware of in children with bow legs and knock knees:

1. More than 10 cm between the malleoli.
2. A family history of skeletal abnormality.
3. Asymmetry.
4. Abnormally short stature.

If one of these features is present there may be a serious developmental abnormality or a dislocated hip. If none then the child will probably develop normally.

In-toe gait

The commonest problem seen in a children's orthopaedic clinic is an in-toe gait. An in-turned foot is very obvious, the child can fall and the gait attracts much comment.

There are three causes of an in-toe gait:

1. Anteversion of the femoral neck.
2. Metatarsus adductus.
3. Outward curved tibiae.

Anteversion of the femoral neck

The most common cause is abnormal rotation at the hip due to excessive anteversion of the neck of the femur relative to its shaft. This allows a greater range of internal rotation than external (Fig. 21.3). Abnormalities of rotation are much more obvious with the leg straight than with the hip and knee flexed.

In an adult, the ranges of internal and external rotation of the hip are roughly the same but in a child there may be 90° of internal rotation and only 30° of external rotation. Such a child will walk with the foot in the middle of the range of motion, i.e. in 30° of internal rotation, and will be able to squat with the legs turned outwards. It is not unusual for one of the parents to recall doing the same thing when young, which makes reassurance easy.

Treatment

No treatment, whether by splintage or operation, is helpful. If the patient has no external rotation at all, a rotational osteotomy of the femur may be required when growth is complete. Apart from this, nothing is needed except firm reassurance that the shape of the femur will gradually change so that the range of internal and external rotation approach each other. The position continues improving until 10 years of age.

Metatarsus adductus

Metatarsus adductus also causes an in-toe gait and is dealt with under foot deformities below.

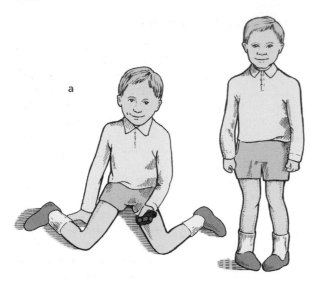

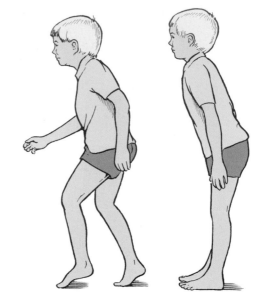

Fig. 21.4 Toe-walkers walk on tiptoe and lean slightly forward when standing.

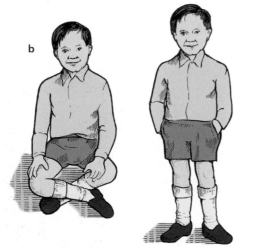

Fig. 21.3 Anteversion and retroversion of the femoral neck: (a) children with anteversion of the femoral neck can sit with their feet out beside them and walk with the toes turned in; (b) children with retroversion can sit with the legs crossed and walk with the toes turned out.

Outward curved tibiae

Outward curved tibiae can also cause an in-toe gait. No treatment is required.

Out-toe gait

Retroversion of the femoral neck

A smaller number of children have a greater range of external rotation than internal and walk with

their feet turned out 'like Charlie Chaplin'. These children can also sit with their legs crossed, impossible for children with excessive internal rotation. External rotation of the leg is also seen in DDH and this must be excluded before reassuring the parents. As always, check the rest of the child for deformities.

Treatment

As with internal rotation of the hip, firm reassurance is all that is required.

Toe-walkers

In some children, the Achilles tendon is tight and restricts dorsiflexion of the ankle so that the child walks on tiptoe and cannot stand with the heels flat (Fig. 21.4).

The feet and ankles appear normal at first glance and the parents may already have been reassured that 'there is nothing wrong' by the time they reach an orthopaedic clinic. On careful examination, dorsiflexion of the ankle is restricted or absent, the child cannot squat with the heels to the ground and stands with a characteristic forward stoop. If they attempt to stand upright, the children fall over backwards. The signs are worse when the child is barefoot.

Untreated, the Achilles tendon will usually stretch enough to acquire a reasonable gait but the patient will usually have a 'bouncing' gait because they have to rise on tiptoe when the body's weight passes in front of the foot.

It must be remembered that hyperactive children and patients with mild cerebral palsy may also walk on their toes. *Be sure to exclude neurological abnormalities in toe-walkers!*

Treatment

Serial plasters are sometimes effective but lengthening of the Achilles tendon is often required.

Tight hamstrings

If the child has tight hamstrings which prevent forward flexion, suspect spondylolisthesis (p. 457). Radiographs of the lumbosacral spine are essential in any child with tight hamstrings or calf muscles.

Foot deformities

Foot deformities (Fig. 21.5) **can be divided into two groups:**

1. Forefoot deformities, more common and usually trivial.
2. Hindfoot deformities, less common and more serious.

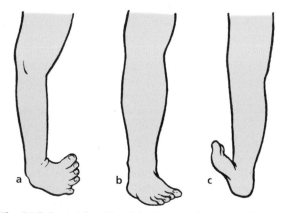

Fig. 21.5 Foot deformities: (a) talipes equinovarus with a wasted calf; (b) metatarsus adductus; (c) talipes calcaneovalgus.

Metatarsus adductus

The commonest forefoot deformity is metatarsus adductus or hooked forefoot, which is usually noticed at about the age of 6 months when children begin to pull themselves upright. The deformity occurs at the midtarsal joint (Fig. 21.6a) and the hindfoot is completely normal. This can be confirmed by covering the forefoot while examining the hindfoot. When this is done, the foot looks entirely normal (Fig. 21.6b).

The cause is not known but an attractive suggestion is that the forefoot is pushed inwards by the child while sleeping face down with their bottom in the air, a position only stable if the feet are pointing towards each other. It is certainly true that the condition begins to correct when the child is too 'bottom-heavy' to sleep in this position, usually at the age of about 18 months.

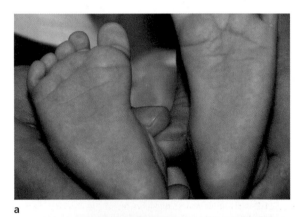

a

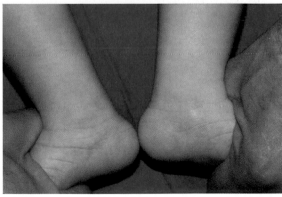

b

Fig. 21.6 Metatarsus adductus. The deformity arises in the middle of the foot (a). If the forefoot is covered over (b), the foot cannot be distinguished from normal.

The position of the foot makes walking difficult as children trip over their own feet. This causes a characteristic scuff mark at the anterolateral corner of the shoes. The position of the foot also produces an in-toe gait and makes a coexisting in-toe gait of femoral anteversion more obvious.

Treatment

Treatment begins by reassuring the parents that the child does not have a club foot and that the deformity corrects itself spontaneously in over 90% of patients.

Before the age of 3 years, no active treatment is required apart from gentle stretching of the medial side of the forefoot by holding the heel in one hand and the forefoot in the other. This should be done twice daily when dressing or bathing the child.

After the age of 3, treatment depends on the mobility of the foot. If gentle pressure corrects the deformity completely, observation can be continued, but if it cannot be corrected, serial casts are needed. A below-knee cast is applied in the position of maximum correction and changed at 2 week intervals to achieve a gradual correction. If serial casts are unsuccessful and the deformity is still marked by the age of 6, surgical correction may be necessary.

Congenital talipes equinovarus

The most common type of club foot, congenital talipes equinovarus (CTEV), is a deformity of the whole foot, which is pulled downwards (equinus) and inwards (varus) (Fig. 21.7).

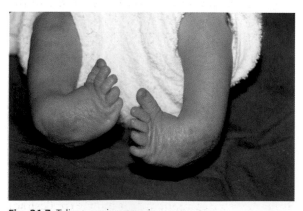

Fig. 21.7 Talipes equinovarus in a neonate.

The condition has been recognized for centuries but remains an enigma. The demi-god Vulcan, who injured his foot when cast from heaven, is depicted with a club foot. The poet Byron also had a club foot.

As far as we know, the condition is caused by failure of growth in the posteromedial muscles of the calf, particularly tibialis posterior, the toe flexors, gastrocnemius and soleus. The muscles are entirely normal in all other respects but are simply too small for the patient. The bones of the forefoot, and sometimes the tibia and fibula, may be shorter than those of the opposite side. The condition is more common if a relative is affected or there is any other genetic abnormality.

Because the muscles on the medial side of the foot and calf are too short, the foot is pulled downwards and inwards with the ankle in flexion. As growth proceeds, the talonavicular joint is distorted, the navicular is pulled off the talus medially and a bony deformity quickly develops as the soft bones of childhood mould themselves to surrounding tissues.

Treatment

No treatment will make the foot and calf completely normal and this should be explained to parents as gently as possible before treatment is begun. It is unkind to lead the parents to believe that a complete cure is possible.

The aims of treatment are twofold:

1. To prevent bony deformity developing.
2. To keep the foot plantigrade; i.e. in such a position that it can be placed flat on the ground.

The Ponseti method of treatment is gaining popularity. This involves sequential gentle manipulation and splinting of the foot with serial casts for a considerable period of time (Fig. 21.8). The treatment is started as soon after birth as possible and continued until the foot is held in the desired position. A tendo Achilles lengthening (percutaneous tenotomy) is often required to achieve a plantigrade foot. Subsequent night braces may need to be worn up to 4 years of age.

If the deformity is still present or is unable to be corrected then an operation is needed to lengthen the structures on the medial side of the foot and calf as well as release of the posterior capsule of the ankle joint. This will produce a good appearance but as growth proceeds the short structures may need to be lengthened again.

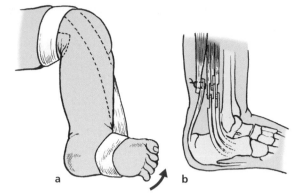

Fig. 21.8 Treatment of CTEV: (a) strapping is applied to pull the foot upwards and outwards; (b) if this fails, the posteromedial structures must be lengthened and the posterior capsule of the ankle divided.

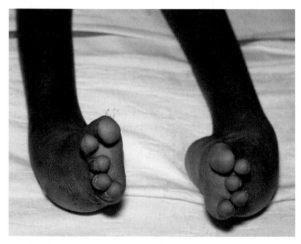

Fig. 21.9 End result of untreated CTEV.

If the deformity cannot be corrected by soft tissue release, the lateral side of the foot may need to be shortened by removing a bony wedge. This would typically be done in the older child, especially if the treatment had been delayed initially.

If the position is still unsatisfactory when growth is complete (Fig. 21.9), a triple arthrodesis will be required to fuse the following three joints (see Fig. 25.3):

1. Calcaneocuboid.
2. Subtalar.
3. Talonavicular.

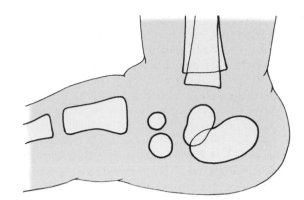

Fig. 21.10 The position of the bones in a child with congenital vertical talus.

Congenital vertical talus

A congenital vertical talus produces a spectacularly flat foot, usually obvious at birth. Radiographs are difficult to interpret in early life but the vertical position of the talus is usually obvious (Fig. 21.10).

Treatment. Although rare, the condition must be recognized and treated promptly by open reduction. This is one type of flat foot for which reassurance is not appropriate.

Talipes calcaneovalgus

A calcaneovalgus foot points upwards and the heel points downwards. The deformity is usually postural and is commonest in large babies delivered of small mothers. The deformity corrects itself within the first 12 months of life without treatment, but firm reassurance that all is well cannot be given until more serious conditions have been excluded, particularly DDH.

Calcaneovalgus deformities are also seen in patients with meningomyelocoele and abnormalities of the cauda equina. A thorough neurological examination of the lower limbs is therefore important.

Flat foot

Flat feet in adults is dealt with on page 442. Two types of flat foot are seen in children:

1. Mobile flat foot
2. Rigid flat foot.

Mobile flat foot

By far the more common type is mobile (or flexible) flat foot. The deformity is only apparent when the child stands with the feet flat to the ground; it disappears when the child is standing on tiptoe or lying relaxed on a couch.

Treatment. Most patients with this condition have generalized ligamentous laxity and require no treatment because the feet become normal as growth proceeds and ligaments become tighter. Special shoes are only needed if the wear on one part of the shoe is excessive, yet shoes with a 3–5 mm inside wedge or firm arch support are often recommended. There is no evidence that they hasten the natural resolution of the deformity but prescribing special shoes may be comforting to parents who then feel that 'something is being done'.

Rigid flat foot

Rigid (or 'spastic') flat foot is present if the deformity does not disappear when the child stands on tiptoe or lies flat. The rigidity is due partly to joint abnormalities and partly to spasm of the surrounding muscles. Further investigation is needed to exclude abnormal tarsal coalitions (p. 434) and other structural deformities.

Treatment depends on the underlying pathology. Special shoes or operation may be needed.

Children's shoes

Much nonsense is talked about children's shoes as a cause of foot deformity. Two points are worth considering:

1. Deformed feet occur in developing countries where shoes are not worn at all.
2. Attempts to correct foot deformity by diligent external splintage are generally unsuccessful.

It is therefore difficult to understand how a comfortable shoe worn for perhaps 12 h a day can lead to a permanent alteration of growth. Nevertheless, it is important that children should wear good shoes with the following features (Fig. 21.11):

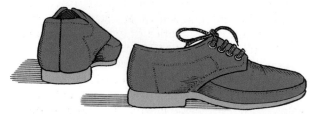

Fig. 21.11 A good child's shoe. The heel is flat on the ground, support for the heel is firm and the inner side of the shoe is well supported. There is ample room for growth.

1. A firm heel to prevent the hindfoot rolling into inversion or eversion.
2. A firm medial edge to support the longitudinal arch.
3. A firm flat sole.

Such a shoe will support the foot and give stable contact with the ground.

Developmental dysplasia of the hip (DDH)

Previously known as congenital dislocation of the hip, this is a serious condition if not diagnosed and treated within the first months of life. The incidence varies from race to race but is approximately 1.5 per 1000 live births in European nations. Girls are affected eight times more often than boys, the left hip is affected more often than the right, and the incidence is higher if a relative is affected. One-third of dislocated hips have an abnormality of the opposite hip as well.

Diagnosis

The diagnosis is made by clinical examination at the routine postnatal examination, assisted by ultrasound examination. Radiographs are unhelpful because the femoral head does not start to calcify until the age of 10 weeks, often later. Several tests are described (Barlow's, Ortolani's, von Rosen's), all very similar.

Clinical examination. The child is laid supine, without nappies, and the femur held between the thumb and forefinger (Fig. 21.12). The hip is abducted and the femoral head moved backwards and forwards relative to the acetabulum; i.e. up and down relative to the couch. If the hip is unstable, an unmistakable thud or jolt is felt as the femur moves in and out of the acetabulum.

Correctly performed, this test will identify almost every unstable hip, but there are two exceptions. The first is a very small group in which the femoral head slips slowly out of the acetabulum during the first year of life, and the second is the very unusual hip that is irreducible at birth.

Abnormal clicks are found in about 20 per 1000 live births at the immediate postnatal examination, but fall to about 6 per 1000 after 2 weeks.

Ultrasound examination allows the hips to be placed in one of four categories. In most centres the examination is advised in 'high risk' hips; i.e. babies with a click on clinical examination, a family history of DDH, or other predisposing factor.

If ultrasound shows the hip to be dislocated or the acetabular roof to be sloping, a splint or harness is applied and retained until ultrasound shows the hip is reduced.

It is better to treat 100 patients needlessly in this way than miss one patient with DDH, even though incorrectly applied splintage which holds the hip in excess abduction can cause aseptic necrosis of the femoral head.

Treatment

Treatment depends on the time of diagnosis – the sooner the diagnosis, the easier the treatment.

At birth. If DDH is diagnosed within the first week of life, it can be corrected by the child wearing double nappies or using a harness which holds the hips abducted and flexed (Fig. 21.13). One study showed that the condition was far commoner in North American Indians, who wrapped their babies in a papoose, than in racially identical Eskimos who carried their babies on their backs with the hips abducted and flexed.

An appliance such as the Cambridge splint, Pavlik harness or von Rosen splint holds the hips in the same position and will achieve a stable hip if worn correctly for 12 weeks. The pelvis is then examined radiologically or with ultrasound to confirm that the

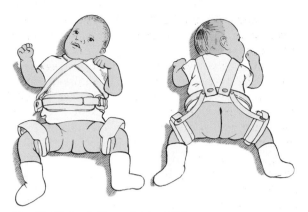

Fig. 21.13 Cambridge splint for DDH.

hip is reduced. If the plain radiograph is not conclusive, an arthrogram is performed (Fig. 21.14). If the hip is satisfactory at 12 weeks, the joint is likely to be virtually normal but the child should be reviewed regularly until skeletal maturity. The patient can then be discharged but should be urged to check her or his own children's and grandchildren's hips for dislocation.

At 2 months. If the condition is not diagnosed at birth it may be identified at routine examination 8 weeks later, when it should be apparent from the restriction of hip abduction. DDH diagnosed at this age can be managed conservatively with a brace traction or plaster immobilization.

At 12–18 months. If the dislocation is not found at the 8 week examination the diagnosis will probably be missed until the age of 12–18 months, when the child begins to walk with a limp and a rolling gait. The diagnosis can be confirmed on clinical examination because there will be shortening of the limb, the foot will be externally rotated, the skin creases asymmetrical and the Trendelenburg sign positive (Fig. 21.15).

At this stage the hip cannot be made perfect but a series of operations will usually achieve a stable joint, although at the price of great physical and emotional upset for the child and the family.

Because the prognosis is so much better if the diagnosis is made early, special care should be taken with the neonatal examination. A missed DDH is a disaster. The only patients who can lead a moderately normal life with a dislocated hip are those with both hips dislocated, because their problem is then symmetrical (Fig. 21.16).

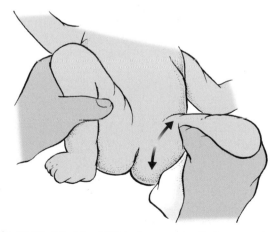

Fig. 21.12 A test for DDH in the neonate. Backward and forward pressure on the femur in full flexion and abduction can move the head of the femur in and out of the acetabulum.

355

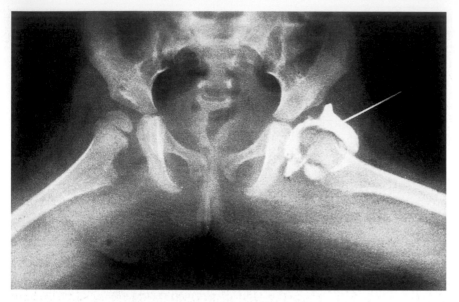

Fig. 21.14 Arthrogram of a congenitally dislocated hip after reduction. Note that the acetabulum is well formed but not as well calcified as the healthy side.

Neurological disorders

Spina bifida and meningomyelocoele

Meningomyelocoele is a congenital anomaly of the spinal cord in which there is defective tubulation of the neural plate, which remains open (Fig. 21.17). Neural tissues, including the roots and long tracts, lie visible on the child's back and do not function. The lesion is often surrounded by hair (see Fig. 21.17). The extent of the lesion is variable and it may be associated with the Arnold–Chiari malformation and hydrocephalus.

Treatment

The problems of meningomyelocoele are enormous. Paediatricians, urologists and neurosurgeons are all as much involved as orthopaedic surgeons.

The management of the orthopaedic problems is complex and is determined as much by the intellectual potential of the child as by the deformity. If the child has mental impairment and is unlikely to manage anything more than a wheelchair existence, it is unkind to inflict operation, calipers and intensive physiotherapy. These cause just as much emotional strain as they would to a normal child or an adult and it may be wiser to help the child come to terms with a wheelchair existence.

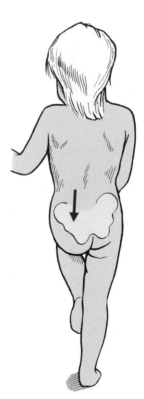

Fig. 21.15 Positive Trendelenburg test at the age of 15 months in a child with a dislocated left hip.

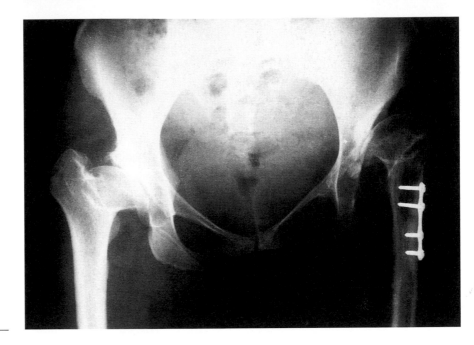

Fig. 21.16 Bilateral DDH. The left hip remains dislocated despite an osteotomy to attempt reduction. Both femoral heads have dysplasia from damage due to splinting in extreme abduction. This damage can be avoided.

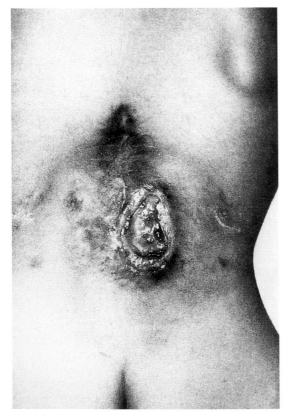

Fig. 21.17 A meningomyelocoele.

Other children with myelomeningocoele have normal intellectual attainment and drive and can easily overcome these difficulties. As with so much of orthopaedics, it is the patient that must be treated, not the pathology.

The appropriate treatment for the individual child can be selected during the first 2 years of life, and decisions made then will determine future policy. In general, the best approach is a realistic assessment of the child's potential and minimal surgery to prevent deformity.

Diastematomyelia

Diastematomyelia is dealt with on page 460.

Cerebral palsy

Cerebral palsy is caused by a lesion of the immature brain, often sustained at birth. It leads to a variety of neurological disorders, including spastic diplegia and choreoathetosis.

Clinical features

The principal feature is loss of voluntary control of the muscles. The commonest pattern is increased tone in the flexor muscle groups on one side pro-

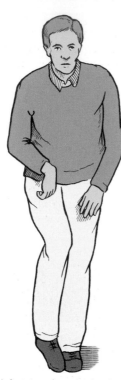

Fig. 21.18 The deformity of cerebral palsy in an adult. The flexor groups of the elbow, wrist, fingers, hip and ankle all have increased tone, which is not balanced by the opposing extensor groups.

ducing a spastic hemiparesis, or spasticity of both lower limbs. Spinal deformities are also seen. In spastic hemiparesis the lower limb is usually more seriously affected than the upper (Fig. 21.18). Mental retardation, athetosis and other abnormalities may also be present.

Examination

Because the flexor muscles are tight the limbs are pulled into characteristic positions. The foot is held in equinus, the knees are flexed and the hips adducted and flexed. The arm is held across the body, with the wrist and elbow flexed.

If the patient is relaxed the spasm in the flexors can easily be overcome by gentle manipulation but returns as soon as the limb is released or the child becomes agitated.

Treatment

Conservative treatment is important and the parents need much care and support. Physiotherapy helps to relieve muscle spasm and makes the best use of normal muscles. Calipers support the limbs and control unwanted movements.

If conservative treatment fails, operation is required to relieve flexor spasm by the following means:

1. Denervating muscles.
2. Lengthening tendons.
3. Moving muscle attachments.

In older patients, joints can be stabilized and bony deformities corrected by osteotomy or arthrodesis.

Selecting treatment is difficult and the whole patient must be considered. The equinus deformity of the foot, for example, is easily corrected by lengthening the Achilles tendon but the child may depend on that equinus deformity to compensate for the associated flexion deformities at the hip and the knee. In short, the deformity does not need to be corrected simply because it is there, but only if correction will improve the function of the limb as a whole.

Adductor spasm can lead to progressive subluxation of the hip and make it difficult to clean the perineum. The spasm can be relieved by dividing the adductor tendons and the obturator nerve. There may be a place for botulinum toxin injections to eradicate the spasm in some cases.

Poliomyelitis

Poliomyelitis, or infantile paralysis, causes deformities in children and should be a piece of history. Immunization is very effective if properly done, yet the disease is still seen.

The condition differs from cerebral palsy in two ways:

1. The paralysis is flaccid, not spastic.
2. Any muscle can be involved and the condition does not affect flexor muscles more than extensors. Individual nerve roots are involved.

Treatment

The aim of treatment is to produce a balanced limb with stable joints.

Conservative. Physiotherapy is important to overcome contractures and rehabilitate muscles; calipers or braces will often stabilize a flail limb but they are not strong enough to control active and unopposed muscles.

Operative. Operation may be required to make unaffected normal muscles work in a balanced way. If, for example, all the knee extensors are paralysed but all the flexors are working normally, one or more hamstrings can be transferred to the quadriceps tendon to act as extensors. If muscle balance cannot be achieved, the joint will need to be arthrodesed to make it stable.

Congenital deformities

A host of minor congenital deformities exist but not all require treatment and it is usually advisable to defer operation until growth is complete (Figs 21.19, 21.20). In deciding whether or not to operate, remember that function is more important than appearance; to turn a painless digit that works well but looks odd into a useless one that hurts but looks perfect is a poor exchange.

Fortunately, it is seldom necessary to correct a deformity until growth is complete, by which time the patient will be able to make her or his own decision.

Hammer toe (or mallet toe)

Fixed flexion deformity of the distal interphalangeal joint of the second toe is a familial disorder that can cause pressure problems at the tip of the toe (Fig. 21.21a).

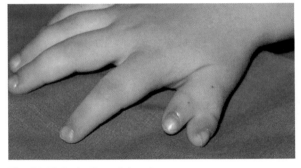

Fig. 21.19 Reduplicated thumb.

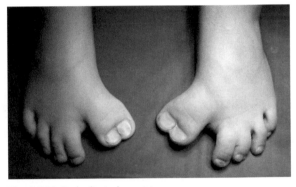

Fig. 21.20 Reduplicated great toes.

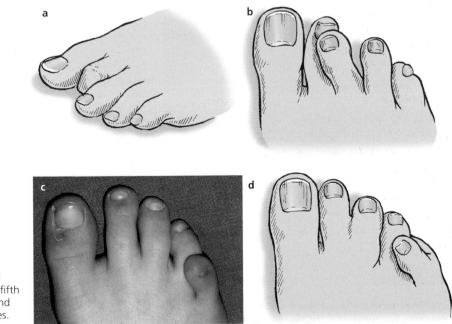

Fig. 21.21 (a) Mallet toe deformity; (b) crossed second and third toes; (c) overriding fifth toe; (d) overriding fifth toe and webbed second and third toes.

Treatment

If the symptoms warrant it, the toe can be straightened or the tip amputated when growth is finished. Before skeletal maturity, simple flexor tenotomy will relieve the deformity.

Crossed second and third toes

The second and third toes sometimes cross over each other and cause difficulty with shoe wear (Fig. 21.21b).

Treatment

No disability is likely from this deformity and correction is seldom needed.

Overriding fifth toe (digiti quinti varus)

In this condition the little toe lies transversely across the top of the fourth toe, producing a curious appearance and making shoe wear difficult (Fig. 21.21c, d).

Treatment

The deformity may need correction in early adolescence if the symptoms justify it. The operation,

Butler's procedure, is radical and involves dissecting the toe free until it is held only by vessels and nerves. The toe is then 'reimplanted' in the correct position. Less radical procedures are ineffective.

Lobster claw hand

Lobster claw hand (Fig. 21.22) is inherited as an autosomal dominant and involves dysplasia of the middle rays of the hand and foot, producing a bizarre appearance that rarely interferes with function.

Absence of parts (Fig. 21.23)

The absence of a limb is known as amelia and is extremely rare. Absence of part of a limb is more common and is known as phocomelia. This term has nothing to do with 'focal' and means that the limbs look like the flippers of a seal. Phocomelia can arise from many causes but the best known in recent years was the drug thalidomide.

Any limb can be involved to any degree, but proximal focal femoral deficiency creates special difficulties with weight-bearing.

Treatment is by braces and appliances.

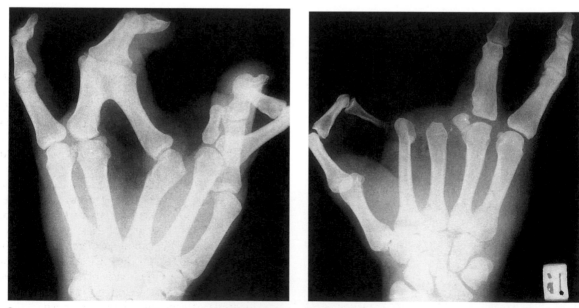

a   b

Fig. 21.22 (a), (b) Lobster claw hand.

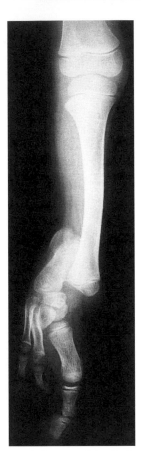

Fig. 21.23 Congenital absence of the fibula.

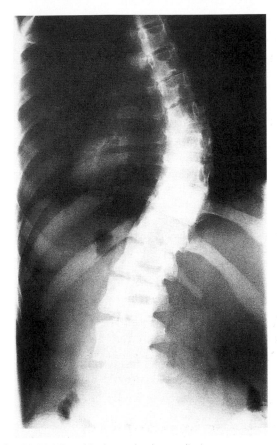

Fig. 21.24 Idiopathic thoracolumbar scoliosis.

Scoliosis

Very few patients have scoliosis requiring treatment but the condition attracts much attention. There are several types.

Types of scoliosis

1. Non-structural (postural) curves due, for example, to limb inequality. There is no rotation of the vertebrae with these curves.
2. Structural curves, which have rotation and sometimes wedging of the vertebrae.

Structural curves can be subdivided into four groups:

1. Idiopathic scoliosis.
2. Congenital and infantile.
3. Neuromuscular.
4. Miscellaneous.

Idiopathic scoliosis

Idiopathic scoliosis may be infantile (0–3 years), juvenile (3–10 years), adolescent (10 years to maturity), or adult (after maturity), according to the time of onset. Of these, adolescent idiopathic scoliosis is the commonest type (Fig. 21.24). It develops during the adolescent growth spurt, is commoner in girls than boys, and thoracic curves are usually convex to the right. The cause is unknown.

In its mildest form there is a slight curve of the spine, which may pass completely unnoticed or may be part of a more obvious asymmetry. Over 10% of adolescents have some degree of chest asymmetry. In more severe forms the spine can become grossly deformed if not treated, producing the classic hunchback of history. The hunchback of Nôtre Dame is said to have had a facial deformity and this makes neurofibromatosis the most likely diagnosis.

The thoracic spine is most often involved and has the most serious consequences, but deformities of the more flexible lumbar, thoracolumbar and cervical spines are also seen.

Natural history

The deformity appears at the start of the adolescent growth spurt and increases rapidly over the next 2 or 3 years. Progression continues until growth ceases. Some progress to moderate, mild or severe deformity, but some do not progress at all.

Untreated, the deformity may produce no obvious locomotor disability but it may cause cosmetic problems, cardiopulmonary compromise, pain from secondary degenerative changes in the spinal joints and loss of balance when sitting.

Clinical features

There are five important clinical features:

1. The spine is curved. The curve is best seen by asking the child to bend forward and inspecting the contour of the spine from behind (see Fig. 2.6). Structural curves in the spine will be exaggerated and postural curves reduced.
2. The shoulders are not level.
3. The waist is asymmetrical.
4. There is asymmetry of the chest or loin on forward bending.
5. There may be features of an underlying disorder, e.g. café-au-lait patches in neurofibromatosis or hairy patches in spina bifida.

Treatment

Not all deformities become worse but it is wise to review the patients regularly so that those which do progress can be treated promptly. There are three forms of treatment:

1. Corrective casts may stop infantile idiopathic curves progressing if applied early.
2. Braces may stop progression in some curves, but this is an area of controversy. Some evidence suggests that conservative treatment, including braces, has no effect at all and that the patients whose deformity was 'controlled' by devices such as braces were the ones who would not have progressed anyway.
3. Operation may be needed in severe and increasing deformity. The curve can be corrected by instrumentation to the back or front of the spine

and held with internal fixation devices or it can be fused permanently in the corrected position. Both are major surgical undertakings and sometimes followed by serious complications, including paraplegia.

Congenital and infantile scoliosis

Congenital deformities such as hemivertebra give rise to a deformity present at birth. Correction is difficult or impossible.

Infantile idiopathic scoliosis develops during the first 3 years of life, is commoner in boys than in girls, and the thoracic curve is usually convex to the left, the opposite of adolescent idiopathic scoliosis. Ninety per cent of thoracic curves resolve spontaneously but the rest need treatment with braces or internal fixation if severe. Even if no treatment is required, it is sensible to obtain an opinion on the value of a brace in the individual case.

Neuromuscular scoliosis

Neurological imbalance of the spinal muscles from poliomyelitis, spina bifida, neurofibromatosis or other neurological disorders produces a severe scoliosis which cannot always be treated successfully. Braces or internal fixation may be required.

Other conditions

Limb inequality

To have limbs of equal length is rare; there is usually a difference of up to 1 cm. Because the lower limb is about 1 metre long, this represents a 'tolerance' of 1%.

Management of limb inequality

<2 cm at maturity – no treatment.
2–5 cm – raise to shoe.
>5 cm – operation sometimes.

Treatment

Shortening of less than 2 cm is scarcely noticeable, and up to 5 cm can be treated by a raise to the shoe. Shortening greater than 5cm can be treated either by

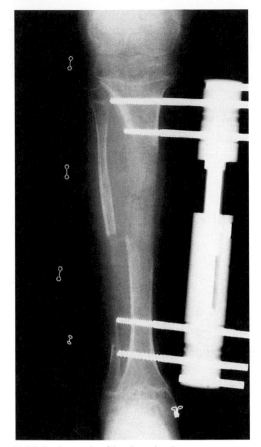

Fig. 21.25 Radiograph of leg lengthening.

interfering with the epiphysis to arrest growth in the longer limb or shortening the longer limb when growth is complete.

Alternatively, the shorter limb can be elongated by distraction apparatus applied either across a transverse cut in the diaphysis or the epiphyseal plate. Operation is not easy and vessels, nerves and tendons may not stretch as easily as the divided bone (Fig. 21.25).

To determine how much the limb must be lengthened, or when growth should be arrested, requires an accurate assessment of the likely difference in limb length when growth is complete. This information is derived from tables and graphs showing the rate of growth of the individual epiphyses at different ages.

Arthrogryposis multiplex congenita

Arthrogryposis is a rare condition characterized by the replacement of striated muscle with fibrous tissue and by soft tissue contractures. The result is a disabling loss of movement in many joints accompanied by a severe talipes and often dislocation of the hip. The degree of involvement is variable.

The elbows are usually fixed in extension and the wrists in flexion. The muscles of respiration are also involved and a few patients die of respiratory insufficiency. The patients are of normal intelligence and usually very determined.

Treatment

Treatment consists of soft tissue release and osteotomy to bring the limbs into the most useful position.

Radial club hand

Congenital anomalies of the hand are less common than the foot but radial club hand is seen and is usually associated with an absent or deficient radius, which allows the hand to 'fall off' the arm.

Treatment

Treatment consists of stabilizing the hand on the ulna, either with a brace or by operation.

Torticollis

Torticollis, or wry-neck, is now seldom seen but once occupied much orthopaedic time. The condition is the result of excessive stretching of the sternomastoid during delivery; improved obstetric care has reduced its incidence dramatically.

The area of damaged muscle contracts to form a firm fibrous mass in the muscle known as a sternomastoid 'tumour'. With growth, the head is pulled progressively over to one side by the tight contracture of sternomastoid (Fig. 21.26).

Treatment

Physiotherapy is only effective in the first year of life. If the deformity persists the sternomastoid must be released from the clavicle and the head held in the corrected position until the patient no longer tilts it. The operation should be done early for two reasons:

1. Growth changes produce a very odd asymmetrical face.

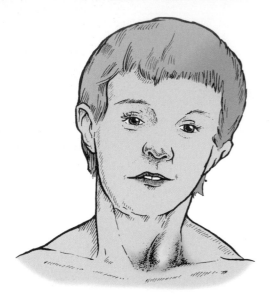

Fig. 21.26 Torticollis due to sternomastoid 'tumour'. Note the asymmetrical eyes and tilted face.

2. The eyes 'learn' to work in one position and the head tends to revert to that position.

Pseudarthrosis of the tibia

Pseudarthrosis of the tibia is a rare condition and should be differentiated from neurofibromatosis. In essence, the middle third of the tibia is deficient and either breaks with trivial injury or is completely absent. The appearances are very similar to an atrophic non-union in an adult and union is just as difficult to achieve.

Children's fractures usually unite rapidly and it is not known why the tibia sometimes behaves in this pernicious manner.

Treatment is by internal fixation and bone grafting. Amputation has been required in the past, but with solid fixation and bone grafting this should be avoided.

Congenital dislocation of the knee

This is a very rare condition consisting of hyperextension of the knee so that the knees appear to be mounted backwards. The condition is not analagous to DDH.

Treatment

Conservative treatment may be effective but open correction is often needed. Gentle manipulation early on is recommended. Open release of the contracted tissue is often needed and disorders of patella–femoral movement are common.

Chapter |22|

Disorders of the shoulder and elbow

By the end of this chapter you should:

- Be able to diagnose a shoulder dislocation and be aware of treatment options in the chronic dislocations.
- Appreciate the importance of arthroscopic surgery for the diagnosis and treatment of intra-articular disorders of both shoulder and elbow.

Shoulder

Recurrent dislocation of the shoulder

Acute dislocations of the shoulder are described on page 192. Although most shoulders in elderly patients remain stable after reduction, some dislocate repeatedly with trivial trauma, especially those with ligamentous laxity. The dislocations can be anterior, posterior, inferior or multidirectional, but anterior dislocation is by far the commonest.

Recurrent anterior dislocation

Recurrent anterior dislocation happens when the shoulder is fully abducted and externally rotated, which brings the head of the humerus against the weak inferior joint capsule (p. 193). This position, in which the arm is above the head and the hand facing forwards, occurs when swimming backstroke, reaching for a ball in a rugby line-out, or reaching into the back seat of a car from the front (Fig. 22.1). Patients with ligamentous laxity or those where there is a Bankart lesion (disruption of the anterior glenoid labrum and capsule) are most at risk.

Occasionally the humeral head may be fractured, giving a flat appearance or a hatchet-like deformity on radiographs (Hill–Sachs lesions).

Treatment

The dislocation can usually be reduced easily and many patients are able to reduce their own shoulders. Some learn to avoid dislocations and do not want operation, but others are disabled by their instability, and surgery must then be considered (e.g. Fig 22.2). Unfortunately, in young patients there is a significant chance of recurrence (up to 90%); recent trials of early surgery in these patients have shown a reasonable reduction in the subsequent dislocation rate.

Methods of correcting recurrent anterior dislocation of the shoulder include:

1. Tightening the inferior pouch of the joint capsule (by open surgery or arthroscopic surgery and/or electrocautery).

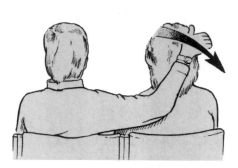

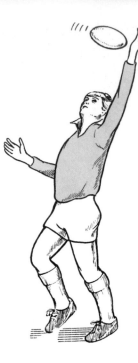

Fig. 22.1 Movements that can dislocate the shoulder.

a

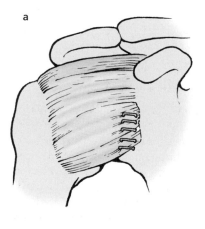

b

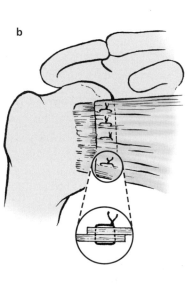

Fig. 22.2 Operations for recurrent dislocation of the shoulder: (a) reattachment of the inferior corner of the capsule; (b) shortening of the subscapularis tendon.

2. Reattaching the glenoid labrum in its correct position (Bankart's operation).

3. Tightening the subscapularis muscle to limit external rotation (Putti–Platt operation).

4. A bone block on the glenoid neck.

5. A combination of these.

After operation, the arm is bandaged to the side for 3 weeks. The forearm can then be released to allow rotation, and physiotherapy begun. The results are generally satisfactory.

Recurrent posterior dislocation

Recurrent posterior dislocation is less common than anterior dislocation and is often seen as a 'party trick' in teenagers with loose joints. The same patients can usually click their jaws and do weird

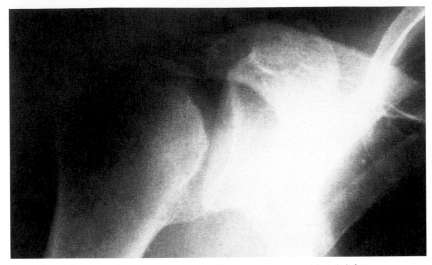

Fig. 22.3 Locked posterior dislocation of the shoulder in a patient with a humeral head defect.

tricks with their thumbs. The humeral head can become 'locked' behind the glenoid (Fig. 22.3).

Acute dislocations are described on page 192.

Treatment

The basis of treatment is to tell the patients not to do it on purpose, in the hope that they will learn to avoid the movements that cause the dislocation. It is very rare for recurrent posterior dislocation to cause enough disability to warrant stabilization. If operation is required then either a posterior bone block or a glenoid osteotomy will be needed. Both these operations are formidable and very unreliable.

Internal derangements of the shoulder

The glenoid labrum, like a meniscus in the knee, can be torn or detached at its rim and cause painful clicking or catching within the joint. Lesions of the superior labrum adjacent to the biceps tendon are described as SLAP lesions (SLAP = superior labrum anterior posterior). These occur when the superior glenoid labrum is avulsed or detached from the glenoid. Loose bodies and irregularities of the articular surface produce similar catching and clicking symptoms. MRI scans and, previously, arthrograms are very useful for identifying the lesion.

Treatment

The vast majority of these lesions are now dealt with arthroscopically. Labral lesions can be reattached with sutures or absorbable fixation devices. Loose bodies and chondral lesions are easily seen and removed with the arthroscope.

Supraspinatus tendinitis

The supraspinatus tendon passes through the narrow tunnel between the acromion and the head of the humerus and may degenerate or become inflamed where it crosses the humeral head (Fig. 22.4). With the resultant impingement between the humeral head and the acromion, the affected area of the tendon swells and causes pain during active abduction. The pain goes as soon as the sensitive area has passed through the tunnel. Because the pain is present in a small arc of movement only, usually between 60 and 120° of abduction, the condition is sometimes known as 'painful arc syndrome'.

The diagnosis can be confirmed by comparing passive movement with active. When the shoulder is moved passively there is no pressure on the tendon and movement is painless. During active movement the tendon is compressed against the humeral head and this is painful.

There are effectively three stages of this tendinitis, depending on the severity of the inflammation: stage 1, microscopic changes in the tendon; stage 2,

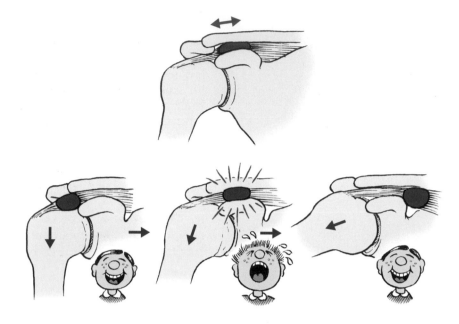

Fig. 22.4 Supraspinatus tendinitis and painful arc syndrome. An inflamed and swollen area of the supraspinatus tendon causes pain as it passes beneath the acromioclavicular joint.

oedema of the tendon; and finally, stage 3, where the tendon starts to rupture and tear.

Treatment

In the early stages, rest and avoidance of activities provoking the inflammation may be sufficient, but with prolonged or severe cases an injection of 25 mg of hydrocortisone acetate and local anaesthetic placed around the tendon (but not into it) is effective in most patients. The injection is given with the arm hanging and the patient sitting and supported. The needle is placed either beneath the acromion from its lateral end or posteriorly in the line of the tendon. In recalcitrant cases that fail to settle with appropriate conservative treatment, or where the supraspinatus tendon has torn, then surgery may be necessary. Arthroscopic (or open) surgery to remove the spur on the under-surface of the acromion or inferior surface of the acromioclavicular joint has a good prognosis, although the recovery for this may be prolonged. Occasionally the acromioclavicular joint needs to be excised. The aim of the surgery is to allow increased room for the inflamed tendon to pass under the acromion without impingement. By removing the cause of the impingement, the tendon will hopefully heal. Where there is a tear of the tendon this can again be repaired to bone or side to side, either arthroscopically or via an open approach.

The advantage of arthroscopic procedures is the shortened recovery time postoperatively.

Acute calcific supraspinatus tendinitis

If the symptoms of supraspinatus tendinitis come on rapidly over a period of hours and the pain is intense, radiographs may show a patch of calcification within the tendon, often adjacent to its insertion on the humeral head. It is frequently described as one of the worst pains imaginable. The patients are usually in the second or third decade of life and the condition is probably a variation of crystal arthropathy (p. 305). Women are affected more often than men.

Treatment

Aspiration can be attempted but injection of hydrocortisone acetate into the calcified area itself brings dramatic relief. The calcified material may need to be excised if these methods fail.

Rupture or tear of supraspinatus tendon

The supraspinatus tendon can rupture spontaneously without causing acute symptoms (Fig. 22.5).

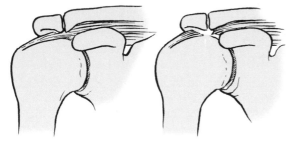

Fig. 22.5 Attrition rupture of the supraspinatus tendon. The supraspinatus tendon becomes worn beneath an osteophyte on the acromioclavicular joint and may rupture.

Cadaver studies show that the tendon is defective in 40% of patients at age 40, 60% at 60 and 80% at 80, but a much smaller percentage of patients have shoulder symptoms. From this it can be concluded that many supraspinatus ruptures are asymptomatic, although some cause intermittent aching in the shoulders after the age of 40.

Gradual attrition of a degenerate and ischaemic tendon on osteophytes on the under-surface of the acromion or the acromioclavicular joint is the likely mechanism (see above).

Treatment

No treatment is required in the asymptomatic, but in those patients with significant weakness of the power of abduction then a debridement of the tendon, repair of the torn portion back to the bone, and a decompression of the impingement may be required. Symptomatic relief with anti-inflammatory drugs and physiotherapy may be effective in some patients.

Frozen shoulder

The main diagnostic feature of frozen shoulder is painful restriction of external rotation. It is a common and troublesome condition in which the shoulder is at first painful, then stiff. The stiffness makes it difficult to bring the hand to the mouth, behind the head to comb hair or behind the back to fasten buttons or hooks.

The cause is not known. There may be a precipitating cause, such as a minor injury, but there is often none. A localized autoimmune response is one possible explanation.

The condition has three distinct stages:

1. *Painful phase.* In the first stage, which can last for about 6 months, there is a painful restriction of movement in all directions. This distinguishes the condition from supraspinatus tendinitis, in which a specific arc of motion is painful during active movement only. The pain gradually subsides as the disease enters its second stage.

2. *Stiff phase.* The shoulder is very stiff, but usually painless with gross restriction of movement. This stage gives 'frozen' shoulder its name and lasts from 6 to 12 months. The pain gradually goes but the stiffness remains.

3. *Recovery phase.* During the next 6 months movement returns slowly but seldom completely.

Treatment

Treatment varies according to the stage of the disease.

Painful phase. Anti-inflammatory drugs are effective and a short course of systemic steroids may be needed for patients with severe pain. Physiotherapy is ineffective during this stage.

Stiff phase. During this phase, physiotherapy to improve the range of movement is occasionally helpful but relief is unpredictable.

Recovery phase. Physiotherapy or manipulation under anaesthetic may produce an increase in movement. Arthroscopic surgery to release the capsule has been shown to speed up the recovery.

Ruptured biceps tendon

The tendon of the long head of biceps, like that of the supraspinatus, is vulnerable at the shoulder and may rupture near its scapular origin (Fig. 22.6). The lesion occurs in older patients with minimal trauma and allows the muscle belly to contract unopposed, forming a firm ball of muscle in the lower part of the upper arm. This is sometimes called the 'Popeye sign' after the well known 'sailor man' (Fig. 22.7).

The condition is always alarming for the patient, who feels something snap in the shoulder. There is an obvious unfamiliar lump, which soon becomes discoloured by subcutaneous bleeding.

Treatment

No treatment is required apart from firm reassurance and explanation. The soft tissue

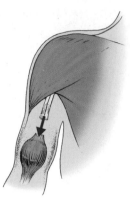

Fig. 22.6 Ruptured biceps tendon allowing the muscle belly to contract into the lower part of the upper arm.

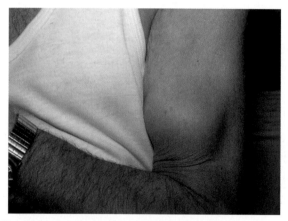

Fig. 22.7 A patient with a ruptured biceps tendon.

swelling and bruising gradually subsides and the short head of biceps continues to function and hypertrophies. Movement of the shoulder is little affected.

Acromioclavicular instability

Acute separation of the acromioclavicular joint may escape diagnosis until the patient presents with acromioclavicular instability. The arm is painful when working in front of the body at shoulder height, as when writing on a blackboard or carrying a tray. The joint itself is seldom tender, but a marked step at the joint is usual and can be abolished by holding the arm to the side, placing a hand under the elbow and lifting the humerus vertically upwards.

The exact clinical features depend upon the extent of the lesion.

Treatment

Surgical treatment is not required unless there is localized tenderness over the joint itself, in which case excision of the outer end of the clavicle may be needed.

Referred pain

Pain around the shoulder, particularly around the supraspinatus muscle, is often referred from the neck. The cervical spine should be examined in any patient who is complaining of pain in the shoulder.

Osteoarthritis of the shoulder

Osteoarthritis of the shoulder causes painful restriction of movement, particularly abduction and forward flexion. Movement of the scapulothoracic joint compensates to some extent, but there is often substantial disability.

Treatment

Conservative treatment with physiotherapy and anti-inflammatory drugs is helpful. Joint replacement is required for severe pain and restriction of movement.

The rheumatoid shoulder

The shoulder is not designed for weight-bearing. It is therefore unfortunate that the elbows and shoulders of patients with rheumatoid arthritis must function as weight-bearing joints when the patient gets out of a chair or uses crutches. To make matters worse, the shoulder is not mechanically stable and has a large synovial cavity, features which make it susceptible to destruction by rheumatoid arthritis.

Treatment

Anti-inflammatory drugs, appliances and aids are the mainstay of treatment but total joint replacement (Fig. 22.8) is required in some patients with painful or disorganized joints. Excision arthroplasty is also possible. The results of shoulder arthroplasty are good in rheumatoid arthritis.

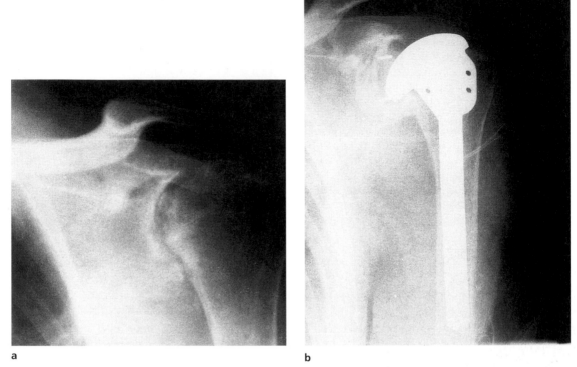

a   b

Fig. 22.8 (a), (b) Rheumatoid arthritis of the shoulder treated by total shoulder replacement.

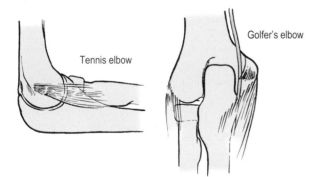

Fig. 22.9 Sites of muscle tears in tennis and golfer's elbow.

Elbow

Tennis elbow

The commonest lesion of the insertion of muscle or tendon onto bone is tennis elbow in which a microscopic tear occurs in or near the insertion of the common extensor tendon on the lateral condyle and humerus (Fig. 22.9). The injury is caused by either a sharp flexion of the wrist while the extensors are contracted or, in the chronic form, by hitting a tennis ball awkwardly during a backhand stroke. It can also be caused by excessive pressure when using a racquet grip which is too small. This overuse injury also occurs in everyday activities such as gardening, lifting and painting.

On examination, the lateral epicondyle is tender, and stressing the extensor origin, by forcing the wrist into flexion with the extensors contracted, reproduces the patient's symptoms (Mills' test).

Treatment

Treatment is by rest, i.e. avoiding contraction of the extensor muscles, by an injection of hydrcortisone acetate into the tender area, or by pulsed ultrasound. It is helpful to inject 2 ml 1% lidocaine into the affected area. This helps to disperse the steroid throughout the damaged area, as well as anaesthetizing it to confirm that the injection has been placed in the correct spot. The first injection has a very approximate success rate of 75%, the second 50%, and the third 25%.

371

If three injections are unsuccessful in relieving the symptoms, a release of the extensor origin from the humerus must be considered, but this is an uncomfortable and unpredictable operation. The muscle is raised from the bone and some surgeons remove a portion of the lateral epicondyle.

Golfer's elbow

Golfer's elbow is a similar condition to tennis elbow, in which the common flexor attachment on the medial epicondyle of the humerus is strained or torn. Classically, the symptoms are precipitated by the golfer striking the ground instead of the ball, thus straining the flexor origin. The condition is less common and the area of tenderness less precise than tennis elbow.

Treatment

Treatment is by steroid injection into the tender area, taking care to avoid the ulnar nerve if conservative treatment has failed. Treatment is less effective than for tennis elbow.

Loose bodies

Loose bodies in the elbow form in three ways:

1. Fragments from osteochondral fractures.
2. From chondral fragments.
3. Osteochondritis dissecans, which is much rarer at the elbow than the knee.

Clinical features

Loose bodies cause mechanical locking of the elbow (Fig. 22.10). Loose bodies in the olecranon fossa limit extension, in the coronoid fossa they limit flexion, and loose bodies stuck between the radius and ulna block pronation and supination.

Treatment

If the symptoms warrant it, the loose body must be removed either arthroscopically or via open procedure but rehabilitation is slow and some loss of movement is possible.

Olecranon bursitis

The olecranon bursa is a normal structure, comparable with the prepatellar bursa at the knee. A normal

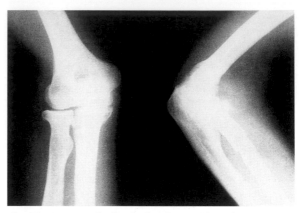

Fig. 22.10 Loose bodies in the elbow with early osteoarthritis.

bursa is small but an inflamed or infected bursa is large, hot and painful.

In the past, olecranon bursitis was known as 'student's elbow', from the notion that students spent much of their time leaning on the elbows poring over textbooks. Today, the condition is seen more often after trauma or a minor penetrating injury. It is also seen in patients with rheumatoid arthritis or gout, both of which can cause inflammation of any vulnerable soft tissue lesion.

Treatment

Infected bursae are treated by antibiotics and drainage, with excision of the bursa if infection recurs. Inflamed but uninfected bursae rarely require operation but excision is sometimes required if the inflammation is recurrent. Anti-inflammatory drugs should be tried first as these often resolve the condition. Gout should be treated or the bursa will recur after excision.

Osteoarthritis

Osteoarthritis of the elbow restricts flexion and extension and is disabling in patients who use their arms strenuously, e.g. blacksmiths, thatchers and steel erectors.

Treatment

Conservative treatment with anti-inflammatory drugs and alteration of daily activity is the treatment of choice whenever possible. Debridement has little to offer because the osteophytes recur after excision, and joint replacement is not effective because the prosthesis almost invariably loosens.

Rheumatoid arthritis

Rheumatoid arthritis can affect both the elbow and the superior radioulnar joint. These must be considered separately.

Elbow

Pain is the main problem in the rheumatoid elbow, but flexion and extension may be restricted and the elbow may eventually become unstable. This is a special problem if the lower limbs are also involved because, like the shoulders, the elbows become weight-bearing joints when the patient uses crutches or pushes up from a chair.

Treatment. If conservative treatment with anti-inflammatory drugs fails to bring relief, surgical synovectomy may be needed. Prosthetic elbow replacements are suitable for patients with joints that are painful and who do not wish to place great physical demands upon their elbows.

Superior radiohumeral joint

The radial head is surrounded by synovium, and involvement of the superior radiohumeral joint is common. Pronation and supination are severely limited but flexion and extension may be unaffected.

Treatment. If conservative treatment is unsuccessful and the symptoms are present only on pronation and supination, excision of the radial head is effective. The operation can be combined with synovectomy of the elbow. Prosthetic replacement of the proximal end of the radius was a popular procedure but is now seldom performed either for rheumatoid arthritis or for fractures.

Case reports

Painful movement of the shoulder is common, especially in the middle-aged athlete.

Patient A

A 42-year-old keen tennis player presented with increasing pain over the right shoulder. He had noticed that over the last few months the shoulder was becoming increasingly painful with most movements above his shoulder height. Movements below shoulder were pain-free. There was no associated history of trauma, but he had recently been doing a lot of DIY activities around the home and remained a keen tennis player.

On examination it was clear that he had a painful arc syndrome with classic pain with abduction of the arm. The shoulder joint itself was stable.

Treatment consisted of non-steroidal anti-inflammatories and physiotherapy to improve the rotator cuff musculature. The pain failed to settle over the next 2 months. A steroid injection into the subacromial bursa relieved the pain and he subsequently went on to an uneventful recovery, returning to playing club tennis.

Patient B

A 58-year-old gentleman who had previously been a keen sportsman presented with increasing pain and weakness of his right shoulder. No other joints were involved and it was clear that he had weakness in the power of abduction and pain with this movement.

Plain radiographs suggested a small spur on the underside of the acromioclavicular joint and sclerosis where the supraspinatous inserts into the humeral head. An MRI scan confirmed a full thickness rotator cuff tear and the patient elected for operative treatment.

The patient underwent an arthroscopic repair of the rotator cuff and excision of the bony spur and an acromioplasty to decrease the risk of future impingement. After an appropriate but slightly prolonged rehabilitation programme, the patient was able to return to normal activities.

Patient C

A 22-year-old previously keen swimmer presented with increasing pain with most over shoulder activities of both shoulders, the right being the most problematic. He described no previous episodes of instability or injury. The pain had failed to settle despite stopping swimming and undergoing physiotherapy.

On examination it was noted that he had a generalized joint hypermobility and it was clear that there was evidence of glenohumeral instability with a positive sulcus sign and some apprehension with external rotation and abduction.

It was felt that this gentleman had glenohumeral instability as a result of the generalized joint hypermobility. He was referred back to physiotherapy for rotator cuff exercises; although this improved his symptoms slightly, he was unable to return to his normal sporting activities. He subsequently went on to have two episodes of instability of the shoulder joint and eventually had an arthroscopic capsular repair.

Summary

These three presentations represent reasonably common presentations of shoulder problems.

Early impingement problems of the rotator cuff can be treated conservatively with physiotherapy and/or injection of the bursa with steroid. Those that fail to resolve or where there is a significant rotator cuff tear may well be treated with arthroscopic surgery and removal of the impingement lesion and repair of the cuff tear. Care should be taken to exclude those patients with a generalized joint hypermobility because these can occasionally present with similar signs, the key being the often generalized joint hypermobility that is often apparent.

Chapter 23

Disorders of the wrist and hand

By the end of this chapter you should be able to:
- Appreciate the effect of rheumatoid arthritis on the small joints of the hand.
- Realize the destructive nature of inflammatory arthropathies and the effect on hand function.
- Understand the difference between the presentation and the clinical features of osteo- and rheumatoid arthritis.
- Diagnose common benign conditions of the hand (ganglia, etc.).
- Remember the importance of infections in the palm, tendon sheaths and pulp spaces.
- Differentiate the causes of clawing of the fingers.
- Remember the neurological supply to the arm and in particular the distribution of nerve fibres.

Rheumatoid arthritis

Wrist

Rheumatoid arthritis affects synovium and the large amount of synovium around the wrist and inferior radioulnar joints makes them especially vulnerable to the disease.

Clinical features

The disease follows the usual pattern. The joint is painful and swollen in the acute attack but then subsides. If the disease cannot be controlled, the mass of synovium on the dorsum of the hand engulfs the extensor tendons and all may rupture (Fig. 23.1).

The tendons which cross the joint also become eroded and eventually rupture. The extensor tendon of the little finger is usually the first to go, but the extensor pollicis longus can also rupture where it runs around Lister's tubercle at the lower end of the radius (Figs 23.2, 23.3). Later the ligaments stretch, bone collapses, the joint becomes unstable and a characteristic deformity develops, with the wrist radially deviated and supinated on the forearm and the fingers in ulnar deviation.

Treatment

Conservative treatment with anti-inflammatory drugs and rest is usually effective but if the synovitis cannot be controlled medically, surgery is needed for the following indications:

1. Synovectomy to remove painful and inflamed synovium if it cannot be controlled by conservative means.

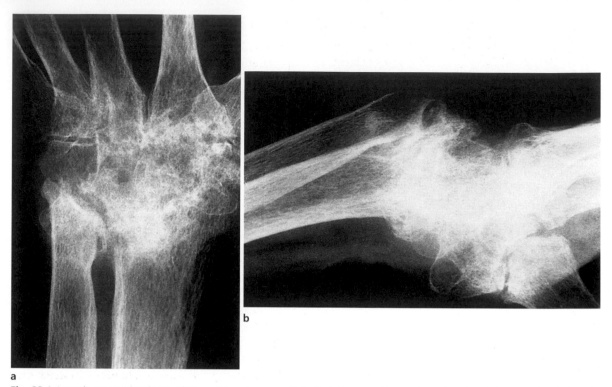

a

b

Fig. 23.1 Late rheumatoid arthritis of the wrist and carpus. Note that the carpal bones have fused and the wrist is ankylosed in flexion.

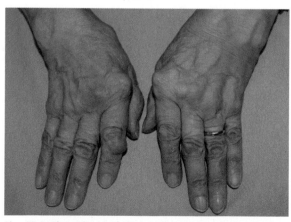

Fig. 23.2 Rheumatoid of the hands with synovial swellings and ulnar deviation.

2. Repair of ruptured tendons.

3. If the lower end of the ulna is unstable it must be excised before it damages the tendons that cross the wrist.

4. Arthrodesis if the wrist joint is unstable. *Note*: Arthrodesis limits flexion and extension of the wrist only, leaving pronation and supination unaffected.

5. Replacement arthroplasty.

Although arthrodesis is contraindicated in multiple joint disease (p. 298), arthrodesis of the wrist in rheumatoid arthritis produces a good result. If both wrists are to be arthrodesed, care should be taken not to fix them both in extension. With both wrists dorsiflexed it is difficult to fasten buttons and personal hygiene is almost impossible. Hold both your own wrists in dorsiflexion and see how inconvenient it is.

Hand

Rheumatoid arthritis of the hand presents many problems and much disability. The disease usually presents with symmetrical painful swelling of the metacarpophalangeal joints caused by synovial proliferation, and is often first visible as in-filling of the valleys between the metacarpal heads (Fig. 23.4). The small joints are destroyed later and fixed deformities develop (Fig. 23.5).

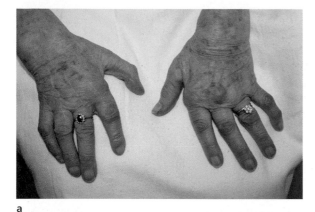

a

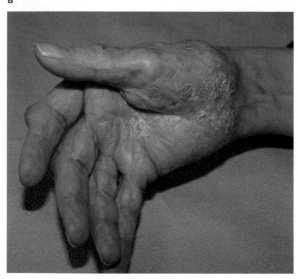

Fig. 23.3 Rheumatoid of the hand: (a) postoperative with correction of m.c.p. joints, synovectomy of wrist; (b) with associated psoriasis in palm.

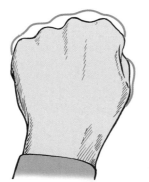

Fig. 23.4 Filling of the 'valleys' between the metacarpal heads in rheumatoid arthritis.

Treatment

Management of the rheumatoid hand is almost a specialty in its own right.

Initial treatment is conservative, with resting splints, occupational therapy and drugs, and is best conducted by a rheumatologist. If rest, night splints and anti-inflammatory drugs do not control symptoms or induce remission, surgical synovectomy may be necessary to remove exuberant synovium from the metacarpophalangeal joints. This will relieve pain but there is no evidence that it minimizes joint destruction.

If conservative measures fail, operation must be considered. This entails a careful and thorough assessment of the patient's disability and a critical estimate of the likely benefit from operation.

Operation is done neither because the disease is there nor because the operation is possible, but to produce a specific improvement in function.

There are several indications for operation:

1. To repair ruptured tendons by using a 'spare' tendon, such as the extensor indicis proprius, or by attaching the ruptured tendons to those that remain intact to produce a common extensor action.

2. To salvage destroyed metacarpophalangeal joints by replacement arthroplasty.

3. To correct other deformities, including the swan-neck deformity that results from tightness of the intrinsic muscles and damage to the volar plate and flexor digitorum sublimis. Dislocation of the extensor tendons may also need correction (Fig. 23.6).

Osteoarthritis

Wrist

Osteoarthritis of the wrist is usually the late result of trauma, often a fractured scaphoid, and causes pain and stiffness of the wrist after use (Fig. 23.7).

Treatment

If the symptoms only occur when the patient is working, a firm wrist support may be sufficient. If this is not effective, arthrodesis is needed. A trial period in plaster before operation will allow the patient to assess the likely result and be convinced

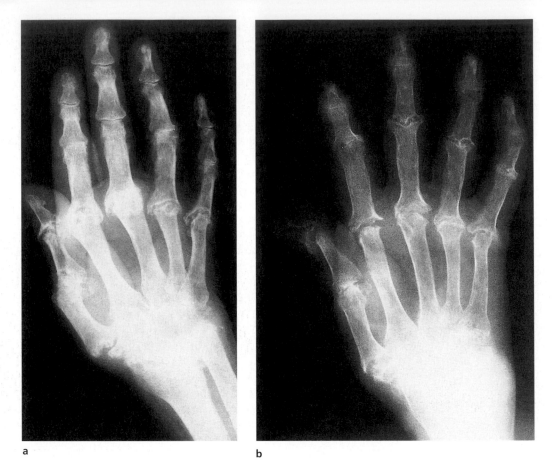

a   b

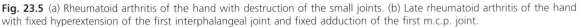

Fig. 23.5 (a) Rheumatoid arthritis of the hand with destruction of the small joints. (b) Late rheumatoid arthritis of the hand with fixed hyperextension of the first interphalangeal joint and fixed adduction of the first m.c.p. joint.

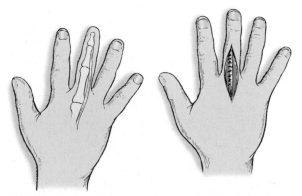

Fig. 23.6 Tendon displacement in rheumatoid arthritis. The extensor tendon can slip off the back of the m.c.p. joint and may need to be replaced.

that pronation and supination really are possible with the wrist fused.

Hand

The trapeziometacarpal joint is affected by osteoarthritis and causes pain on gripping and twisting movements (Fig. 23.8). The joint is tender on palpation, abduction of the thumb is limited, and longitudinal pressure reproduces the symptoms.

Treatment

Conservative treatment includes a support to splint the thumb, anti-inflammatory drugs and restriction of activity. If these measures are unsuccessful, operation may be required.

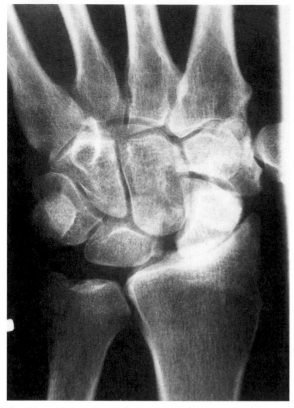

Fig. 23.7 Osteoarthritis of the wrist with narrowing of the radiocarpal joint following perilunate dislocation.

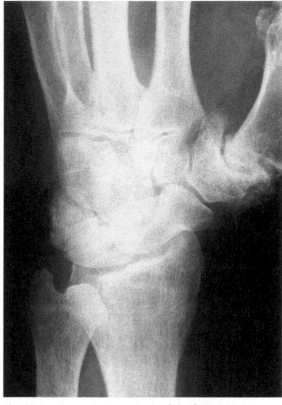

Fig. 23.8 Advanced osteoarthritis of the first carpometacarpal joint.

Excision arthroplasty or interposition arthroplasty by Silastic replacement arthroplasty are the most successful surgical procedures.

Fingers

Generalized osteoarthritis of the interphalangeal joints produces unsightly osteophytic lumps at the margins of the interphalangeal joints (Fig. 23.9). These are called Heberden's nodes if they involve the distal interphalangeal joints and Boucher's nodes if they involve the proximal interphalangeal joints. They are different from the swelling of the interphalangeal joints seen in rheumatoid arthritis.

Treatment

No operative treatment is helpful but physiotherapy may improve function.

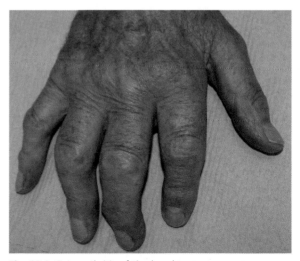

Fig. 23.9 Osteoarthritis of the hand.

Disorders of tendons

De Quervain's tenosynovitis

The extensor pollicis brevis and the abductor pollicis longus pass beneath a tight fibrous bridge just proximal to the radial styloid process and repeated stressing of these tendons by wringing out dish cloths or other twisting movements can cause a localized tenosynovitis (Fig. 23.10). The tendon swells, movements become painful and the fibrous bridge becomes thickened and forms a firm swelling on the lateral side of the radius just proximal to the wrist, which can be alarming. The tendon sheaths sometimes become inflamed above and below the fibrous bridge and make a soft creaking sound with movement.

The diagnosis can be confirmed by stressing the tendons. Ask the patient to grasp the thumb with the other fingers and then push the hand gently into flexion and ulnar deviation. This stretches the affected tendons and reproduces the pain.

Treatment

If elimination of the activity which caused the condition does not produce relief, steroid injection into the tendon sheaths can be helpful. If this is ineffective, the fibrous bridge must be divided surgically.

Extensor tenosynovitis

The extensor tendons, which do not have a tendon sheath, are less vulnerable to tenosynovitis than the flexors but the paratenon can become inflamed. Affected tendons produce the creaking, leathery sensation of muffled crepitus as they move.

Treatment

Rest and splintage are usually effective but steroid injection is sometimes necessary.

Trigger finger

The flexor profundus longus tendon is subjected to friction where it enters its tendon sheath and swelling can occur on the tendon at this point (Fig. 23.11). As the swelling enters the tendon sheath it irritates the opening of the sheath and this can narrow it still further. A vicious circle is therefore established, with the swelling aggravating the constriction and vice versa.

Clinical features

The swelling on the tendon prevents the tendon moving easily and causes a 'pop' as it enters the tendon sheath. The flexors are stronger than the extensors and the tendon becomes stuck in the flexed position. Extension is only possible passively, when it will straighten with a click.

This phenomenon is known as 'triggering' and is usually worse first thing in the morning after sleep-

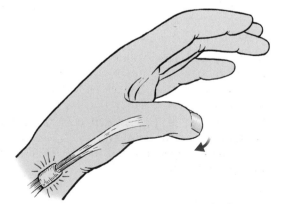

Fig. 23.10 De Quervain's disease. The extensor pollicis brevis and abductor pollicis longus tendons are irritated as they pass beneath a fibrous bridge proximal to the radial styloid.

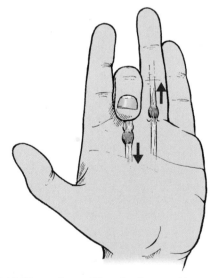

Fig. 23.11 Trigger finger. Triggering is caused by a swelling on the flexor tendon catching as it moves in and out of the opening into the fibrous flexor sheath.

ing with the fingers flexed but improves during the day as soft tissue swelling subsides.

Treatment

The symptoms usually follow unaccustomed repetitive activity and settle with rest and elimination of the cause. If this is ineffective a steroid injection into the tendon sheath is needed.

If the symptoms persist after three injections, the fibrous opening of the flexor tendon sheath must be incised to ease the passage of the tendon swelling. The operation is effective, but only required if all conservative measures have failed.

Trigger thumb

The same phenomenon can occur at the thumb, which can become locked in flexion. The lesion is also seen in infancy, usually before the age of 2.

Treatment

Most can be cured by injection of the tendon sheath with hydrocortisone but open release of the tendon sheath may be needed in children if the condition has not resolved by the age of 4.

Ganglia

A ganglion is a collection of thick fluid, similar to synovial fluid, surrounded by a thin layer of synovium in the soft tissues around joints and tendons. Although these cysts are called ganglia they have no connection with the nervous system.

Synovial fluid is produced by synovial cells, which normally secrete synovial fluid into the joint space. If the cells secrete fluid into the soft tissues rather than the joint cavity then a ganglion results (Fig. 23.12).

The lesions can form around any joint or tendon sheath but do not communicate with the joint space. Some extend inside the sheaths of peripheral nerves and cause peripheral nerve damage. Others extend deep to periosteum and involve bone.

Clinical features

Ganglia usually appear in early adult life and are particularly noticeable on the back of the wrist, associated with the scapholunate ligament. They also occur on the front of the wrist, where they emerge between the flexor tendons and the radial artery.

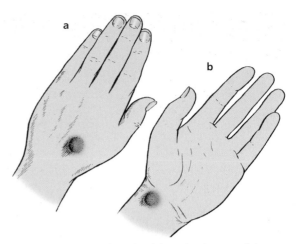

Fig. 23.12 Ganglia at the wrist: (a) on the dorsum of the hand; (b) on the volar aspect of the wrist, beside the radial artery.

Ganglia vary in size, ache after the hand is used, and interfere with its function.

Treatment

Ganglia sometimes rupture or disappear spontaneously after an accidental blow or, according to medical folklore, being 'hit with the family Bible'. If they do not disappear spontaneously and interfere with function, excision is required.

If the ganglion is causing neurological problems, early excision is indicated. If not, operation is best deferred for as long as possible because:

1. The scar is often more unsightly than the ganglion.
2. The soft tissue swelling at the site of operation can be almost as large as the original ganglion and takes up to 6 months to resolve.
3. A new ganglion may form in the place of the original because the area of abnormal synovium produces many small ganglia rather than a single large one.
4. Wide excision of the tissue at the base of the ganglion is needed to minimize the risk of recurrence and the operation causes more discomfort than patients expect.

Pearl ganglia

A variation of the common ganglion occurs in the midline of the flexor tendon sheaths where the

381

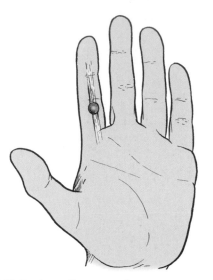

Fig. 23.13 Pearl ganglion – a small tense ganglion may develop on the volar aspect of the flexor sheath at the level of the joint.

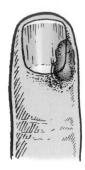

Fig. 23.14 Site of pus in paronychia.

fibres decussate opposite the metacarpophalangeal and interphalangeal joints (Fig. 23.13). These ganglia are small, round, tense and painful when gripping hard objects such as a steering wheel.

Treatment

Pearl ganglia often rupture and disappear after a simple puncture with a hypodermic needle, but they sometimes need excision. At operation they resemble a pearl and have a thin wall. Recurrence is unusual.

Ganglia at the distal interphalangeal joint

Mucous cysts are also seen at the distal interphalangeal joint, where they interfere with the nail bed and sometimes extend into the pulp of the finger. They are unsightly and interfere with the function of the finger.

Treatment

These ganglia seldom respond to conservative treatment and excision may be necessary. They frequently recur.

Infection

Infection in the hand is a serious matter. The function of the hand depends upon smooth soft tissues sliding over each other and anything that causes adhesions between the 'moving parts' has serious consequences. Infection of the hand can be classified as follows:

Infections of the hand

- Nail fold infections (paronychia).
- Pulp space infections or 'whitlow'.
- Web space infections.
- Infections of the tendon sheaths.
- Infections of the deep spaces.

Nail fold infections

Infections of the nail fold, or paronychia, is a common problem (Fig. 23.14). The infection begins with a break in the skin of the nail fold and spreads from there to the subungual space, where it causes severe pain by raising tissue tension. The lesion is seen less often now than in the past, perhaps because people keep their hands cleaner.

Treatment

The lesion should be cleaned, antibiotics administered and the hand elevated (Fig. 23.15). Unless there is a rapid improvement, the edge of the nail should be raised and the pus evacuated, or the proximal half of the nail removed.

This must be done under general or regional anaesthesia; local anaesthetics or ring blocks must

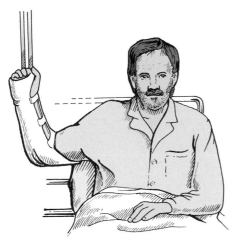

Fig. 23.15 Elevation of the hand for infection.

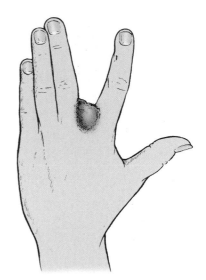

Fig. 23.17 Web space infection.

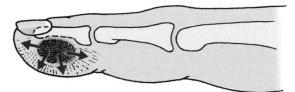

Fig. 23.16 Pulp space infection (whitlow). The spread of pus is limited by fibrous septa and the increased tissue tension causes pain.

never be used in the presence of infection because the injection helps spread the infection.

Pulp space infections

Pulp space infections, often referred to by the ancient name of 'whitlow', usually begin with a penetrating injury (Fig. 23.16).

The pulp has many stout, fibrous septa, which make the pulp of the finger firm but also prevent soft tissue swelling. This in turn means that even a small collection of pus causes severe pain, particularly if the digit is accidentally knocked. The expression 'sticking out like a sore thumb' refers not only to the appearance of the thumb but also to the excruciating pain of a pulp space infection.

Treatment

Treatment is similar to that of paronychia. If rest, antibiotics and elevation do not bring rapid relief, the pus should be released through a transverse or oblique incision in the side of the pulp and not

through a 'fish mouth' incision across the end of the pulp.

Herpetic whitlow

Herpes simplex can cause infection of the pulp space and is common in healthcare workers. Incision makes the condition worse. Beware of nurses and midwives with a whitlow.

Web space infections

The web space between adjacent fingers contains loose tissue, and quite large abscesses can form with little local pain or tissue tension (Fig. 23.17). Penetrating injury is the usual cause.

Treatment

If elevation and adequate antibiotics do not bring rapid relief, a short incision is needed to drain the pus.

Infection of the tendon sheaths

Tendon sheaths infected by spread from the pulp or by penetrating injuries provide an easy route for bacterial spread. The finger quickly becomes painful and is held in slight flexion because the volume of the sheath is greatest in this position. Any movement is excruciating. The extent of the infection is dictated by the anatomy of the tendon sheaths (Fig. 23.18).

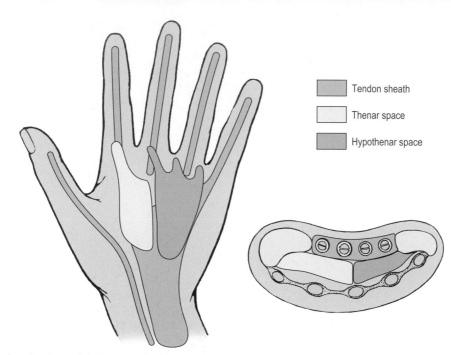

Tendon sheath

Thenar space

Hypothenar space

Fig. 23.18 Tendon sheaths and deep spaces in the palm and fingers. Infection is confined to these spaces initially.

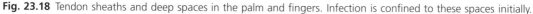

Treatment

The consequences of adhesions in the tendon sheath are worse than paronychia or pulp space infections and more energetic treatment is needed. The patient must be admitted, the arm elevated and antibiotics given in adequate doses. Intravenous antibiotics are advisable.

Unless there is a response within 6 h, the tendon sheath should be opened at each end and then irrigated.

Infection of the deep spaces

There are two spaces in the hand, the thenar and hypothenar spaces, bounded by fascial sheaths that act as bulkheads to prevent the spread of infection (see Fig. 23.18). Infection can follow spread from infection in adjacent structures, penetrating injury, or spread from the web space by way of the lumbricals.

The pain and clinical signs are less dramatic than in the infections described previously because the infection is deeper and there is more room for the infection to spread. The hand is diffusely swollen, finger movement is restricted, and deep pressure over the infected space is painful.

Treatment

The patient should be admitted, the arm elevated and antibiotics given intravenously. Unless there is a rapid response, the appropriate space should be decompressed by an experienced hand surgeon who is familiar with the detailed anatomy of these spaces.

Dupuytren's disease (or 'contracture')

In 1831, Baron Dupuytren, a surgeon in Paris, described a contracture of the hand which begins at the base of the ring or little finger and eventually pulls them into extreme flexion, making it difficult to put on gloves or shake hands (Fig. 23.19). The position of the fingers suggested the contracture was caused by holding the reins of a horse but the condition has survived the horse-drawn carriage and its cause is still unknown.

Pathology

The basic pathology is contracture of the palmar fascia, similar to other fibrous diatheses such as

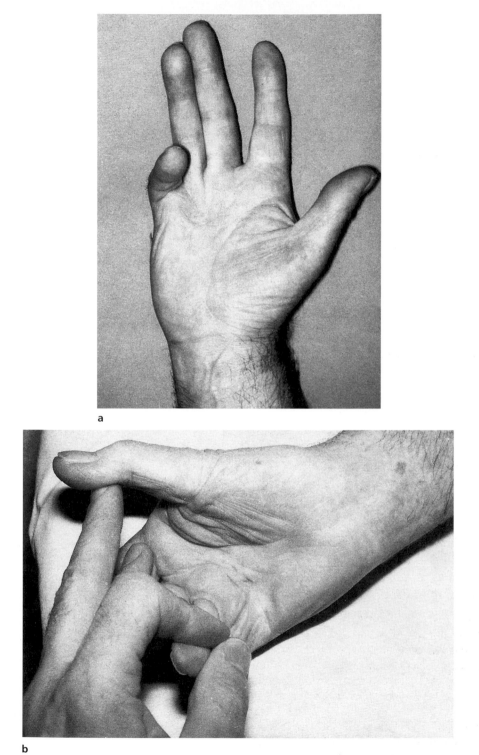

a

b

Fig. 23.19 (a) Dupuytren's contracture affecting the little finger; (b) the thumb is also involved.

Peyronie's disease and retroperitoneal fibrosis. The contracture can also involve the skin.

Clinical features

The condition is very often symmetrical, is commoner in men, may run in families, and is associated with diabetes, epilepsy and alcoholism. The soles of the feet may develop fibrous nodules similar to plantar fibromatosis, and pads of firm fibrous tissue (Garrod's pads) are sometimes seen on the dorsum of the knuckles.

Treatment

There is no effective conservative treatment but the symptoms are not always incapacitating and slight deformities are best left untreated, especially in elderly patients.

Surgical correction is possible by excising the contracted tissue, which is hard and almost cartilaginous in consistency. The success of operation depends on the extent of the contracture and the joints involved. Because of their anatomy (p. 33), the metacarpophalangeal joints can be easily straightened, even if they have been flexed for many years, while the interphalangeal joints quickly stiffen in flexion.

Even if full movement is restored, the contracture can recur or extend as the disease progresses. There is no need to advise operation as long as the patient has no disability and the interphalangeal joints are not involved. There are two indications for operation:

1. More than 30° contracture of the interphalangeal joints.
2. Disability from involvement of the metacarpophalangeal joints.

If the deformity is severe and cannot be corrected, it may be necessary to amputate the affected digit, usually the little finger, through the neck of the metacarpal.

Kienböck's disease

Osteochondritis of the lunate is described on page 328; it may cause pain in the wrist on gripping and at the extremes of the range of movement. A firm splint is usually helpful and operation is seldom needed.

Neurological disorders

Sensory and motor disturbances in the hand are common and differential diagnosis is often difficult. The symptoms may involve the arm as well, but the conditions are described here because they usually present with symptoms in the hand. The following conditions account for the great majority of cases (Fig. 23.20).

Common causes of neurological abnormalities in the upper limb

- Ulnar compression at the elbow.
- Ulnar nerve compression at the wrist.
- Median nerve compression at the wrist (carpal tunnel syndrome).
- Radial nerve lesions.
- Cervical spondylosis.
- Thoracic outlet syndrome.
- Combined lesions.

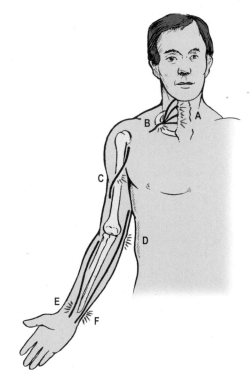

Fig. 23.20 Sites of neurological lesions in the arm: (A) cervical spondylosis; (B) thoracic outlet; (C) radial nerve damage; (D) ulnar nerve compression (E) median nerve compression; (F) ulnar nerve damage.

Ulnar nerve compression

Causes

The ulnar nerve may be compressed where it runs behind the medial epicondyle of the humerus at the elbow (Fig. 23.21). The symptoms are worse with the nerve under tension when the elbow is flexed; prolonged flexion of the elbow when reading or asleep precipitates symptoms.

The condition may arise because of an abnormal valgus angle at the elbow following a supracondylar fracture of the humerus in childhood (p. 200). As the child grows, the valgus deformity increases, the ulnar nerve is stretched and the symptoms develop. This condition is still known by the quaint title of 'tardy ulnar palsy'.

Any other abnormality on the medial side of the elbow, whether the result of trauma or osteoarthritis, may also cause ulnar nerve compression. The symptoms also arise without obvious cause.

Clinical features

The characteristic symptoms are tingling, pain and numbness in the ulnar nerve distribution, which includes the little finger, the ulnar half of the ring finger and the medial side of the hand. The patient may also notice weakness, clumsiness and wasting of the interossei in severe cases.

On examination there is diminished sensibility in the ulnar distribution and sometimes wasting of the intrinsic muscles of the hand. In severe cases the ulnar two or three digits are held in the classic main-en-griffe (claw hand) position associated with loss of intrinsic power.

The ulnar nerve is palpable at the elbow and is sometimes sensitive to light finger pressure. If pressing the nerve does not reproduce the symptoms, the diagnosis can be confirmed by nerve conduction studies, which show a delay at the elbow.

Treatment

Apart from avoiding pressure on the elbow and keeping it straight, there is no conservative treatment for ulnar nerve compression.

If the symptoms become worse, the ulnar nerve can be transposed from its vulnerable position on the convexity of the elbow to a safer place in front of the medial epicondyle. By freeing the nerve from the fibrous tunnel through which it runs behind the medial epicondyle and allowing it to take a 'short cut' across the elbow, the nerve is decompressed and tension is released.

Reducing pressure on the nerve prevents further deterioration but the neurological symptoms do not always recover completely and patients should be warned that the operation is to prevent the symptoms getting worse rather than to relieve them completely.

Ulnar nerve compression at the wrist

The deep parts of the ulnar nerve may be compressed at the wrist as it enters the hand through the canal of Guyon beside the pisiform. The condition is so excessively uncommon that for practical purposes all ulnar nerve problems arise at the elbow.

Treatment

If the symptoms are severe, which is unusual, and the lesion is proven by electrical studies, surgical decompression is required.

Median nerve compression (carpal tunnel syndrome)

Cause

The median nerve enters the hand through the carpal tunnel, a bony trough covered with a stout fibrous roof (the flexor retinaculum) which it shares

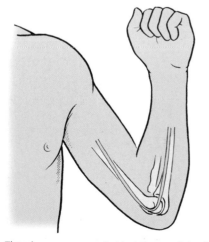

Fig. 23.21 The ulnar nerve runs behind the medial epicondyle and may be irritated after prolonged full flexion.

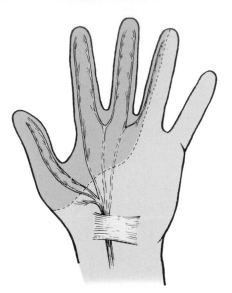

Fig. 23.22 Carpal tunnel syndrome. The median nerve is compressed where it runs beneath the carpal ligament. There may be altered sensibility of the thumb, index, middle and half of the ring finger and wasting of the thenar muscles.

with nine tendons, each covered with two layers of synovium (Fig. 23.22). There is no room in this tight tunnel for the tissues to expand and any swelling of the tendons or the synovium around them is bound to compress the median nerve.

The commonest overall cause of carpal tunnel syndrome is fluid retention, of which the commonest cause is pregnancy. Overuse of the tendons from repeated forceful movements of the wrist, either at work or recreation, is probably the commonest cause of carpal tunnel syndrome referred to orthopaedic clinics. Any condition that causes synovial thickening, including rheumatoid arthritis and Colles' fracture, can also be responsible.

Clinical features

Median nerve compression causes paraesthesia in the median nerve distribution, which in most patients is the front of the thumb, index finger, middle finger and the radial half of the ring finger. The palm is not involved because the palmar branch of the median nerve arises above the wrist.

The symptoms are worse at night and the patient will wake and fling the hand up and down to try and relieve the symptoms. In time, the paraesthesia is replaced by pain proximally as far up as the elbow,

and eventually by numbness in the median distribution.

Most patients notice that the little finger is not affected and those who report that all the fingers are involved should be treated with suspicion.

Differential diagnosis

The differential diagnosis includes peripheral neuropathy, mononeuritis, cervical spondylosis and tumours of the thoracic inlet involving the brachial plexus (p. 186). These are often forgotten because carpal tunnel syndrome is such a common condition. If there is any doubt, the diagnosis can be confirmed by nerve conduction studies.

Conservative treatment

Conservative treatment consists of rest, diuretics and hydrocortisone injection.

Rest and diuretics. The carpal tunnel syndrome of pregnancy disappears after delivery and most other patients recover when the original cause has been eliminated. If symptoms persist, conservative treatment with diuretics and a resting splint at night is usually effective.

Hydrocortisone injection. Injection of hydrocortisone acetate into the carpal tunnel may be effective but if the patient is still troubled after three injections, carpal tunnel decompression is needed.

Operative treatment

Carpal tunnel decompression is a straightforward and reliable operation and recurrence is unusual. The tunnel is decompressed by dividing the flexor retinaculum throughout its length from top to bottom through a longitudinal incision.

Radial nerve lesions

In the upper arm

The radial nerve is vulnerable as it winds around the humerus and can be damaged by pressure against the medial side of the humerus in the axilla. Axillary crutches used wrongly can cause radial palsy, as can pressure against a hard object. The nerve can be compressed while dozing in an armchair or sitting with the arm resting along the back of an adjacent chair (Fig. 23.23).

The characteristic symptom is weakness of the extensors, with a 'drop wrist' on clinical examina-

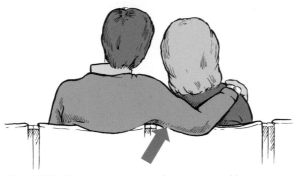

Fig. 23.23 The radial nerve may be compressed by pressure on the back of a chair.

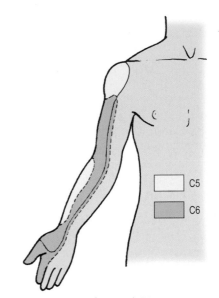

Fig. 23.24 Dermatomes of C5 and C6.

tion. There may be a small area of diminished sensibility on the back of the hand at the base of the thumb in the area supplied by the radial nerve. Paraesthesiae may be felt in the same area when the pressure is relieved.

The radial nerve may also be injured in fractures of the humerus, when the history will suggest the diagnosis.

Posterior interosseous nerve

The posterior interosseous nerve is vulnerable where it winds around the neck of the radius, as the common peroneal nerve is at the neck of the fibula. The interosseous nerve does not run between the radius and ulna, despite its name. It is comparable with the common peroneal nerve and is only called interosseous because it runs on the interosseous membrane.

The commonest cause of injury is trauma and the position of the nerve must never be forgotten when operating on the lateral side of the elbow. If the nerve is damaged at this point there will be weakness of all the wrist and finger extensors but there is seldom any sensory impairment.

Lateral cutaneous nerve of the forearm

The lateral cutaneous nerve of the forearm is also very vulnerable and its continuation into the hand has the doubtful distinction of being one of the few cutaneous nerves that can be palpated. If the extensor pollicis longus is contracted, the nerve can be felt by drawing a thumb nail along the tendon until a tingling sensation is felt in the hand.

Treatment

Operation is only required for mechanical entrapment or irritation of the nerve by adhesions or bone spurs around a fracture.

Cervical spondylosis

The cervical nerve roots can be compressed or irritated as they leave the cervical spine through the nerve root canals. Typically, the patient will have sensory symptoms confined to a single dermatome, usually the C5 or C6 dermatome (Fig. 23.24). The distribution of the sensory symptoms should point to the diagnosis but it may be hard to find any objective neurological impairment and EMG studies are often needed to exclude damage to the median, ulnar and radial nerves. The motor symptoms are usually overshadowed by the sensory symptoms. Weakness may be absent because most muscles in the forearm are innervated by several roots.

Treatment

See page 446.

Thoracic outlet

Pressure on the lowest cervical roots as they cross the first rib or a fibrous cervical rib at the thoracic outlet can cause pain down the inner side of the forearm and hand in the T1 distribution.

Treatment

Removal of a cervical rib sometimes relieves the symptoms but the operation is best undertaken by a thoracic surgeon accustomed to operating in this region. An intrathoracic tumour can cause the same symptoms and signs.

Tumours of the thoracic inlet

Apical lung tumours can involve both the brachial plexus and cervical sympathetic chain. Although rare, it is important to consider this diagnosis and exclude it radiologically.

Combined lesions

More than one of these conditions can exist in combination and diagnosis is then more difficult. If a patient with carpal tunnel syndrome also has cervical spondylosis involving the C5 root, there will be altered sensibility on the radial side of the forearm as well as the hand and electrical studies may be helpful but not conclusive.

Treatment

In such patients it is wise to treat only one condition at a time and to stress to the patient that it will require more than one form of treatment to relieve all the symptoms. The cervical spondylosis may be relieved by physiotherapy, for example, while carpal tunnel decompression is needed to relieve carpal tunnel symptoms.

Case reports

Contractures and obvious clawing of the hand can be caused by a number of different conditions.

Patient A

A 53-year-old diabetic gentleman with a history of alcohol abuse presented in the Orthopaedic Clinic with clawing of the little and ring finger of the left hand. This had been a gradual process over the past 10 or 15 years and he had noticed a thickening of the skin in the palm of his hand.

On presentation he was unable to fully extend the fingers and it was obvious that there were nodules in the skin and tethering of the skin in the palm of the hand. The metacarpophalangeal and interphalangeal joint motion was severely restricted, but there was no loss of skin sensitivity and he had normal vascularity of the hand.

A diagnosis of Dupuytren's contracture was made and he was referred for surgery to correct the deformity as this was impacting on his day-to-day activities.

Patient B

A 30-year-old worker had been involved in an industrial accident, sustaining a significant injury to the left elbow. He had a comminuted fracture of the distal humerus, which had been plated and this had subsequently healed. He had, however, noticed postoperatively that there was a loss of feeling on the little and ring finger of that hand and he had a clawing of these two fingers.

Examination confirmed normal median nerve sensibility, but an absence of the ulnar nerve function.

Patient C

A 46-year-old gentleman presented to the Orthopaedic Department with a catching sensation when flexing the middle finger. He was able to flex the finger, but this would catch within the palm and on extending the finger there was an audible and popping sensation in the palm. He had always been able to fully extend the finger, but over the last few weeks this had become more difficult and painful.

On examination he had a palpable nodule over the metacarpophalangeal joint and this was causing a trigger finger abnormality. When flexing the finger the nodule on the flexor tendon passed under the A1 pulley, getting trapped proximally and stopping the finger from extending fully. On forceful extension this nodule passed back through under the A1 pulley allowing the finger to extend. This was not associated with any neurovascular problems in the rest of the hand.

This was treated with an injection of a steroid into the flexor tendon sheath, but this failed to resolve the symptoms completely and he underwent a release of the A1 pulley.

Summary

Clawing of the fingers of the hand can be for a number of reasons. It is important to look for general health problems including smoking, alcohol abuse or diabetes as these can be associated with Dupuytren's contracture.

On examination of the hand it is important to identify whether there is a neural element, both motor and sensory, in the presentation. Remember that trigger fingers may be purely mechanical with neither an inflammatory process in the skin nor as a result of neurovascular problems.

Chapter |24|

Disorders of the hip and knee

By the end of this chapter you should be able to:
- Make a clear diagnosis of arthritic change in hip and knee.
- Recommend the correct early conservative treatment in these cases.
- Be aware of the operative options for a destroyed joint, but not forget the complications of this surgery.
- Be aware of the value but also the limitations of arthroscopic surgery in arthritis.
- Remember again the destructive nature of infections in both normal and replaced joints.
- Appreciate the impact of arthroscopic surgery on treatment of ligamentous, meniscal and chondral lesions.
- Be cautious about the treatment of anterior knee pain in the adolescent.

Osteoarthritis of the hip

Clinical features

Osteoarthritis of the hip is one of the commonest causes of disability in the western world. The condition is essentially mechanical wearing out of the hip joint rather than a disease and can be caused by many things. Trauma, obesity and previous infection can all be followed by osteoarthritis but there is probably a genetic element as well. The disease is much less often seen in Asiatic races.

The characteristic symptoms are:

1. Pain.
2. Loss of hip movement.
3. Abnormal gait.

Pain. The pain is worse on weight-bearing and movement of the hip but also occurs at rest and disturbs sleep. The pain is dull and aching in character at first but becomes sharper as the disease progresses.

The pain is usually felt in the groin but pain down the outer side of the thigh is also common. Some patients also have pain low in the thigh, around the knee, and become convinced that the trouble lies in the knee, not the hip. Referred pain of this type is a well-known diagnostic pitfall but still confounds the unwary.

Loss of movement. Movement is lost because osteophytes form around the joint and change the shape of the joint surfaces. As movement is lost, a flexion, adduction and external rotation deformity develops. The flexion deformity is compensated for by hyper-extension of the lumbar spine, and this can cause backache. The adduction deformity causes apparent shortening of the leg and patients often complain that 'my leg is getting shorter'.

The stiffness makes it difficult to tie shoe-laces, put on socks or cut toenails.

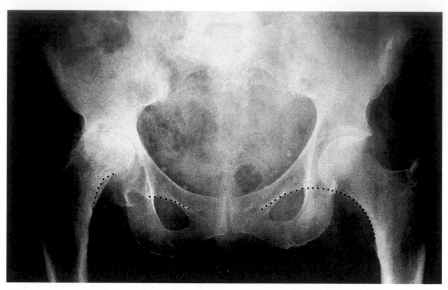

Fig. 24.1 Osteoarthritis of the hip showing joint space narrowing, cyst formation, subchondral sclerosis, osteophytes, thickening of the femoral head and bone destruction. Shenton's line (dotted) shows collapse of the femoral head.

Abnormal gait. The limp is due partly to the restriction of movement in the joint, and partly to an antalgic gait (p. 25); i.e. walking so that the load on the hip joint is reduced. The limp is usually observed by other people rather than the patient but a few are more worried by the limp than anything else.

Clinical examination

Patients with osteoarthritis of the hip are ideal subjects for the clinical section of final medical examinations, and it is only the most foolhardy student who will attend the examination without being able to examine the hip easily and confidently.

Movements. The technique of examination is described on p. 24. Examination will usually show apparent shortening of the affected limb and a fixed flexion deformity detectable by Thomas' test (p. 25).

Radiology

Osteoarthritic hips show characteristic radiological changes (Fig. 24.1).

Radiological changes in osteoarthritis of the hip

1. Narrowing of the joint space.
2. Cyst formation in the femoral head and the acetabulum.
3. Sclerosis of subchondral bone.
4. Osteophyte formation.
5. Subcortical thickening on the medial side of the femoral neck.
6. If there is bone destruction as well, Shenton's line will be disturbed, indicating true shortening of the limb.

Pathology

Osteoarthritis of the hip begins with fibrillation of the articular surface and the formation of wear particles. The wear particles are swept to the side of the joint where they irritate the synovium and are responsible for some of the patient's pain and the formation of osteophytes.

As the disease progresses, articular cartilage is lost, subchondral bone is exposed and the bone surfaces become eburnated (Fig. 24.2). Grooves form in the joint surfaces and the hip is gradually converted

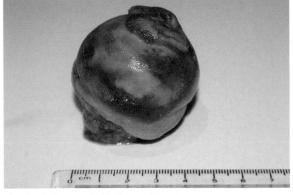

Fig. 24.2 Osteoarthritic femoral head.

from a ball and socket into a roller bearing. Later, cysts form in the bone and the femoral head may collapse.

Untreated, the hip becomes fixed in flexion, adduction and external rotation, a position which interferes seriously with mobility.

Treatment

The conservative treatment of osteoarthritis of the hip includes the following:

Conservative treatment of osteoarthritis of the hip

1. Anti-inflammatory drugs.
2. Weight reduction.
3. A stick, which is only helpful if it is held in the opposite hand and used correctly.
4. A raise to the shoe of the shorter limb to correct the apparent shortening and relieve the abnormal strain on the lumbar spine and opposite hip.
5. Aids to daily living to help the patient put on shoes and stockings and pick up dropped articles.

All these measures are important and must be considered, even if not adopted, before operation is recommended. There is some evidence that an arthroscopic washout and debridement is useful in the early stages. The results of this in established osteoarthritis of the elderly are poor.

Rheumatoid arthritis of the hip

As elsewhere, rheumatoid arthritis destroys bone, but the osteophytes and sclerosis of osteoarthritis

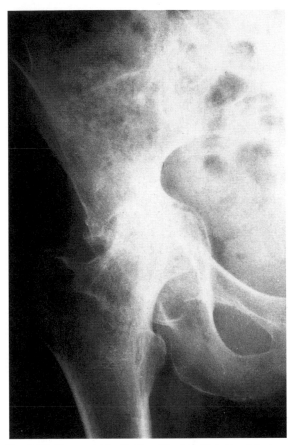

Fig. 24.3 Rheumatoid arthritis of the hip. Note the thinning of the medial wall.

are usually absent. Instead, the femoral head is gradually eroded or collapses suddenly, resulting in true shortening of the leg (Fig. 24.3).

Treatment

If conservative measures fail, joint replacement is the only effective treatment. Rheumatoid patients do well because their activity is limited by disease elsewhere and also because they are generally lightweight.

Total hip replacement

Total hip replacement is the most popular operation for osteoarthritis of the hip and consists of replacing both surfaces of the joint with artificial materials (Fig. 24.4). The acetabulum is reamed out to take a cup and the femoral head replaced with a metal ball attached to a stem inserted in the femoral shaft. A resurfacing component that does not use a long

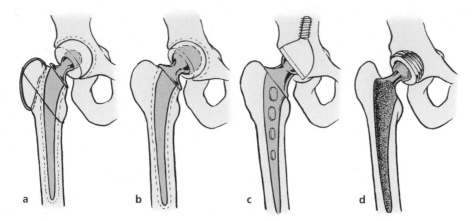

Fig. 24.4 Types of total hip replacement: (a) Charnley hip replacement with greater trochanter reattachment; (b) Müller type replacement with larger femoral head; (c) ring-type replacement using a long, threaded acetabular component without cement; (d) uncemented prosthesis with sintered surfaces and screw-in acetabular prosthesis.

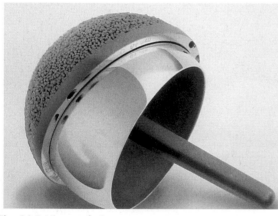

Fig. 24.5 Hip resurfacing components.

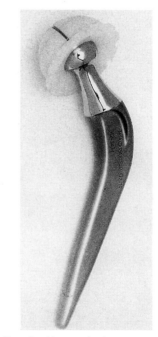

Fig. 24.6 A Charnley hip prosthesis.

stem has recently been introduced and is often used in younger patients to prevent bone loss (Fig. 24.5).

There are many types of hip replacement but most have a femoral component made of either stainless steel or a chrome cobalt molybdenum alloy and a cup made of high density polyethylene. Both components are usually fixed to the skeleton with cold curing acrylic cement (pp. 49, 299). Metal on metal articulation is possible and reduces the amount of wear debris within the hip capsule, as do ceramic bearings.

Some prostheses are inserted without cement, fixation relying on bone growing into irregularities on the surface of the component. The size and shape of the pores into which bone can grow is critical in securing fixation. A covering of hydroxyapatite may enhance this ingrowth; ceramic components are also used and new designs are continually being introduced.

Of the many different types of hip replacement, the Charnley low friction arthroplasty, the Exeter and the Stanmore are the best known (Fig. 24.6, 24.7).

The friction in most total hip prostheses is about 40 times greater than that of a normal healthy hip and this imposes a strain on the fixation of the

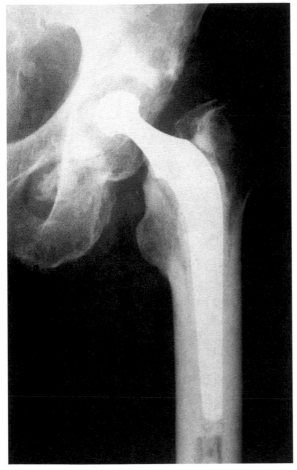

Fig. 24.7 A Charnley total hip replacement.

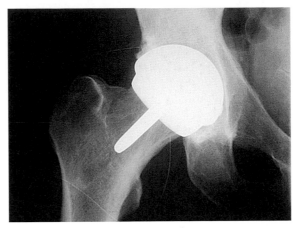

Fig. 24.8 A metal on metal hip resurfacing component.

- *Ceramic*. The bearing surfaces are made of aluminium oxide. Mechanical characteristics are good but the components can crack and ceramic particles may be irritant.
- *Resurfacing*. Use of a metal on metal articulation without a long femoral stem (Fig. 24.8).

Results

The results of total hip replacement are spectacular, with good or excellent results in approximately 98% of patients. The operation is most successful in relieving pain but some restoration of movement and an improved gait can also be expected.

The results are so good that the operation has revolutionized hip surgery and brought treatment to many who would otherwise have been untreatable. This has in turn brought great pressure on the resources available for orthopaedic surgery.

Indications

The ideal patient for total hip replacement is a lightweight elderly patient who has severe pain and places few demands on the hip. The most unsuitable is a young, heavy, active man who wants to play football and return to heavy work. Between these two extremes the degree of pain and disability is weighed against the patient's age and physical requirements but, in general, total hip replacement should not be offered to the following types of patient:

1. Those under the age of 60.
2. Those who are obese.

components to bone. Furthermore, the rigid femoral stem causes stress risers in the femoral shaft.

Types of total hip prosthesis

- *Cemented*. In this, the most commonly used type, the components are fixed to bone with an acrylic cement. The acrylic cement can cause bone destruction if the components become loose, e.g. Charnley. Designed by Sir John Charnley, this prosthesis has been used since the late 1960s. It is made of stainless steel, has a small femoral head, a high density polyethylene cup and is secured with acrylic cement.
- *Hybrid*. In this, only one of the components is fixed by cement.
- *Isoelastic*. The femoral stem is designed to have the same flexibility as bone in order to minimize stress risers within the femoral shaft. These have not been shown to offer any great advantage.

3. Those involved in physically demanding activities.

Technique

The operation can be done in several ways and through several approaches. These include:

1. The anterolateral approach, between tensor fasciae latae and the glutei.
2. The posterior approach through the posterior capsule.
3. The Charnley approach with detachment of the greater trochanter.
4. Detachment of the glutei and a portion of the vastus lateralis muscle.

With all these approaches the principle is the same. The acetabular surface is prepared by removing all debris and soft tissue and the femoral head is removed. The acetabulum is then replaced with a prosthetic component, which is fixed either mechanically or with bone cement. The femoral component is then inserted and similarly secured.

Prevention of infection

Infection in a prosthetic hip is a disaster and great care must be taken to prevent it occurring during operation by the following measures:

1. Meticulous asepsis during operation, or
2. Prophylactic antibiotics, or
3. A combination of the two.

Aseptic techniques. Meticulous asepsis in an operating enclosure with ultraclean air changed continuously and impervious operating gowns with individual exhaust systems for expired air (Fig. 24.9) can reduce the infection rate to 0.2%, but the operations may also be done in a standard operating theatre.

Prophylactic antibiotics used in a standard operating theatre will produce a similar infection rate to the operating enclosure. A regimen of flucloxacillin 500 mg started with the premedication and continued for three doses is effective. If the patient is allergic to penicillin, vancomycin may be used.

Combining antibiotics with a clean air enclosure can reduce the infection rate still further.

Catheterization. Inserting catheters immediately after operation runs the risk of infection. If it cannot be avoided, catheterization should be done gently with complete sterility and covered with an appropriate antibacterial drug.

Cross-infection. Patients with clean joint replacements should not be nursed in the same ward as those with abscesses, colostomies or open infection.

Postoperative care

Some surgeons prefer to hold the hip in abduction by placing a wedge-shaped pillow between the patient's thighs for 2 days. This is particularly helpful if a Charnley hip prosthesis with a small femoral head has been used.

The suction drains are usually removed after 2 days, when the patient may sit out of bed. They should not sit in a low chair because this flexes the hips beyond 90° and can, in some circumstances, cause the hip to dislocate. Most patients should mobilize the next day with a frame and be walking reasonably with elbow crutches, ready for discharge, after 4–5 days. By then the patients should be able to climb stairs and be able to cope with many activities of daily living.

Between 6 and 12 weeks after the operation most patients have little pain from their hip and an improved range of motion that allows them to resume normal activities. However, heavy work, especially lifting and jumping, should be avoided indefinitely in case it stresses the bone–cement interface.

Failure

Not all hip replacements are successful and it is estimated that between 0.5% and 1% of all hip prostheses in position fail each year because of infection or loosening (Fig. 24.10).

Early infection around a total hip replacement almost invariably leads to failure and special care is needed to avoid infection at the time of operation.

Late infection can also occur later via the bloodstream from infections in the urinary tract or elsewhere.

The organisms responsible for infection around total hip replacements include many normally regarded as non-pathogenic, e.g. *Staphylococcus epidermidis*. The explanation is unknown but it may be that these bacteria flourish in the unusual tissue that surrounds prosthetic materials (glycocalyx), or that the minute amount of metallic salts leaving the prostheses inhibits macrophage activity.

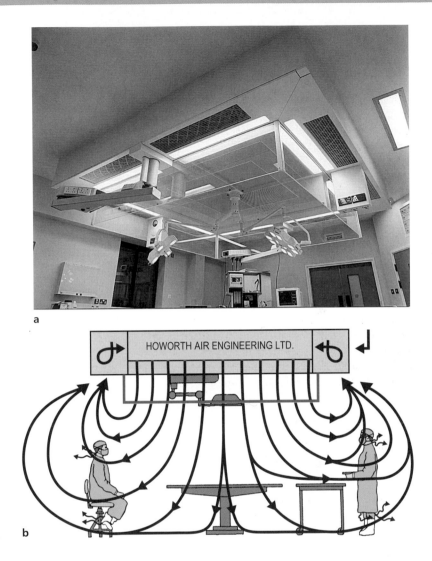

a

HOWORTH AIR ENGINEERING LTD.

b

Fig. 24.9 (a) Modern version of the world's first clean air enclosure for surgery – the Charnley Howorth Exflow Ultra-Clean Air System. (b) The flow of air using an ultraclean system with exponential flow. By kind permission of Howorth Airtech.

Treatment of infection. It is possible to remove the prosthesis with all the infected debris and replace the prosthesis with another. This is often successful but, if not, the prosthesis must be removed and the operation converted to an excision arthroplasty.

Loosening. Acrylic cement is strong in compression but weak in shear and torque. It causes little soft tissue reaction as long as it is intact but in particulate form it initiates a foreign body reaction that destroys bone. These two factors put together mean that violent twisting stresses may split the cement and allow the two surfaces of acrylic to 'fret', creating wear particles which destroy bone, cause more loosening, more fractures in the cement, and failure of the bone–cement interface.

In many ways, a hip prosthesis can be compared with a fibreglass patch on an old car; the repair is perfect as long as the car remains in the garage but it will loosen if driven hard over a bumpy road. The analogy is apt because the cement used in hip surgery is similar to that used for car repairs.

From the clinical standpoint, loosening usually affects the femoral component in active and overweight patients and causes pain on weight-bearing and hip movement.

Pain in the thigh usually indicates loosening of the femoral component, pain in the groin loosening of the acetabular component. The patient does not feel the components moving within the bone until the loosening is very severe indeed.

399

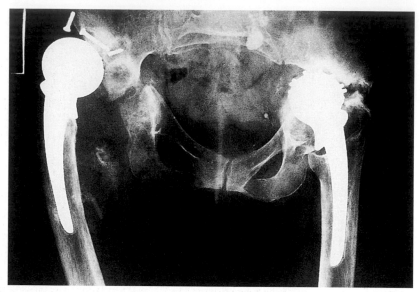

Fig. 24.10 Early McKee–Farrar prosthesis with loosening and fracture of the pelvis.

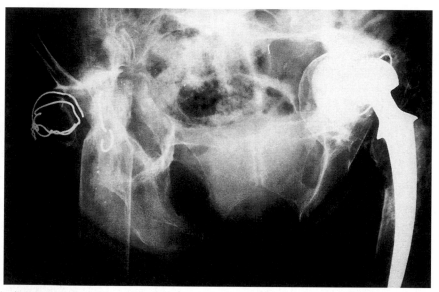

Fig. 24.11 Porotic rheumatoid bone. The prosthetic components have been removed from the right hip and the bone has fractured around the cement on the left.

Treatment of loosening. Replacement of the loose component with another may be successful, but the operation is more difficult and less reliable than a primary hip replacement. Excision arthroplasty may be needed (Fig. 24.11) as a salvage procedure.

Other complications

Other complications include fracture of the components (Fig. 24.12), dislocation (Fig. 24.13) and excessive new bone formation (Fig. 24.14).

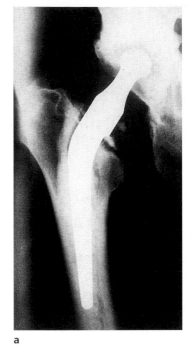
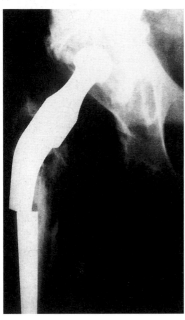

Fig. 24.12 Fracture of a femoral component. (a) Note the 'windscreen wiper' gap between the cement and prosthesis; (b) the component has fractured.

a

b

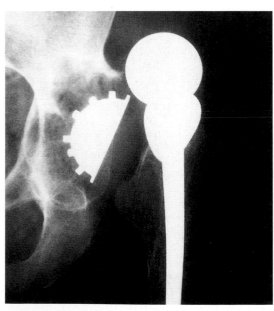

Fig. 24.13 Dislocation of a prosthesis. The cup was placed too steeply.

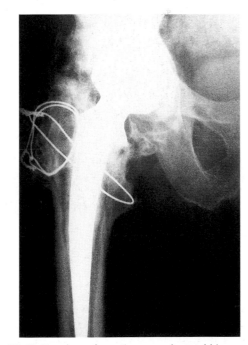

Fig. 24.14 New bone formation around a total hip prosthesis.

Investigation of a painful hip prosthesis

A painful hip prosthesis needs investigation by the following means:

- Radiographs.
- Blood tests.
- Isotope scans.
- Aspiration.

Radiographs. A transradiant line is seen around a loose or infected prosthesis, with scalloping of the deep surface of the cortex where it has been eroded by the foreign body reaction or infection.

Blood tests. Infection around hip prostheses is not dramatic and the white cell count is almost always normal. The ESR is usually raised to between 30 and 50 mm/h in both loosening and infection and does not differentiate between the two. The polymerase chain reaction to detect microscopic parts of the bacterial DNA may be the most sensitive.

Isotope scan. Technetium-99m scans show areas of activity in both loosening and infection and a gallium or indium scan may show areas of infection (Fig. 24.15).

Aspiration. Aspiration of the fluid around the prosthesis is helpful if a bacterium is retrieved but a sterile aspirate does not exclude infection. This procedure should be done with full sterile precautions in the operating theatre.

Revision hip replacement

Replacing (revising) a hip replacement is more difficult than the original procedure. Technical problems include dissecting through tissue that has abnormal anatomy. Dense scar tissue may contain the femoral and sciatic nerves.

Removing the prosthesis and the bone cement is difficult. Bone cement is harder than bone and the femur may be split as the cement is removed from the depth of the shaft. There is likely to be such extensive bone loss in both the femur and acetabulum that the standard prostheses do not fit.

Care must be taken to be as certain as possible that the wound is not infected. Tissues can be examined by Gram staining during the procedure but a negative finding does not exclude infection. If it seems likely that infection is present, it is wise to remove all foreign material, irrigate thoroughly, pack the wound with antibiotic-impregnated beads and close it. Antibiotics should be given systemically for at least 8 weeks, by which time any residual infection should be under control. The new prosthesis can then be inserted at a second operation.

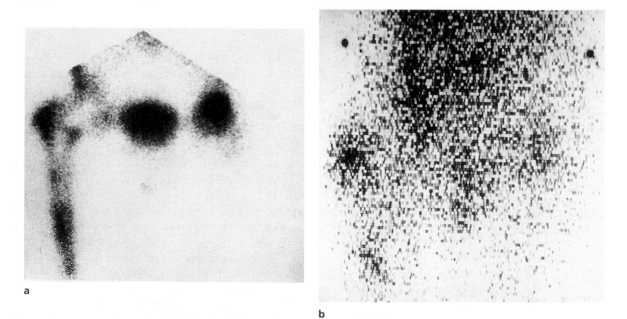

a

b

Fig. 24.15 (a) Technetium-99m bone scan showing loosening or infection around the femoral components. (b) Gallium scan showing activity around the tip of the prosthesis and the greater trochanter, suggesting infection.

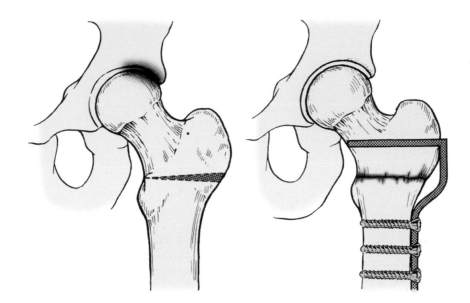

Fig. 24.16 Osteotomy for osteoarthritis of the hip. A wedge is taken from the femur to alter load bearing across the hip.

Bone loss can be made good by bone grafting either with autograft bone from the patient or allograft. A specially constructed 'custom' prosthesis may have to be prepared for the individual patient and these are always larger than the original; they are also more expensive. Moreover, fixation of the prosthesis is difficult and requires meticulous technique.

For all these reasons, revision surgery of the hip and other joints is a formidable procedure in terms of technique, surgical time and expense.

Other operations for osteoarthritis

Osteotomy

Before total hip replacement was available, femoral osteotomy was commonly done to realign the femur so that the load was taken by a different area of bone (Fig. 24.16). In this respect, the operation was similar in principle to moving an area of worn carpet away from the door. Osteotomy also affects the venous drainage of bone, and perhaps allows micro-fractures to heal.

Results of osteotomy are satisfactory in about 75% of patients 2 years after operation, but many have pain relief for much longer. The operation is indicated for younger patients who are unsuitable for total hip replacement. Acetabular rotational osteotomies work in the same way.

Excision arthroplasty

Excision arthroplasty was developed by Girdlestone as a primary procedure for osteoarthritis and is still known as Girdlestone's operation. The hip joint is replaced with a fibrous ankylosis and is similar to Keller's operation and other excision arthroplasties.

The operation converts a painful but stable joint into one that is unstable but less painful. The limb is shortened but function of the limb is improved. Today, the operation is done as a salvage procedure for failed total hip replacement and not as a primary procedure.

Arthrodesis

Arthrodesis of the hip leaves a solid hip that will last a lifetime and is indicated for gross destruction of the hip in a young patient, e.g. after a motorcycle accident (Fig. 24.17). The alternative operation in such a patient is a total hip replacement, which is doomed to failure in a young and active adult.

The operation has the advantage that an arthrodesis can be revised to a total hip replacement but hip replacement can only be revised to another hip replacement or excision arthroplasty.

Arthrodesis also has the disadvantage that the movement lost at the hip is made up for by excessive movement of the lumbar spine and the knee, which then become worn and present problems of their own.

Hemiarthroplasty

Prosthetic replacement of the femoral head alone was once used as a treatment for osteoarthritis of the hip but was unsuccessful because the degenerate acetabulum was eroded by the metal head of the prosthesis. The operation is successful when used as the treatment for fractures of the femoral neck because the acetabulum is healthy in these patients.

Interposition arthroplasty

Cup, or mould, arthroplasty was a standard operation for osteoarthritis of the hip before total hip replacement was introduced, but has now been superseded.

Surface replacement arthroplasty, in which both joint surfaces were replaced but the femoral shaft left intact, was comparable with a mould arthroplasty. The operation was introduced in the 1980s but the results were poor and it became obsolete. New designs of such prostheses are promising (see Figs 24.5, 24.8).

Other hip conditions

Protrusio acetabuli

Protrusio acetabuli is a strange condition for which no cause is known (Fig. 24.18). The medial wall of the acetabulum becomes paper-thin and the head migrates medially. The result is a hip that is virtually ankylosed in the neutral position.

Treatment. Untreated, the patient loses both rotation and abduction and in effect has bilateral hip arthrodesis. No treatment is effective except joint replacement.

Ankylosing spondylitis

Ankylosing spondylitis causes stiffness of the spine and large weight-bearing joints, including

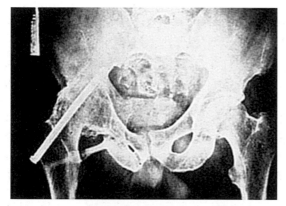

Fig. 24.17 An extra-articular arthrodesis of the hip.

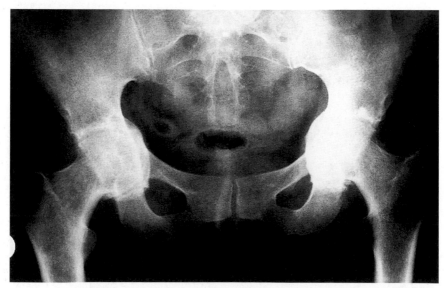

Fig. 24.18 Bilateral protrusio acetabuli.

the hip. The HLAb27 gene is often found in association with this condition.

Treatment. It is tempting to restore joint movement by total hip replacement but the hips may stiffen again with a bony ankylosis around the components. Apart from general conservative management to improve the function of the joint, there is no effective treatment for ankylosing spondylitis of the hip.

Infections

Tuberculosis of the hip was a common cause of hip disease in the past and many older patients still have destroyed or ankylosed hips as a result. Total hip replacement produces a good result. The theoretical risk that the mycobacteria could be lying dormant at the hip and be reactivated at the time of operation does not appear to be justified in practice.

Trochanteric bursitis

The trochanteric bursa lies between the greater trochanter and the insertion of the abductors and, like other bursae, can become inflamed and swollen. Some patients have an acute calcific bursitis comparable with acute calcific supraspinatus tendinitis.

On clinical examination the pain is localized to the greater trochanter and the bursa is tender. Passive hip movements are full but active abduction and abduction against resistance are painful. Radiographs may show a puff of calcification arising from the apex of the greater trochanter.

Treatment. A steroid injection into the bursa usually produces immediate relief of symptoms.

Septic arthritis

Acute septic arthritis is a rare condition today and therefore often escapes diagnosis when it does occur.

Treatment. Left untreated for even 24 h, the articular cartilage of the hip is destroyed and late osteoarthritis becomes almost inevitable. Accordingly, any child with an acute illness and a painful hip should be considered to have septic arthritis until proved otherwise.

The treatment consists of intravenous antibiotics after blood culture specimens have been sent to the laboratory, and immediate exploration of the hip.

Septic arthritis in adults is rare, but gonococcal arthritis is sometimes seen. In debilitated patients, diabetics and those taking steroids, septic arthritis is not uncommon.

Irritable hip (transient synovitis)

This condition is of unknown aetiology. It may occur 2–3 weeks after a viral upper respiratory tract infection. It is important to exclude sepsis of the hip and, in approximately 4% of cases, Perthes' disease. The condition usually settles spontaneously over 2–3 days.

Treatment. No treatment is required apart from reassurance and analgesics but the condition is important because its presentation is similar to that of acute septic arthritis. It is therefore prudent to admit children with irritable hips to hospital if there is any suspicion of systemic illness or pyrexia, so that systemic antibiotics can be administered without delay. Ultrasound scans of the hip and aspiration of the joint are used to differentiate the two conditions and can be used on an outpatient basis.

Snapping hip

Odd thuds and bangs can arise from normal hips and cause much anxiety, although they are seldom of serious significance. The commonest type is due to the iliotibial tract snapping across the greater trochanter when the patient stands on the affected leg while flexing and extending the knee (Fig. 24.19).

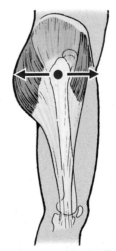

Fig. 24.19 Snapping hip caused by the iliotibial band flicking across the greater trochanter.

A thud can also be felt by some patients when the hip is flexed in external rotation, but not internal rotation.

Treatment. Apart from reassuring the patient that they are not dislocating the hip – a frequent anxiety – no treatment is required for these hips.

Osteoarthritis of the knee

Clinical features

Osteoarthritis of the knee can follow trauma, infection, meniscectomy, ligament injury or any other insult to the joint, but it also occurs without any obvious cause.

The medial compartment is more often affected than the lateral and a varus deformity develops as the medial compartment becomes worn (Figs 24.20, 24.21). As the varus increases, more load is taken by the medial compartment, the wear becomes greater, the deformity worse and the disease progresses rapidly (Fig. 24.22). On examination, a valgus strain will open up the medial side as the tibia returns to

its normal position. This is due to wear of the medial compartment, not to the medial ligament being lax.

As the condition progresses, osteophytes form around the joint, cysts develop in the femur and tibia, and crepitus is felt when the knee is moved.

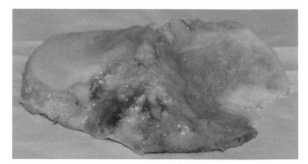

Fig. 24.21 The upper surface of the tibia removed at total knee replacement. The medial plateau has exposed bone and grooves, and is surrounded by osteophytes. The lateral plateau is almost normal. Note that it is convex upwards, not concave.

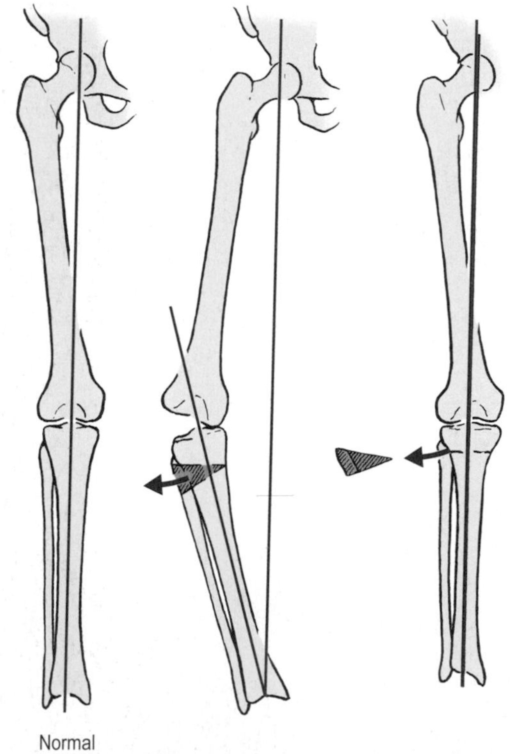

Normal

Fig. 24.20 Corrective osteotomy for osteoarthritis of the knee. The aim of the procedure is to place the hip, knee and ankle in correct alignment.

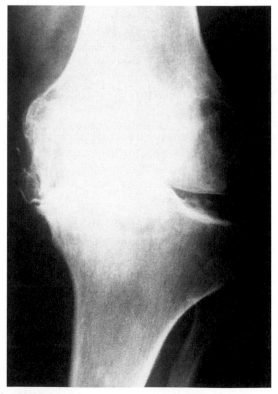

Fig. 24.22 Medial compartment osteoarthritis. Note the narrowing of the medial compartment, widening of the lateral compartment and a varus deformity.

The features of osteoarthritis of the lateral compartment are the opposite and a valgus deformity develops.

Treatment

Conservative treatment should always be tried before suggesting operation.

Many patients with early osteoarthritis experience a little aching after long walks and require only anti-inflammatory drugs. Some find that it is helpful to take the tablets before the anticipated exercise, e.g. before the weekend golf match or long shopping expeditions.

In more advanced disease the usual conservative measures of a stick, weight reduction, restriction of activity, analgesics and anti-inflammatory drugs are all helpful. Only when these measures fail should operation be considered.

Tibial osteotomy

Tibial osteotomy can correct the varus deformity of medial compartment osteoarthritis and break the vicious circle which leads to progressive wear and collapse by adjusting the line of weight-bearing so that the healthy compartment takes more weight (Fig. 24.23). The operation is most useful in patients with a worn medial compartment and a healthy lateral compartment.

Disadvantages are that the operation is a major inconvenience to the patient and is not always effective. The osteotomy takes 6–8 weeks to unite and the underlying osteoarthritis remains. Nevertheless,

about 75% of patients are content with the knee 2 years later and the operation conserves bone stock so that a knee replacement can be performed later if it becomes necessary. Later conversion to a total knee replacement is often difficult.

Low femoral osteotomy

For patients with a valgus deformity greater than 10° a low femoral osteotomy is preferable to a high tibial osteotomy.

When the lateral compartment is worn, there is usually more bone loss from the femoral condyle than the tibial plateau and correcting the deformity by tibial osteotomy leaves a knee joint that is no longer parallel with the ground. This can lead to further problems. The operation is done by removing a wedge of bone based medially from the lower part of the femur and securing the fragments with a blade plate (Fig. 24.24). Early mobilization and

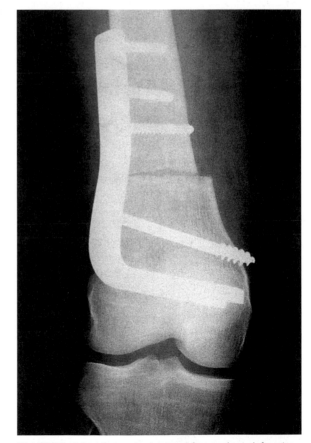

Fig. 24.24 A low femoral osteotomy for a valgus deformity internally fixed with blade plate and screws.

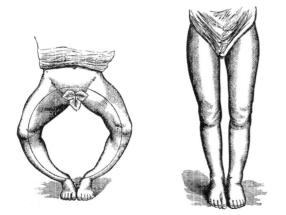

Fig. 24.23 Corrective osteotomy. From: MacEwen, William (1880) *Osteotomy*, J & A Churchill, London. By kind permission of the Wellcome Institute Library, London.

weight-bearing is possible but the plate should be removed approximately 1 year after operation.

Total knee replacement

Total knee replacement is a greater technical challenge than total hip replacement. Whereas the hip can move in any direction and rotate about its axis, the knee has a maximum of 150° flexion in one plane only.

This has a number of implications. The fixation is subjected to far more stress than the hip, making loosening more likely, and the prostheses are designed to minimize the forces on the interface between the patient and the prosthesis.

Placement of the prosthesis must be more accurate than in the hip and even 3° of malalignment can lead to failure. To add to these difficulties, the prostheses are larger and more superficial than a hip prosthesis.

Treatment of a failed total knee replacement is also less straightforward (Fig. 24.25). A failed hip replacement can be salvaged by converting it to an excision arthroplasty but excision of the knee produces a very poor result indeed and the joint must be arthrodesed.

The potential for making the patient worse rather than better is therefore considerable.

Results. The criteria for a good result from knee replacement are less ambitious than for total hip replacement. A successful knee replacement offers the following:

1. A knee that will straighten.
2. Flexion to 100° so that the patient can rise from a chair.
3. A leg that will take the patient's weight while standing.
4. A stable joint.

Five years after operation, the result is still as good as this in approximately 90% of patients.

Total knee prostheses can be considered in four groups and may either be secured with acrylic cement or left uncemented (Fig. 24.26):

1. Unconstrained prostheses.
2. Semiconstrained surface replacements.
3. Mobile bearing prostheses.
4. Fully constrained (hinges).

They can also be considered as unicompartmental or total replacement prostheses. Unicompartmental prostheses replace the medial or lateral compartment when the other is healthy. Total knee replacements replace both the medial and lateral compartments and usually the patellofemoral joint as well.

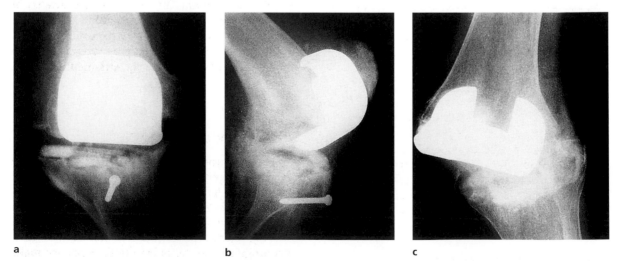

a   b   c

Fig. 24.25 Failed total knee replacement. (a), (b) The bone has collapsed beneath the tibial plateau and the femoral component has come completely away from the femur. (c) The medial side of the joint has become disrupted and the prosthesis has dislocated. The operation was done beneath a stiff hip.

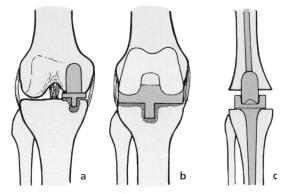

Fig. 24.26 Types of total knee replacement: (a) unicompartmental arthroplasty; (b) unconstrained total knee replacement; (c) constrained hinge total knee replacement.

Unconstrained prostheses consist of metal and plastic components secured separately to the femoral and tibial surfaces of each compartment. The components simply resurface the joint and do not contribute any stability to the joint. They should only be used when the joint is stable and the ligaments intact. They are suitable for early disease or disease of one compartment only and may be revised to another surface replacement (Fig. 24.27).

Semiconstrained prostheses replace the whole of both joint surfaces and the patella and contribute to the stability of the joint by their shape. This means that the fixation to the skeleton is exposed to greater forces (Fig. 24.28). The amount of stability they offer varies from one design to another.

Semiconstrained prostheses are more suitable than unconstrained prostheses for more advanced disease.

Mobile bearing prostheses allow the plastic insert to move on the flat tibial tray, thereby hopefully reducing the wear.

Fully constrained prostheses (hinges). Hinged knees are constrained; i.e. the two parts are firmly linked mechanically. For a grossly unstable joint with poor bone stock, a hinge offers a sound and stable limb (Fig. 24.29). The disadvantages are that extensive bone resection is required, making revision difficult (Fig. 24.30). If the prosthesis is removed for loosening or infection, two hollow trumpets of bone remain, arthrodesis is almost impossible and amputation is sometimes the only solution.

Revision knee replacement

Revision replacement of a prosthesis is more difficult at the knee than the hip for three reasons:

1. Soft tissue tension must be restored to eliminate varus and valgus instability.
2. Loosening and infection both cause bone loss. This means that the new prosthesis must be larger than the old.
3. The extensor mechanism must remain intact.

Revision often involves the use of a 'custom-made' prosthesis for the individual patient. These are sometimes supplied in modular form and assembled during operation.

If the knee is to be revised for infection, the original prosthesis and cement must be removed and infection eradicated. This may involve replacing the prosthesis with a mass of antibiotic-impregnated acrylic cement for between 6 and 12 weeks, during which time the knee will be unstable and the patient may be unable to walk. The new prosthesis can be inserted when the infection has been eliminated but antibiotics should be given for several weeks or months after operation. Even then, the infection may recur.

Amputation must sometimes be considered if the knee cannot be salvaged.

Arthrodesis

Arthrodesis of the knee, like other arthrodeses, is a reliable operation that lasts a lifetime. The operation allows the patient to walk comfortably but makes it impossible to sit comfortably and difficult to climb out of a car or bath. The operation is indicated in badly damaged knees in young adults.

Arthrodesis is achieved by compressing the two bone surfaces together, usually by external fixation devices, or a plate, or with an intramedullary nail (Fig. 24.31).

Debridement and lavage

Arthroscopic joint debridement to remove loose tags of meniscus, osteophytes and articular cartilage debris while leaving the meniscal rim intact produces a satisfactory result in about 75% of patients with early osteoarthritis. Arthroscopy also allows a thorough inspection of the joint surfaces so that a firm prognosis can be offered but it does not make the osteoarthritis regress.

Debridement is not an alternative to osteotomy or joint replacement.

409

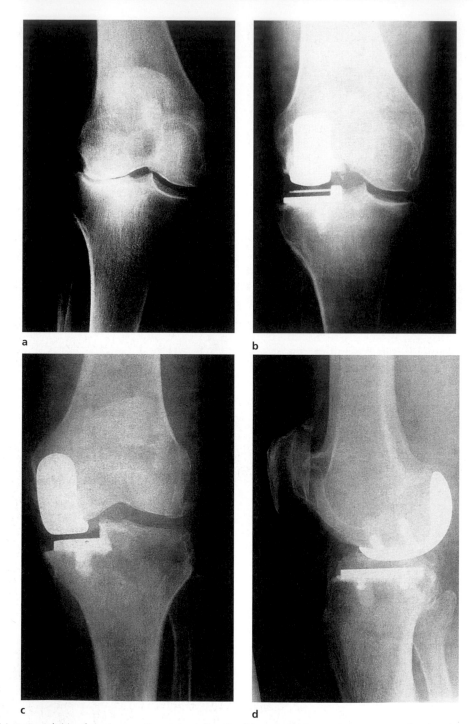

Fig. 24.27 (a) Osteoarthritis of the knee with valgus deformity; (b) corrected by a unicompartmental arthroplasty; (c) anteroposterior and (d) lateral view of a different type of prosthesis inserted for a varus deformity.

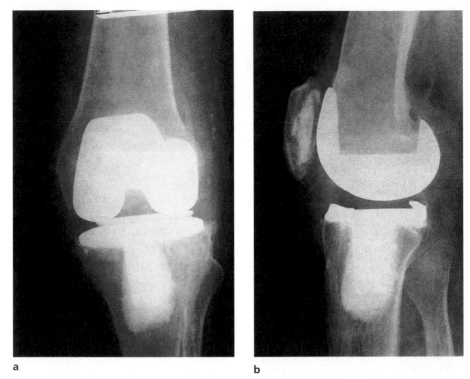

Fig. 24.28 (a), (b) An Insall–Burstein total knee replacement.

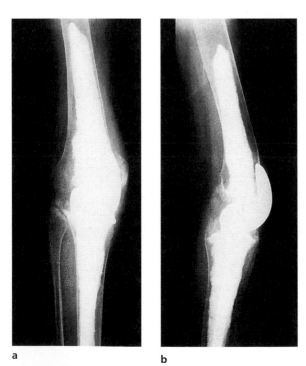

Fig. 24.29 (a), (b) A Stanmore hinge total knee replacement.

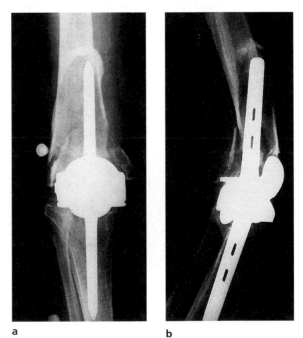

Fig. 24.30 (a), (b) A failed Walldius total knee replacement. The femur has fractured and both femoral and tibial components have worked through the bone.

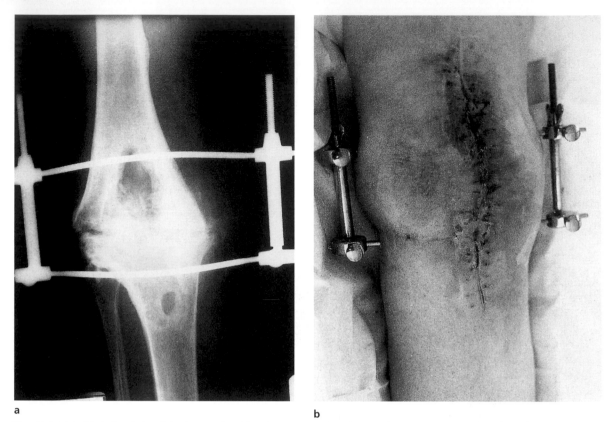

a
b

Fig. 24.31 (a), (b) Arthrodesis of the knee using Charnley compression clamps. The operation was done for infection following total knee replacement.

Management of osteoarthritis of the knee

The following is a very rough guide to the management of osteoarthritis of the knee:

1. Recurrent effusions, little or no deformity and near normal radiographs with or without mechanical symptoms – conservative treatment with NSAIDs, weight reduction, physiotherapy.

2. As above, if conservative treatment has failed – arthroscopic debridement.

3. Increasing deformity and disability in patients under the age of 60 – osteotomy.

4. Increasing deformity with disease confined to only one compartment, over the age of 60 – unicompartmental joint replacement.

5. Deformity and disease involving two or more compartments, over the age of 60 – total joint replacement with unconstrained prosthesis.

6. Gross instability and collapse, over the age of 70 – total joint replacement with constrained prosthesis if necessary.

Rheumatoid arthritis of the knee

The treatment of acute rheumatoid arthritis is conservative but synovectomy may be needed if the synovial disease cannot be controlled medically (Fig. 24.32).

In patients over the age of 60, synovectomy can be done chemically or with a radioisotope such as yttrium. The indications for surgical synovectomy are becoming much less common as medical management improves, but it is still required for young patients with uncontrolled disease.

Synovectomy is now usually performed arthroscopically to minimize surgical trauma.

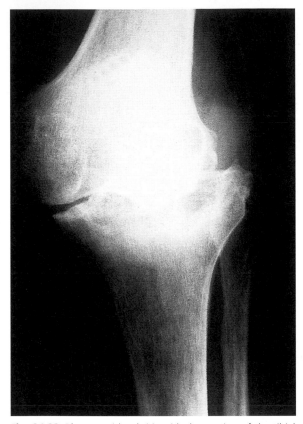

Fig. 24.32 Rheumatoid arthritis with destruction of the tibial plateau and a valgus deformity.

Treatment

As the disease progresses, bone is destroyed, deformities develop and salvage procedures become necessary. Osteotomy is not helpful and joint replacement is usually required.

Septic arthritis of the knee

Septic arthritis of the knee has several causes (p. 314):

1. Penetrating injuries.
2. Spread from osteomyelitis of the lower end of the femur or upper end of the tibia.
3. Systemic infection, e.g. septicaemia or gonococcal infections.

Treatment

Septic arthritis of the knee is managed in the same way as in other joints, with rest, adequate antibiotics and irrigation. Suction drainage is particularly suitable for septic arthritis at the knee, and thorough lavage combined with arthroscopy is effective.

Internal derangements of the knee

The term 'internal derangement of the knee' is a common provisional diagnosis for any patient with mechanical symptoms in the knee. The initials 'IDK' also stand for 'I don't know' and the temptation to use these initials instead of making a complete diagnosis must be avoided.

There are many causes of internal derangements of the knee.

Common internal derangements of the knee

- Meniscus lesions
- Loose bodies
- Chondral separations
- Osteochondritis dissecans.

Meniscus lesions

Meniscus lesions are the commonest internal derangements. Although the menisci are damaged by trauma, they are included in this section because the trauma responsible is often so trivial that the patient cannot remember any injury at all. Because of this, patients with meniscal injuries are most often seen in orthopaedic clinics and not accident departments.

Function of the meniscus

The menisci are important parts of the load-bearing mechanism of the knee and they absorb the downward thrust of the convex femoral condyles (Fig. 24.33). The menisci are so effective that, if they are removed, the force taken by the articular cartilage on peak loading increases by about five times. Meniscectomy therefore exposes the articular cartilage to much greater forces than normal, and evidence of degenerative osteoarthritis is seen in 75% of patients 10 years after total meniscectomy.

If degenerative osteoarthritis is already present at the time of meniscectomy, the degeneration will progress much more rapidly, and it is therefore

413

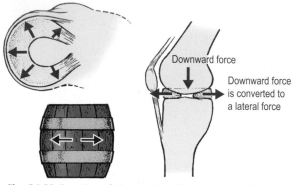

Fig. 24.33 Function of the menisci. The menisci act like hoops on a barrel.

important to conserve as much meniscal tissue as possible in degenerative joints.

The menisci are constructed a little like ligaments but they are curved and their ground substance is stiffer. When a meniscus tears, a mobile gristly fragment is produced inside the knee which pops in and out of the joint and blocks movement.

The characteristic symptoms of a meniscal lesion are caused by movement of the meniscal fragment in the joint and include recurrent locking and unlocking of the knee; i.e. mechanical obstruction of movement followed by a return to normal. The original tear and the subsequent locking usually occur with little applied violence and are often the result of twisting on the bent knee, or even from turning over in bed.

Patients use 'locking' to describe episodes of severe pain, or even collapsing of the knee. It is curious that the word is not applied in this way to other joints. 'Locking' means mechanical 'jamming' of the joint, and nothing more.

Meniscal tears

Several types of meniscal tear are seen (Fig. 24.34). A circumferential tear creates a long fragment attached at each end which can swing over into the intercondylar notch. The movement of the fragment is likened to a bucket handle and these fragments are known as bucket handle fragments (Fig. 24.35).

Flaps and pedunculated fragments do not cause mechanical locking but they move in and out of the joint space and can sometimes be felt in the medial or lateral gutter of the knee.

On the lateral side, complex oblique tears based on the popliteus tunnel occur and are called 'parrot beak' tears because of their shape. These tears result from a sharp twisting injury when the lateral compartment is loaded. They do not occur in the medial compartment because it does not have a popliteus tunnel.

Discoid menisci

In approximately 5% of people the lateral meniscus is congenitally abnormal, lacking its normal crescentic shape. The meniscus in these patients may be truly circular, or discoid, but is more often shaped like a half-moon. The meniscus may also be thicker than normal.

Intact discoid menisci seldom cause symptoms, but in children they may be responsible for a block to extension or a loud clunk when the knee is straightened. Discoid menisci may become torn and cause mechanical symptoms like other meniscal tears, or undergo 'cystic' change which causes a dull aching pain in the knee.

'Cystic' menisci

Meniscal tissue can undergo a myxoid degeneration, which converts the normal firm meniscal tissue to a soft and friable mass (Fig. 24.36). The lateral meniscus is affected far more often than the medial.

The classic symptoms of a cystic meniscus are a dull, aching pain in the lateral side of the knee 'like toothache in the knee', often worse at night. No conservative treatment is effective.

Meniscal cysts

Degeneration of the menisci must be distinguished from ganglia on the lateral joint line. Ganglia can develop anywhere and need only to be excised without opening the joint.

A true cyst in a degenerate meniscus may communicate with the knee by a horizontal fissure, sometimes called a 'fish mouth' tear.

Treatment

Because of the importance of the meniscus in load-bearing it is essential that the meniscus is left undisturbed until the diagnosis has been confirmed by arthroscopy or MRI. Clinical diagnosis alone is accurate in only 70% of patients.

Tears. When the diagnosis is confirmed, the loose fragment should be excised, leaving as much healthy

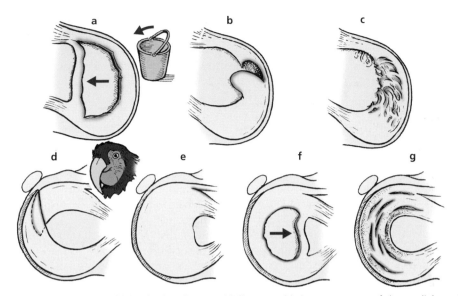

Fig. 24.34 Types of meniscal lesion: (a) bucket-handle tear; (b) flap tear; (c) degenerate tear of the medial meniscus; (d) oblique 'parrot-beak' tear of the lateral meniscus; (e) discoid lateral meniscus; (f) locked bucket-handle tear of the lateral meniscus; (g) cystic or myxoid degeneration of the lateral meniscus.

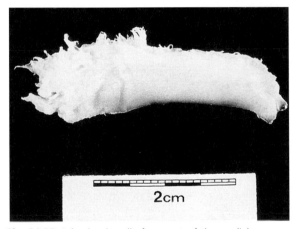

Fig. 24.35 A bucket-handle fragment of the medial meniscus.

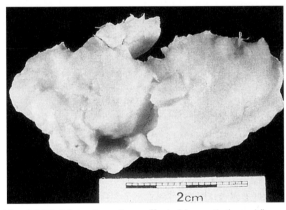

Fig. 24.36 A lateral meniscus affected by cystic (myxoid) degeneration.

meniscal tissue as possible. The operation is almost always undertaken arthroscopically because this allows a precise diagnosis and careful excision of the lesion with preservation of all intact tissue (Fig. 24.37). Patients can return to light work 1 week after arthroscopic meniscectomy, and heavy work within 2 weeks.

Open meniscectomy gives equally good long-term results but the initial rehabilitation is slower and patients may be unable to return to work for as long as 3 months. The only indication for open menis-cectomy is the inability of the surgeon to perform arthroscopic meniscectomy.

Reattachment is suitable for peripheral tears that leave the meniscus intact but mobile. Such tears are most often seen in patients with anterior cruciate ligament ruptures.

Discoid menisci. Conservative surgery is important in the management of discoid menisci, which are commonly seen in children, because total lateral meniscectomy in a child leads to early osteoarthritis. Symptomatic discoid menisci should be treated by excision of any torn fragments.

415

Cystic menisci must be treated by excision of the affected tissue, which often means total meniscectomy. If only a small area is affected, excision of the damaged area alone is sufficient but healthy tissue can undergo degeneration later.

Loose bodies

Loose bodies (Fig. 24.38) which float around the knee and obstruct movement can arise from osteochondritis dissecans, synovial chondromatosis, osteochondral fractures or localized separation of the articular cartilage. They can also grow in the synovial fluid, which is an excellent tissue culture medium. Patients with loose bodies give a classic account of a loose fragment in the knee and will usually be able to describe its size and shape. Loose bodies are sometimes called joint mice – a good analogy because they can be recognized instantly but disappear and may then be impossible to find again.

Radiographs are less helpful than might be imagined and at least two views in different planes are essential (Fig. 24.39). Twenty five percent of loose bodies are transradiant, and not all isolated areas of calcification in the knee are due to loose bodies. Some are firmly fixed to synovium and the fabella can be confused with a loose body by the unwary.

Loose bodies should not be called 'foreign bodies'. Foreign bodies, including bullets and bits of gravel, come from outside the body and are rare in joints.

Treatment

Removing the loose fragment is the only reliable way to relieve symptoms.

Osteochondral lesions

Many different pathological processes can affect the femoral condyles. The conditions themselves are

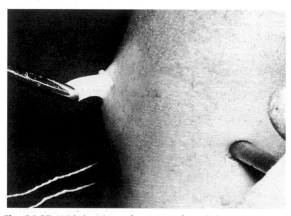

Fig. 24.37 Withdrawing a fragment of medial meniscus from the knee by arthroscopic surgery.

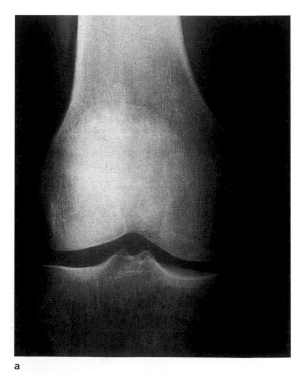

a

Fig. 24.39 (a) Osteochondritis dissecans of the knee. Can you see the crater or the fragment? (See Fig. 24.39 (b) for the answer.)

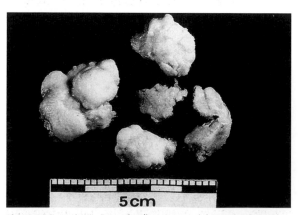

5 cm

Fig. 24.38 Multiple loose bodies removed from the knee.

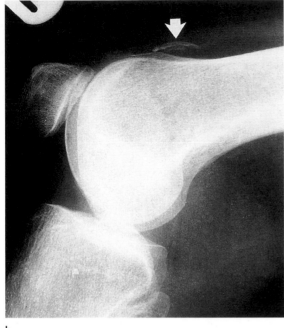

b

Fig. 24.39 (b) The loose body (*arrowed*) is lying in the suprapatellar pouch.

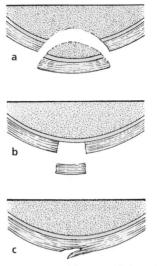

Fig. 24.40 (a) Osteochondral fracture of the articular surface involving articular cartilage and bone; (b) full thickness chondral separation of articular cartilage without involving bone; (c) partial thickness flap of articular cartilage.

separate, are treated differently and have different prognoses. They are not all different types of osteochondritis dissecans, however beguiling such an impressive Latin diagnosis may be.

There are five main types of osteochondral lesion:

1. Osteochondral fractures.
2. Chondral flaps and separations.
3. Osteochondritis dissecans.
4. Spontaneous osteonecrosis.
5. Osteochondritis dissecans of the lateral condyle.

Osteochondral fractures

In adolescents and young adults, twisting movements of the knee or a direct blow can detach a segment of bone and articular cartilage (Fig. 24.40). Patients can usually remember the moment of detachment and the incident is usually accompanied by a haemarthrosis.

Treatment

Fragments can be reattached if they are large enough to take a screw. Many osteochondral fragments pass undiagnosed and wander freely around the joint as a loose body. The bed of the defect eventually heals with fibrocartilage and the fragment rounds off.

Chondral separations and flaps

Osteochondral fractures are rare after the age of 30 but fragments of articular cartilage can separate from the underlying bone (Fig. 24.41). Radiographs do not show these fragments because articular cartilage is transradiant, but they can be found arthroscopically.

Partial thickness separations, or chondral flaps, also occur and can mimic the symptoms of a meniscal tear. These occur in a slightly older age group.

Osteochondral fractures most commonly occur between 10 and 25 years, separations between 25 and 40, and flaps over the age of 40.

Treatment

Some chondral flaps are ground away by the action of the joint and the symptoms then disappear.

Chondral separations do not heal perfectly, however they are treated. Removal of the flap may help but this leaves a large area of bone exposed. An autologous chondrocyte transplantation may help cover this defect, as may a mosaicplasty. This involves moving a core of chondral surface and bone from one part of the knee to the defect.

417

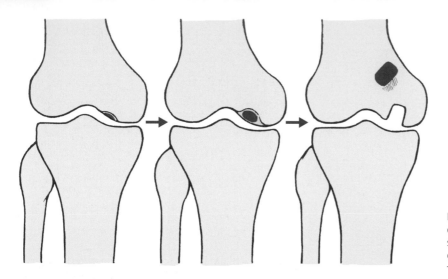

Fig. 24.41 Progression of osteochondritis dissecans from a small lesion on the medial femoral condyle to loose body formation.

Osteochondritis dissecans

Osteochondritis dissecans (not desiccans – the fragment does not dry up but dissects out) involves the medial femoral condyle and presents with pain between the ages of 8 and 12 years (Fig. 24.42). Boys are more often involved than girls, in a ratio of 6:1. The pain is worse when walking and on hyperextension.

On clinical examination there may be tenderness just medial to the patellar ligament and pain on hyperextension. The pain is sometimes more marked with the foot in internal rotation than external rotation.

Radiographs in the very early stages show only a small irregularity of the medial condyle. As growth proceeds, the irregularity develops into an area of bone separated from the rest of the condyle by a transradiant line. There may be several 'fragments' lying in the crater on the condyle. The articular surface overlying the lesion is intact at first, but after skeletal maturity the fragments may become loose and separate as a loose body within the knee.

Treatment

Conservative. Many fragments unite spontaneously without treatment and there is no evidence that the application of a cast increases the chances of natural union. Operation should not be considered unless the patient has been observed for at least 6 months,

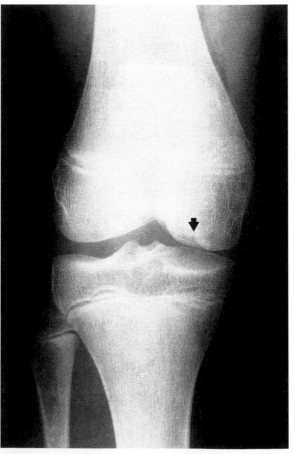

Fig. 24.42 Osteochondritis dissecans before skeletal maturity.

continues to have pain, and has no sign of radiological union.

Operative treatment. The lesion can be made to unite in approximately 90% of cases by drilling holes through the articular surface overlying the lesion into the medial femoral condyle. This can be done under arthroscopic control.

If the articular surface is broken and the fragment is loose it may be secured with a small screw or several pins. There are many techniques for performing this procedure.

Once the fragment has separated as a loose body a permanent defect remains on the articular surface. The fragment must be removed as a loose body and attempts to replace it are usually unsuccessful.

Spontaneous osteonecrosis

The cancellous bone in the weight-bearing area of the medial femoral condyle may undergo necrosis in patients over the age of 50. No cause is known. The cancellous bone is involved but the articular cartilage and cortex remain intact until they collapse into the defect. The condition is accompanied by pain and an increasing varus deformity.

Treatment

The lesion can be debrided arthroscopically and this produces a temporary benefit. Osteotomy may be helpful in transferring weight to the healthy lateral compartment but joint replacement is usually required in the long term.

Osteochondritis of the lateral femoral condyle

Large segments of the weight-bearing area of the lateral femoral condyle may separate from the rest of the condyle in early adult life. The condition differs from 'classic' osteochondritis dissecans, described above, in the age of the patients affected, the shape of the lesion, and the outcome. The cause is not known but the outcome is poor.

Treatment

The loose fragments require excision because the bone is too soft to be replaced.

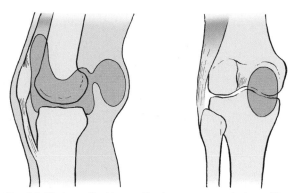

Fig. 24.43 A popliteal bursa. The bursa communicates with the synovial cavity of the knee.

Other knee disorders

Popliteal cysts

The synovial cavity of the knee often extends into the popliteal fossa through defects in the posterior capsule, of which the commonest lies just above the head of gastrocnemius (Figs 24.43, 24.44). The result is a swelling at the back of the knee, which is uncomfortable more than painful and limits flexion. The pain is worse after walking and may be confused with intermittent claudication.

Popliteal cysts are usually an indication of pathology in the rest of the knee rather than a disorder in their own right. Rheumatoid arthritis, gout and tuberculosis can all produce a large painful popliteal swelling but osteoarthrosis and trauma are more common. Beware of calling these cysts 'Baker's cysts'. In 1877, William Morrant Baker described massive swellings that extended down to the ankle. The original Baker's cysts were probably tuberculous or rheumatoid in origin and are very rare nowadays.

Popliteal cysts also occur in children and present as a firm or hard swelling in the popliteal fossa. The swelling often arouses the fear of malignancy but this anxiety can easily be allayed by transilluminating the lesion to demonstrate that it consists of fluid only.

Natural history

Untreated, popliteal cysts do one of three things:

1. Disappear gradually.
2. Rupture suddenly, when they mimic a deep vein thrombosis. The calf becomes hot, tender and red

419

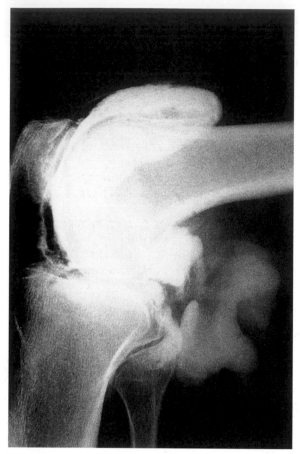

Fig. 24.44 An arthrogram showing a ruptured popliteal cyst with contrast medium leaking into the soft tissues of the calf.

and the patient may be admitted under the physicians and given anticoagulants. An arthrogram will confirm the diagnosis by showing the synovial leak into the calf.

3. Become so tense and painful that excision is required.

Treatment

Because most popliteal cysts disappear spontaneously, operation is seldom required. The joint should be investigated to exclude gout, rheumatoid arthritis or an internal derangement and any underlying cause treated. The patient should be warned that the cyst may rupture, so that they can avoid needless anticoagulation. If the cyst does rupture, rest and analgesics are all that is needed.

Excising a popliteal cyst is an extensive procedure, involving a dissection of the popliteal fossa; recurrence of the cyst is possible.

Ligamentous instability

Anterior cruciate instability

Clinical features

Patients with anterior cruciate instability give a very characteristic history, beginning with a violent injury in which the patient felt something break in the knee when tackled or twisting awkwardly (p. 259). Most patients remember the incident vividly, even many years later. The knee swelled after the injury and the swelling gradually subsided. Ever since then the knee collapses when the patient puts weight on it and twists and, although able to run fast in straight lines, he or she must slow down to turn corners.

Some patients only have symptoms when the knee is under great stress on the football field but some knees are so unstable that they collapse if the patient turns round when walking over a level floor, while walking over cobbles or uneven ground is quite impossible.

Roughly one patient in three needs reconstruction following anterior cruciate rupture. The remainder are evenly divided between those who have occasional minor problems and those who have no symptoms whatever.

Comparison with meniscal injuries. The history of anterior cruciate instability is very different from a meniscus lesion.

Differences between anterior cruciate rupture and meniscal lesions

1. Cruciate symptoms are caused by a high speed twisting or a deceleration injury with the knee almost straight, the meniscus lesion by low speed movements with the knee bent.
2. Patients stop playing after a cruciate injury.
3. Ligament injuries usually follow a memorable injury, meniscal injuries seldom do.
4. Menisci can lock the knee and block extension, but ligament injuries cause collapsing.

The diagnosis can be difficult if the patient has both a meniscal tear and an anterior cruciate injury, with locking as well as collapsing, but the two elements can be separated if the history is taken intelligently.

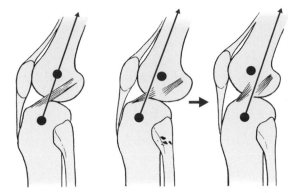

Fig. 24.45 Mechanism of the 'pivot shift' phenomenon. If the anterior cruciate ligament is ruptured, the short arched lateral tibial plateau can slip in front of the femoral condyle. As the knee is flexed, the iliotibial tract moves behind the axis of rotation and the bones reduce with a thud.

Mechanics

The instability is caused by the odd design of the lateral compartment of the knee, which consists of two convex surfaces that slip off each other when the compartment is loaded. Only the anterior cruciate holds the lateral condyle and the lateral plateau in the correct relationship (Fig. 24.45).

Clinical examination

Testing for anterior cruciate laxity is difficult. The hamstrings must be fully relaxed to elicit the anterior drawer sign, but even with the hamstrings tight, Lachman's test (p. 29) is usually positive. The pivot shift test, in which the knee is flexed while loading the lateral compartment, will reproduce the patient's symptoms, but the test is difficult and requires considerable experience.

Treatment

Conservative treatment cannot restore the integrity of the ligament but it can restore function.

Physiotherapy should be directed to building up the hamstrings so that they will help pull the tibia backwards on the femur and help make good the deficiency of the cruciate. Quadriceps exercises work in the opposite direction and may be counterproductive.

Many patients are content to adjust their life to their disability by giving up violent sports, and this should always be discussed with the patient.

Surgical treatment. If the symptoms interfere with everyday activities and conservative measures have failed, reconstruction of the anterior cruciate may be needed. This is a complex operation requiring much rehabilitation and at least 6 months away from sport. Two types of operation are available:

1. Replacement of the anterior cruciate, either with natural tissue or an allograft.

2. An extracapsular repair using the iliotibial tract.

The treatment of choice is an intra-articular reconstruction using the middle third of the patellar tendon or a four-strand hamstring graft. The use of an extra-articular reconstruction using the iliotibial tract may play a part in stabilizing the lateral structures.

The results remain satisfactory in about 80% of patients 5 years after operation.

Prosthetic ligaments have been described and discarded since about 1918. None has remained on the market for more than a few years because the long-term results are poor.

Chronic posterior cruciate instability

Posterior cruciate ruptures cause fewer problems than anterior cruciate injuries, but when they do, they are often intractable.

The usual symptoms of posterior cruciate deficiency are a feeling of unsteadiness when descending slopes or putting weight on the bent knee.

The posterior cruciate is ruptured in two ways:

1. A blow to the front of the knee in flexion.

2. Hyperextension.

If the patient gives a history of such an injury, or has a scar at the upper end of the tibia consistent with a blow, posterior cruciate rupture should be suspected.

Clinical examination

The injury can be distinguished from anterior cruciate rupture because the posterior sag sign is positive (Fig. 24.46). This can look a little like an anterior drawer sign but is easily distinguished by observing the knee from the side.

Treatment

Quadriceps function can compensate for posterior cruciate instability. Operation is difficult, unreliable and indicated only if the symptoms are disabling. Many well-known athletes have returned to their

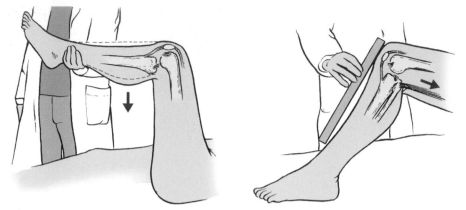

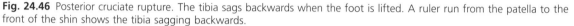

Fig. 24.46 Posterior cruciate rupture. The tibia sags backwards when the foot is lifted. A ruler run from the patella to the front of the shin shows the tibia sagging backwards.

former level of achievement after conservative treatment alone.

Medial ligament instability

For practical purposes, rupture of the medial collateral ligament alone does not cause symptoms unless it is accompanied by an anterior cruciate rupture. Management of the acute injury is described on page 261.

Patients with medial ligament injuries experience unsteadiness when the leg is caught awkwardly by a sideways blow to the foot.

Treatment

Reconstruction is difficult. The symptoms in most patients are due to the associated anterior cruciate ligament injury and are relieved by anterior cruciate reconstruction.

Anterior knee pain

Patellofemoral joint

Pain at the front of the knee usually comes from the patellofemoral joint, which is quite separate from the tibiofemoral joint. This joint is stressed when the knee is flexed under load, as when squatting or descending stairs, but there are many other causes (Fig. 24.47).

The mechanics of the joint means that it takes up to seven times the weight of the body when loaded in flexion and it is therefore exposed to enormous stresses. The pain is felt around the knee cap and patients usually indicate the site of the pain by rubbing the palm of the hand over the knee cap. The pain can be serious enough to curtail sports or even make it difficult to climb stairs.

The articular surface may be abnormal but pain can also arise from structures around the joint.

Adolescent anterior knee pain

Anterior knee pain is a particular problem in adolescence. Girls between 13 and 15 years old are most often affected and the pain may be so severe that they are unable to take part in sports or even move between classrooms at school.

On clinical examination there are usually very few physical signs but the patella may be tender to the touch. A few have reflex sympathetic dystrophy (p. 309) in the early stages before the colour changes are present.

In many patients, no cause can be found but a plausible explanation is that during the adolescent growth spurt the load on the joint increases suddenly because of the rapid rise in body weight and muscle power. This, combined with the lengthening of the lower limb bones, which increases the leverage applied to the knee, increases the load across the patellofemoral joint very markedly.

The great majority of adolescents with anterior knee pain recover spontaneously without treatment. Provided there is no mechanical element to their symptoms, such as clicking, collapsing or an effu-

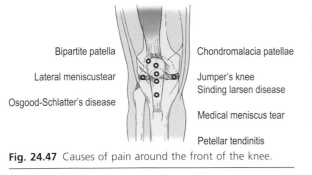

Bipartite patella

Lateral meniscus tear

Osgood-Schlatter's disease

Chondromalacia patellae

Jumper's knee
Sinding larsen disease

Medical meniscus tear

Petellar tendinitis

Fig. 24.47 Causes of pain around the front of the knee.

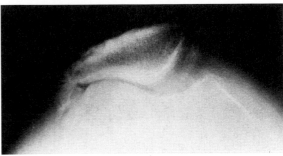

Fig. 24.48 Osteoarthritis of the patellofemoral joint, involving the lateral facet of the patella.

sion, a gradual recovery can be expected over a period of 1 or 2 years.

Treatment

If there are no mechanical symptoms or signs and the radiograph is normal, the patient can safely be observed at regular intervals, perhaps every 6 months, until the symptoms settle.

Physiotherapy is unlikely to be helpful and may aggravate the pain. Operation, including arthroscopy, should be avoided at all costs. It is not possible to see pain down an arthroscope and the trauma of any procedure may precipitate reflex sympathetic dystrophy.

If it is necessary to exclude an internal derangement, MRI is preferable to arthroscopy. The mainstay of treatment is sympathy and regular reassurance until the pain resolves.

Chondromalacia patellae

Beware of the term 'chondromalacia patellae': it means only softening of the articular cartilage of the patella but is commonly used as a synonym for anterior knee pain in an adolescent.

Because the stresses on the patellofemoral joint are so great, some areas of articular cartilage are overloaded and become soft and swollen. This condition is known as chondromalacia patellae and is probably reversible in early cases. In some patients, the softened surface develops fissures and begins to break up, producing a condition which is, in effect, early osteoarthritis.

Chondromalacia patellae is only one cause of anterior knee pain – there are many others.

Treatment

The patient should be treated like other adolescents with anterior knee pain (see above) unless they develop definite crepitus or clicking under the patella. They will then require arthroscopic surgery to smooth irregularities on the patellar surface. The prognosis for patellae with articular surface irregularities is poor and many develop patellofemoral osteoarthritis later.

Lateral pressure syndrome

In a few patients the patella does not sit as firmly in the femoral trochlea as it should. Instead, it tilts so that the lateral facet runs along the lateral edge of the femoral trochlea.

On examination the pain is localized to the lateral edge of the patella. Untreated, such patellae will probably develop patellofemoral osteoarthritis of the type shown in Figure 24.48.

Treatment

There is no reliable conservative treatment. If the symptoms persist for more than 6 months, lateral release to divide the lateral structures of the extensor retinaculum may be needed. This procedure allows the patella to resume its correct position and relieves pain in about 75% of patients, but it requires vigorous physiotherapy afterwards and recovery is often slow.

Note: Lateral release does not help undiagnosed anterior knee pain or chondromalacia patellae.

Synovial shelf syndrome (plica)

A fold of synovium, the medial synovial shelf, lies against the medial femoral condyle in flexion and

423

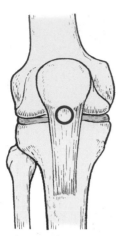

Fig. 24.49 Jumper's knee. The lower pole of the patella is tender at the centre of the patellar tendon attachment.

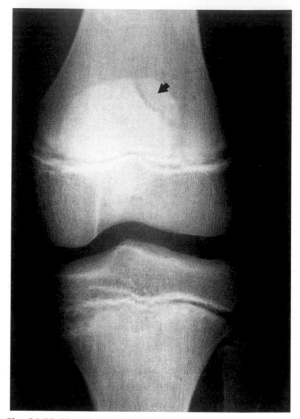

Fig. 24.50 Bipartite patella.

can be irritated by trauma or prolonged pressure against the condyle. If the shelf is the cause of pain, the patient will point to it with an index finger.

Treatment

If the symptoms do not settle with time, they can be relieved by excising the synovial shelf arthroscopically.

Jumper's knee

Jumper's knee is similar to tennis elbow (p. 371) and occurs at the insertion of the patellar ligament onto the lower pole of the patella (Fig. 24.49). The patient cannot jump vigorously and athletic performance is affected.

Treatment

Treatment is similar to tennis elbow. If three injections of hydrocortisone acetate at the site of pain (but not into the tendon) are unsuccessful, the area must be explored and the tissues drilled or scarified. Return to sport is unusual within 6 months of this procedure.

Bipartite patella

Some patellae have a separate fragment at the supero-lateral corner but it is not agreed whether this is congenital or acquired (Fig. 24.50). The condition is often bilateral.

Treatment

Operation is seldom needed but, if the separated fragment is painful or tender, excision of the separated fragment or a lateral release of the extensor mechanism will usually relieve pain.

Patellofemoral osteoarthritis

If the patellar surface develops osteoarthritis, the patient will be unable to bend the knee under load without pain. The rough areas cause crepitus, which is felt as an unpleasant grating 'like broken biscuits in the knee' when the patellofemoral joint is loaded, and in some patients the crepitus is audible. The lateral facet is affected more than the medial (see Fig. 24.48) and the condition is common in patients over the age of 40.

Treatment

No conservative treatment is really effective, apart from weight reduction, analgesics, and anti-inflammatory drugs. If the pain is severe, patellectomy will be needed to replace the rough surface of the patella with smooth tendon. After removing the patella, the tendon is carefully repaired and physiotherapy begun to restore joint movement and quadriceps strength.

The tibiofemoral joint is not involved in patellofemoral osteoarthritis and the two joints can be considered separately. It must be remembered, however, that if the tibiofemoral joint is badly affected by osteoarthritis a patellectomy will make a total knee replacement very difficult.

Anterior knee pain in the obese patient

Because the patellofemoral joint takes about seven times body weight during flexion, obese patients are particularly vulnerable to patellofemoral pain. Many of these patients have pushed the articular surface of the patella past its design limits and have done irreparable damage to their joint.

Treatment

No treatment is effective and it is folly to advise operation in such a patient unless their weight can be brought within normal limits.

Housemaid's knee (prepatellar bursitis)

The prepatellar bursa is a normal structure which allows the skin to slide easily over the patella as the knee is flexed (Fig. 24.51). If the bursa becomes infected, injured or inflamed, fluid will accumulate inside the bursa and a swelling will appear in front of the patella in a characteristic position, which distinguishes it from an effusion of the knee. Sometimes a small fibrinous body forms in the bursa and causes severe pain on kneeling.

In days past, before mechanization, housemaids spent much of their working days kneeling and leaning slightly forwards while scrubbing floors and doing other household tasks. Today, 'housemaid's knee' is an occupational hazard of carpet layers, tilers and roofers, all of whom should use protective pads when kneeling.

Treatment

The swelling usually subsides with rest but in some patients an injection of hydrocortisone acetate into

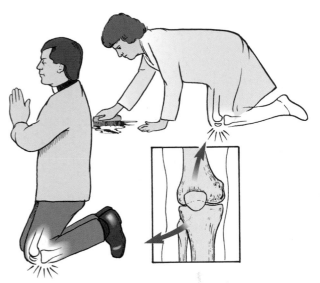

Fig. 24.51 Housemaid's knee and clergyman's knee. Housemaid's knee affects the prepatellar bursa; clergyman's knee affects the infrapatellar bursa.

the bursa is needed. If this is ineffective and the swelling recurs, excision is required. Patients with gout are particularly susceptible to prepatellar bursitis, as well as olecranon bursitis (p. 372) and the bursitis is likely to remain or recur unless the gout is treated.

Clergyman's knee (infrapatellar bursitis)

The infrapatellar bursa, which lies in front of the tibial tubercle, can also be inflamed. The condition is called clergyman's knee because priests kneel in a more upright position than housemaids and take the load on the tibial tubercle instead of the patella.

Treatment

Treatment is the same as for prepatellar bursitis.

Patellar instability

The patellofemoral joint has little mechanical congruity and the patellar ligament is not in the same straight line as the quadriceps. The angle between the patellar ligament and the quadriceps is about 20° in the normal population and this angle is known as the Q angle (Fig. 24.52).

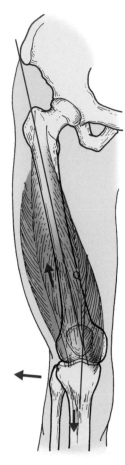

Fig. 24.52 The 'Q' angle: (a) the extensor mechanism does not run in a straight line from origin to insertion; (b) a lateral force is applied to the patella when the quadriceps contracts.

Because the Q angle exists, a lateral force is applied to the patella every time the quadriceps contracts. This lateral force is resisted by three things:

1. The median ridge of the patella sitting in the femoral trochlea.
2. The tightness of the medial structures.
3. The lateral edge of the femoral trochlea.

If any of these features is abnormal, e.g. an abnormally small or high patella (patella alta), generalized ligamentous laxity or dysplasia of the lateral condyle of the femur, patellar instability is likely.

Recurrent dislocation of the patella

Recurrent dislocation of the patella is a problem during adolescence, especially in girls because they have looser ligaments and smaller bones than boys. The dislocation is usually caused by a twisting movement of the knee in slight flexion and each generation appears to develop its own dance designed to displace the patella (see Fig. 14.30).

The patient usually knows if the patella has slipped out of place but if it reduces quickly the condition can be mistaken for an internal derangement. Other patients will say that their knee dislocates and this can be misleading.

Treatment

If the patella has dislocated three times and the patient has stopped growing, surgical stabilization is indicated. (Management of acute dislocations is described on page 256).

Stability can be achieved in several ways:

1. Releasing the lateral structures.
2. Realigning the quadriceps mechanism by transferring the tibial tubercle medially, thus reducing the Q angle.
3. Moving the tibial tubercle distally to bring the patella lower down in the femoral trochlea.
4. Tightening medial structures.

The choice of operation depends on the anatomical problem to be treated. Knees with normal anatomy and ligaments usually require only a lateral release but medial tibial tubercle transposition is needed if there is abnormal ligamentous laxity. Those with a small high patella require distal and medial transposition of the tibial tubercle combined with lateral release and perhaps medial plication.

Habitual and congenital dislocation of the patella

Habitual and congenital dislocation of the patella are different from recurrent dislocation (Fig. 24.53). In habitual dislocation the patella dislocates with every flexion of the knee, often because of abnormal tightness of the lateral structures. This may be the result of fibrosis following trauma, or injections into the vastus lateralis in the neonatal period.

Congenital dislocation of the patella is extremely rare and usually requires extensive surgery for its correction. The principles involved are the same as those for recurrent dislocation of the patella.

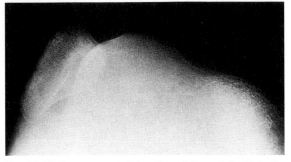

Fig. 24.53 A permanent dislocation of the patella. Note the abnormal shape of the patella and the intercondylar groove.

Osgood–Schlatter's disease and Sinding Larsen's disease

These conditions also cause pain at the front of the knee and are described on pages 328 and 331.

Case reports

These cases represent the decision making process in hip replacement surgery.

Patient A

A 48-year-old male patient presented to the orthopaedic surgeon with increasing rest and night pain in the right hip. He had previously been a keen athlete. He did not recall a specific history of trauma, but there was a strong family history of joint related problems with both his father and elder brother having had hip replacements.

Over the past 2 years he had had increasing pain and discomfort of such severity that he was unable to carry out his normal day-to-day activities. He had modified his lifestyle by stopping sport, losing weight and taking appropriate analgesics and using a walking stick when needed. Despite this, the pain was unacceptable and the orthopaedic surgeon discussed with him the operative treatment of the significant osteoarthritic degeneration in the hip.

He subsequently underwent a resurfacing total hip replacement after having been made aware of the risks and results of this procedure.

Patient B

A 78-year-old retired gentleman presented to the orthopaedic surgeon with increasing pain and discomfort in the right hip. As with Case A, conservative management had not helped sufficiently and it was felt that he needed a hip replacement.

He subsequently underwent a cemented Exeter total hip replacement.

Case C

A 22-year-old lady presented to the orthopaedic surgeon with a similar complaint of increasing pain and discomfort in the right hip. There was no clear history of a developmental dysplasia of the hip, but she had always recounted a 'clicky' hip and subsequent increasing pain.

Plain radiographs confirmed an acetabular dysplasia and an abnormal femoral neck shaft angle. It appeared that the hip was gradually progressing to an osteoarthritic hip and it was felt initially that she should have a hip arthroscopy to assess the chondral surfaces and labrum.

She subsequently went on to have a rotational acetabular osteotomy to cover the femoral head in the hope that this would prolong the life of the hip.

Summary

These three cases indicate different methods of management. In a very young patient it is important to try and preserve hip function for as long as possible.

In the middle-aged patient, when the symptoms are truly unacceptable and the patient has definitely failed conservative management then a hip replacement can be contemplated, but there are significant risks with this procedure. A resurfacing procedure may be beneficial as there is less resection of bone and this may, therefore, help in the long-term when this joint fails and a revision is contemplated.

In the elderly patient, again when conservative treatment has failed, a simple cemented total arthroplasty is indicated. The results of this are excellent in over 95% of cases.

Chapter |25|

Disorders of the ankle and foot

By the end of this chapter you should be able to:

- Remember the injuries of the ankle mortise (bony and ligamentous).
- Appreciate the difficulty in returning a patient with destructive foot lesions (e.g. rheumatoid arthritis) to normal function.
- Diagnose simple bunions and understand the indications for treatment.
- Be aware of the different types of toe deformity.

Ankle

Osteoarthritis of the ankle

Osteoarthritis of the ankle can follow any damage to the joint. The damage may be a single injury such as a fracture, repeated minor trauma, or any other insult to the joint, including infection.

Clinical features

As the degeneration proceeds, osteophytes form on the neck of the talus and obstruct joint movement. Dorsiflexion is usually the first to be affected. The patient gradually becomes aware that they cannot walk comfortably barefoot. This is because the heel of the shoe allows the ankle to be held in slight flexion.

Later, as the osteophytes on the neck of the talus and the anterior lip of the tibia enlarge, the ankle becomes progressively stiffer and it becomes painful to walk, even in normal shoes. At this point the patient will usually seek advice.

Footballer's ankle

Footballer's ankle occurs in habitual footballers and is caused by repeated strains of the anterior capsule (Fig. 25.1). Bone gradually builds up at each end of the anterior capsular fibres, producing osteophytes which restrict movement. The condition is indistinguishable from early osteoarthritis.

Conservative treatment

There are three forms of conservative treatment:

1. A raise to the heel of the shoe will take pressure off the anterior osteophytes.
2. A normal working boot may reduce the angular forces at the ankle.
3. Anti-inflammatory drugs.

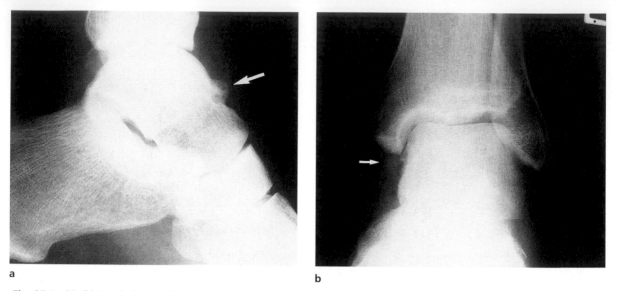

Fig. 25.1 (a), (b) 'Footballer's ankle'. Early osteoarthritic change with osteophytes and new bone formation (*arrowed*).

If these simple measures are ineffective, operation must be considered.

Operative treatment

Operative treatment is seldom required but three procedures are available:

1. Excision of osteophytes and arthroscopic debridement.
2. Arthrodesis.
3. Joint replacement.

Excision of osteophytes from the neck of the talus and the anterior margin of the tibia will improve extension and may relieve symptoms for many years, particularly in footballer's ankle, but recurrence is likely if the patient continues to play.

Arthrodesis. If pain is severe, arthrodesis may be needed. Arthrodesis of the ankle only abolishes flexion and extension. Inversion and eversion, which occur at the subtalar joint, and supination and pronation, which occur at the midtarsal joint, are unaffected. Rehabilitation after arthrodesis of the ankle is slow, and patients should be warned that it takes 2 years to achieve the final result.

The ankle is usually arthrodesed in slight flexion to accommodate the heel of a normal shoe, although this makes it difficult to walk barefoot. The opera-

tion is unsuitable for women who wish to wear heels of a varying height.

Joint replacement is possible, but unsuccessful with present prostheses.

Osteochondritis dissecans and osteochondral fractures

A small fragment of talus may separate from the body as a loose fragment by a similar process to that seen at the knee (p. 326). Osteochondral fractures of the talus also occur (Fig. 25.2).

Treatment

If the loose bodies are painful or cause mechanical symptoms then they need to be removed, either arthroscopically or by arthrotomy.

Aseptic necrosis

Aseptic necrosis of the body of the talus may follow fractures through its neck (p. 276). The end result is a loss of height of the talus and a stiff ankle. Left untreated the ankle becomes progressively stiffer but usually becomes painless after a few years. Arthrodesis is not possible because the bone on the talar side of the ankle is dead. Prosthetic replace-

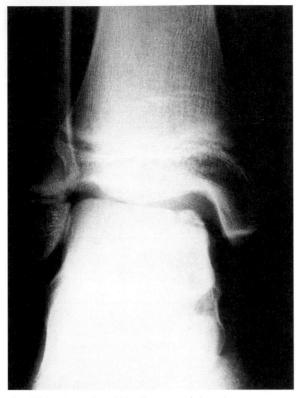

Fig. 25.2 Osteochondritis dissecans of the talus.

ment is not possible and the disability has to be accepted.

Treatment

There is no active treatment for this condition apart from analgesics and a firm boot to support the ankle.

Rheumatoid arthritis

The bone destruction of rheumatoid arthritis produces a foot and ankle that are unstable as well as painful. Because bone is lost, the ligaments no longer hold the bones in the correct position, the foot rolls into valgus at the subtalar joint and the forces at the ankle produce wear on the lateral side. This in turn leads to a valgus deformity.

Treatment

The unstable valgus ankle of rheumatoid is difficult to manage. Conservative treatment should always

be tried before operation. The following measures may help:

1. Ankle supports or surgical footwear to control the deformity, but these are often ineffective.
2. Arthrodesis, which is usually effective despite the poor bone texture.
3. Total ankle replacement, which is less reliable than joint replacement elsewhere.
4. Osteotomy to correct the alignment of the foot and ankle, but the deformity can recur.

Patients with rheumatoid arthritis of the ankle generally have other joints involved as well and the whole problem must be considered.

Ligamentous instability

Damage to the ligaments of the ankle from sprains may make the ankle liable to recurrent episodes of minor instability. The patient may complain that he or she keeps 'turning the ankle over' with trivial injury, but clinical and radiological examination are normal. Stress radiographs will demonstrate the opening of the joint and from this pattern the ligaments involved can be deduced.

The lateral collateral ligament, and in particular the anterior talar fibular ligament, is the most common site of injury but the anterior capsule can also be involved.

Treatment

The symptoms can often be relieved by exercises to improve the postural reflexes and strengthen the postural muscles around the ankle. If this is ineffective, operation may be needed to reinforce the lateral side of the ankle by rerouting the peroneus brevis tendon or by a free graft of plantaris. Direct suture methods and shortening of the lateral ligaments can give good results.

Tarsal tunnel syndrome

The medial plantar nerve enters the foot after passing beneath the medial ligament of the ankle, which it shares with the posterior tibial and flexor tendons. The anatomy is comparable with the carpal tunnel at the wrist and the medial plantar nerve is vulnerable to compression by swelling of the tendons or space-occupying lesions such as ganglia. The symptoms of 'tarsal tunnel syndrome' include pain and paraesthesia in the distribution of the medial plantar nerve.

431

This condition is extremely rare, but should be considered in patients with neurological symptoms in the hindfoot.

Treatment

Decompression of the tunnel is needed only if there is definite proof by electrical studies that the nerve is compressed within the tunnel.

Foot

Subtalar joint

The subtalar joint allows inversion and eversion. Damage to the talus or fractures of the calcaneum can restrict eversion and inversion and make it difficult or painful to walk over rough ground.

Injuries to the subtalar joint commonly result from a fracture of the calcaneum in a fall onto the heel, a common injury in building workers. Ironically, these are the very people who need a good subtalar joint to walk over rough ground.

Treatment

Injuries to the subtalar joint can take at least 2 years to reach their final state and any decision on operation should be deferred until this time has been reached. Until then, support to the ankle and subtalar joint with a firm boot to restrict inversion and eversion will produce some relief and may allow the patient to walk over rough ground.

If the joint is still painful after 2 years, subtalar fusion may be required. Like ankle arthrodesis, it may take 2 years to achieve the final result.

Midtarsal joint

The midtarsal joint lies between the calcaneum proximally and the cuboid and navicular bones distally and, with the tarsometatarsal joint, allows pronation and supination of the forefoot on the hindfoot. Because the subtalar, midtarsal and tarsometatarsal joints are so closely connected, damage to one can impair the function of the other two.

The joint can be damaged by trauma (p. 278), talipes equinovarus (p. 352) and other foot defor-

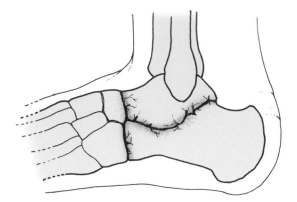

Fig. 25.3 Triple fusion. Three joints are fused – calcaneocuboid, talonavicular and subtalar.

mities. The result is painful restriction of movement in the foot, detectable on clinical examination (p. 31).

Treatment

Conservative treatment with a firm shoe or boot is often effective, but if pain or deformity cannot be controlled, a triple fusion may be required.

Triple fusion is an arthrodesis of all three joints (talonavicular, calcaneocuboid and subtalar) and converts the tarsus into a solid block of bone (Fig. 25.3). Ankle movement and midtarsal movements are not affected, but inversion and eversion are abolished. The operation is often used as the definitive treatment for the residual deformity of talipes when the patient has reached adult life.

Pantalar arthrodesis. If the triple fusion is accompanied by an ankle arthrodesis, the operation is known as a pantalar arthrodesis and may be required if the talus has been damaged by trauma or avascular necrosis.

Köhler's disease

Köhler's disease is a vascular osteochondritis which causes collapse of the navicular and is comparable with Perthes' disease at the hip and Kienböck's disease at the wrist. The joint becomes painful and the affected bone is tender. Radiographs show that the bone becomes dense, collapses and gradually reforms over a period of 2–3 years. The shape of the reformed bone is different from the original, but frequently produces an excellent functional result.

Treatment

No treatment is required.

Sever's disease

Sever's disease is a traction apophysitis at the insertion of the Achilles tendon comparable with Osgood–Schlatter's and Sinding Larsen's diseases at the knee. The condition occurs most often in boys about the age of 12 and causes pain and tenderness at the insertion of the Achilles tendon onto the calcaneum.

Treatment

The symptoms usually resolve within 12 months and no treatment is required apart from a slight raise to the heel of the shoe to take tension off the Achilles tendon.

Achilles tendinitis and paratenonitis

The paratenon around the Achilles tendon may be irritated by repeated friction. The condition is common in athletes.

Treatment

If rest, a raise to the heel and attention to athletic technique do not help, a steroid injection into the space between the tendon and paratenon – *but not into the tendon itself* – may be helpful.

In very resistant cases the paratenon will need to be freed from the tendon surgically.

Partial rupture of the Achilles tendon

The central fibres of the Achilles tendon sometimes rupture without breaking the continuity of the tendon. In such patients, the 'squeeze' test (p. 276) is negative and the tendon will have a tender, fusiform swelling in its midportion.

Treatment

The symptoms usually resolve over 12–18 months and a raise to the heel is helpful. If the symptoms persist after this time, the tendon may need to be explored. A cyst or softened area of tendon will often be found in the centre of the tendon corresponding to the site of the rupture of the original central fibres.

Flexor and peroneal tendonitis

The peroneal and flexor tendons have flexor sheaths and are sometimes affected by tenosynovitis where the tendons run round the corner from the calf into the foot, particularly if there has been trauma to the ankle or subtalar joints.

Treatment

Anti-inflammatory drugs and steroid injection into the tendon sheaths are usually effective.

Recurrent subluxation of the peroneal tendons

The peroneal tendons run in a shallow groove behind the lateral malleolus and may become unstable. If this occurs, the tendons will flick out of their groove and lie in front of the malleolus. The ankle feels unstable and the patient may stumble.

Treatment

Conservative treatment is rarely effective. If the symptoms warrant it the tendons should be stabilized by a bone block to deepen the groove in which they run.

Plantar fasciitis

Plantar fasciitis is a common and troublesome condition caused by a strain of the attachment of the plantar fascia to the calcaneum, and causes pain when the patient puts the foot to the ground when walking (Fig. 25.4).

Clinical examination will show a very tender spot at its calcaneal insertion and radiographs may show a spur of bone at the same site but no other abnormality (Fig. 25.5).

Treatment

A small heel raise and a pad worn in the shoe will usually relieve symptoms if the pad is firm and not too soft. Physiotherapy with stretching of the Achilles and the plantar fascia is the treatment of choice. Steroid injection is often advised, but is always painful and often ineffective. Excision of the heel

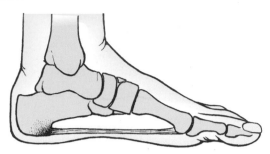

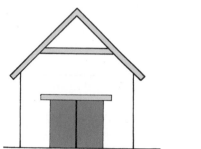

Fig. 25.4 Plantar fasciitis. The plantar fascia supports the medial arch of the foot like a tie-bar and its posterior attachment may be painful.

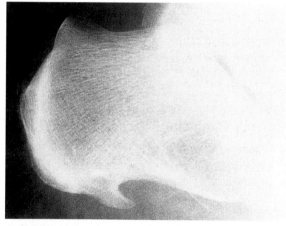

Fig. 25.5 A plantar spur.

spur seen on the radiographs is tempting but not generally successful. (Remember that 10% of the normal population have a spur visible on X-ray and of these, only 10% are symptomatic.)

'Heel bumps'

Heel bumps (Haglund's deformity) or exostoses occur just lateral to the Achilles tendon and cause

particular worry to teenagers, in whom they interfere with shoe wear.

The bumps appear about the age of 11 and usually stop hurting when growth is complete.

Treatment

If the bumps are particularly large and painful, they need to be excised, but this is a troublesome operation. The excision must include the underlying bony lump and the resulting scar and soft tissue swelling may be almost as troublesome as the original bump. Calcaneal osteotomy is an alternative.

Talonavicular bar

The talus, navicular and the other tarsal bones are occasionally linked by a bar of bone. These bars, which are congenital anomalies, prevent all subtalar movement and cause pain when the foot is twisted.

In some patients, the 'bar' is of fibrous tissue instead of bone and some movement is then possible, although still abnormal.

Treatment

The symptoms usually subside as growth proceeds and can be controlled by supportive footwear. In a very few cases, the bar will need to be excised.

Ganglia

The joints on the dorsum of the foot are superficial and, as on the back of the hand, ganglia can cause troublesome symptoms. Before making the diagnosis be sure that the swelling is not the muscle belly of the extensor hallucis brevis, which can look very like a ganglion, lipoma or a soft tissue tumour.

Treatment

Excision is only needed if the ganglion is persistent, tender and painful. As in the hand, the scar and postoperative swelling may be as much trouble as the original ganglion. Pain may last for 6 months after operation.

Dorsal exostosis

The dorsum of the foot is a common site for an exostosis, particularly at the junction of the

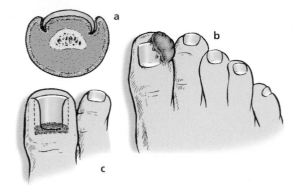

Fig. 25.6 Ingrowing toenail: (a) the nail curls into the pulp; (b) the surrounding tissues become swollen and inflamed, perhaps infected; (c) if conservative treatment is unsuccessful, the whole of the nail and nail-forming area must be removed.

navicular and cuneiform bones. The swelling interferes with shoe wear and a bursa may develop over it.

Treatment

If the swelling is troublesome then it should be excised.

Ingrowing toenail

Toenails are curved, not flat, and the edges can dig into the pulp of the toe (Fig. 25.6). The medial edge of the big toenail is most often affected and will dig into the pulp of the toe, causing soft tissue damage with every step. The damaged area can then become infected, producing a chronic infected granulomatous lesion along the medial side of the big toenail.

Treatment

Conservative treatment. This is usually effective and consists of three measures:

1. Regular cleaning.
2. Placing a small pledget of cotton wool beneath the edge of the nail (Fig. 25.7a).
3. Allowing the nail to grow beyond the end of the toe. Cutting it as short as possible leaves a spike which digs into the pulp even more, but letting the nail grow beyond the end of the toe takes the tip of the nail away from the vulnerable soft tissue.

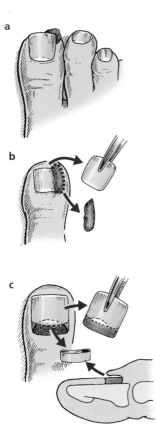

Fig. 25.7 Treatment of an ingrowing toenail: (a) protection of sharp corner with wisp of cotton wool; (b) avulsion of the toenail and excision of inflamed tissue; (c) Zadik's operation to remove the nail and nail-forming tissue.

Operative treatment. If conservative measures fail, one of the following operations may be needed:

1. Avulsion of the toenail.
2. Wedge excision.
3. Ablation of the nail and nail bed.

Avulsion of the nail exposes the infected area and relieves the pressure upon it. The infection will subside but the operation does not change the shape of the nail and the problem often recurs when the nail has regrown.

Wedge excision is more radical than avulsion. As well as avulsing the nail the infected and inflamed groove on the medial side of the toe is excised and the medial third of the nail bed removed (Fig. 25.7b). This prevents the medial third of the nail regrowing and allows the wound to heal. The resulting nail is narrower than normal.

Ablation of the nail and nail bed. If the problem recurs after wedge excision the nail and nail-forming

435

tissue should be removed. This operation, called Zadik's operation, leaves a fibrous scar in place of the toenail (Fig. 25.7c).

The operation is more difficult than it sounds because the fold from which the nail grows is shaped like an envelope and the corners must be meticulously excised. If this is not done a horn of nail will form at each corner of the nail bed and will need to be removed at a second operation. Recurrence can be minimized by applying phenol to the site of the nail-forming tissue. Phenol is also useful in preventing recurrence after segmental wedge excision.

Anaesthetic. If the toe is not infected, the operation can be performed under local anaesthetic using a ring block of plain lidocaine. Lidocaine with added adrenaline (epinephrine) should never be used on a digit because it causes arterial spasm, leading to ischaemia, and gangrene, leading to amputation. Apart from this, infiltration of local anaesthetic can spread the infection. If there is any sign of infection the operation should be performed under general anaesthetic.

Onychogryphosis

In the elderly, the big toenail can become so thickened and deformed that it resembles a talon (Fig. 25.8).

Treatment

Cutting such a nail is difficult because it is very hard and excision may be needed. In onychogryphosis,

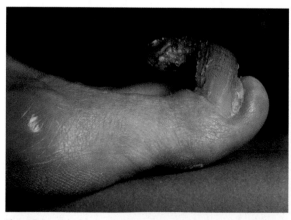

Fig. 25.8 Onychogryphosis.

the nail forms from the nail bed as well as the nail fold and the whole area must be removed.

Hallux rigidus

Hallux rigidus, which means 'stiff big toe', is the result of osteoarthritis confined to the first metatarsophalangeal joint (Fig. 25.9). The cause is not known but is probably some insult to the joint sustained in early life because patients in the second and third decades have the appearances of osteoarthritis appropriate to someone 50 years older. No other joints are affected and the patient's anxiety that this is the first sign of a widespread crippling arthritis can be allayed.

Clinical features

As the joint surfaces become worn, an osteophyte forms on the head of the first metatarsal and dorsiflexion is restricted. The toe gradually becomes more rigid and is eventually fixed in flexion. This has three consequences:

1. The patient can only walk comfortably in bare feet and women find that they cannot wear high heels.
2. The stride becomes shorter because extension of the toe at the end of the stride is lost.
3. The patient learns to avoid stressing the big toe by rolling the weight of the body around the outer edge of the foot instead of over the metatarsal heads. This abnormal gait can cause pain in the ankle and knee.

On examination, osteophytes can be felt around the first metatarsal head and the shoe will show excessive wear under the tip of the big toe.

Conservative treatment

Conservative treatment consists of wearing low-heeled shoes and a metatarsal bar fixed to the sole of the shoe so that it takes the strain off the first metatarsophalangeal joint. The metatarsal bar is uncomfortable to walk on and sometimes makes the patient trip. If these measures are unsuccessful, operation may be required.

Operative treatment

Excision of the osteophytes and osteotomy of the proximal phalanx is sometimes helpful but the symptoms recur with time.

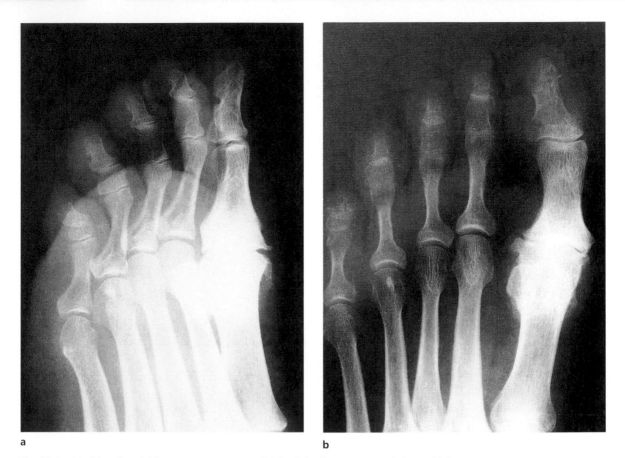

a b

Fig. 25.9 (a), (b) Hallux rigidus. Premature osteoarthritis of the first metatarsophalangeal joint.

Excision arthroplasty (Keller's operation) is sometimes effective, but the resulting pseudarthrosis may also stiffen (Fig. 25.10).

Arthrodesis is reliable, but the final position of the toe makes the choice of shoe wear difficult and the operation is usually suitable only for men. The toe should be fixed in slight dorsiflexion and adducted to permit normal walking and shoe wear.

Interposition arthroplasty with a Silastic spacer is often advised but, like any operation in which a foreign body is retained, can be followed by pain and inflammation.

Hallux valgus

The cause of hallux valgus (Fig. 25.11) is unknown and much nonsense is talked about the evils of pointed shoes and high heels. The condition tends to run in families and is seen in primitive tribes who walk barefoot. There is no evidence at all that shoe

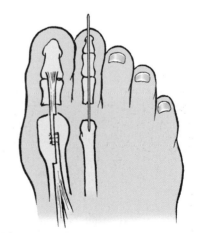

Fig. 25.10 Keller's operation for hallux valgus and correction of the second toe. The exostosis on the first metatarsal has been levelled, the base of the proximal phalanx excised and the tendon lengthened. The position of the second toe has been corrected with a longitudinal Kirschner wire.

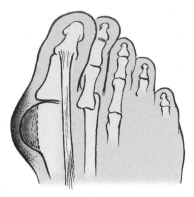

Fig. 25.11 Pathology of late hallux valgus. The big toe lies in valgus and the second toe may override it or lie beneath it. The second metatarsophalangeal joint dislocates. The extensor hallucis longus tendon acts as a bowstring accentuating the deformity. An inflamed bursa develops over an exostosis on the first metatarsal head.

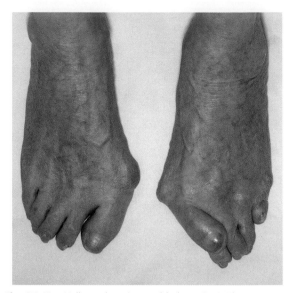

Fig. 25.12 Hallux valgus in an elderly patient. The great toe is overriding the second toe.

wear has any influence, either good or bad, on the development of hallux valgus, although bad shoes can probably aggravate the problem if it is already there.

Two main groups of patients are affected by hallux valgus. In the first group, which consists of adolescents and young adults, the condition is often familial and the primary pathology is a varus first metatarsal. The articular surfaces are intact in these patients.

The second group consists of elderly women, and occasionally men, with degenerative changes in the first metatarsophalangeal joint, and secondary deformities in the adjoining toes (Figs 25.12, 25.13). These two groups are very different and should be treated differently.

Conservative treatment

There is no conservative management which corrects the deformity. Sponge pads and splints may be comfortable, but they do not arrest the progress of the condition.

Surgical shoes are helpful in the old and infirm patient, for whom surgical correction is not appropriate, but these shoes are unacceptable to younger patients.

Operative treatment

Several operations are available (Fig. 25.14):

1. Metatarsal osteotomy.
2. Exostectomy.

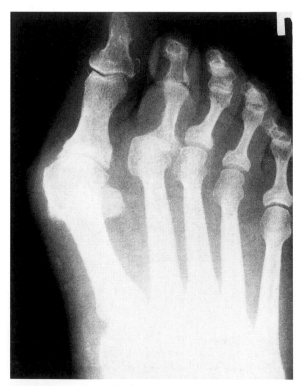

Fig. 25.13 Radiograph of a patient with hallux valgus and early osteoarthritis in the first metatarsophalangeal joint with dislocation of the second metatarsophalangeal joint.

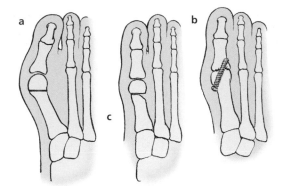

Fig. 25.14 (a) Metatarsal osteotomy for correction of metatarsus primus varus and hallux valgus in a young patient. (b) Arthrodesis of the first metatarsophalangeal joint.

3. Excision arthroplasty (Keller's operation).

4. Arthrodesis.

Metatarsal osteotomy is the most popular operation in younger patients and corrects the deformity by moving the whole toe and metatarsal head laterally. The head must also be moved slightly inferiorly to balance the load taken by the metatarsal heads. This procedure is indicated in young patients with intact joints.

Exostectomy. If the main complaint is the bony swelling over the metatarsal head, it is reasonable to excise it but the patient must be warned that the deformity is likely to progress.

Excision arthroplasty or Keller's operation (see Fig. 25.10) produces a toe that is slightly shorter and more 'floppy' than normal. Shortening the toe also has the disadvantage that it allows the sesamoids to slip backwards and leaves the metatarsal head unsupported, which in turn causes pain in the forefoot. The operation is useful for older patients with arthritic joints and secondary deformities.

Arthrodesis is sometimes recommended for hallux valgus but is most useful in men with secondary deformities of the other toes (Fig. 25.14b).

Choice of treatment. Management depends largely upon the age of the patient. Deformities in adolescence are usually the result of a varus first metatarsal, with the toe lying in valgus to compensate. At this age the condition is likely to progress rapidly; no conservative treatment is effective and metatarsal osteotomy is required.

In older patients the main problem is often an exostosis and bursa overlying the metatarsal head. This bump, with its bursa, is popularly called a

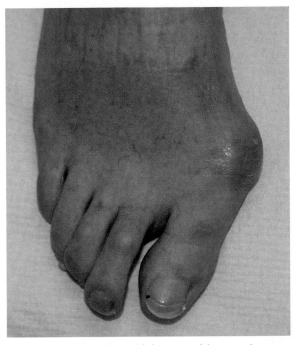

Fig. 25.15 Hallux valgus with bursa overlying prominent joint.

bunion and may become red, painful or infected (see below).

If there is a varus metatarsal the exostosis and the bursa should be excised and an osteotomy performed. If there is no varus metatarsal or if there is degenerate osteoarthritis as well as hallux valgus, an exostectomy and excision arthroplasty is better.

Bunions

Patients complain of 'bunions' but the word means different things to different people (Fig. 25.15). Strictly speaking, a bunion is a bursa over an unduly prominent first metatarsal head or an exostosis on the metatarsal.

The bursa can become infected and the infection can spread to the first metatarsophalangeal joint. In patients with diabetes this may lead to gangrene; in patients with rheumatoid arthritis the skin may be very slow to heal.

Treatment

A soft felt pad and comfortable shoes will solve the problem for many patients. If this fails, operation must be considered.

'Bunionectomy', to remove the bump and bursa, is a good operation if there is no hallux valgus. If hallux valgus is present, excision of the bunion alone is not enough and may actually make the deformity worse.

Secondary deformities

Lateral displacement of the other toes

A valgus hallux can push the other toes laterally, sometimes until the big toe lies transversely across the foot with the others resting on it.

Treatment

Although correction of all these deformities is possible, surgical shoes may be preferable to extensive corrective surgery in an elderly patient with a gross deformity.

Dislocated second toe

Subluxation of the second metatarsophalangeal joint with flexion at the proximal interphalangeal (p.i.p.) joint is a common deformity. In some patients, the toe dislocates with the p.i.p. joint fixed in flexion and the proximal phalanx lying on the dorsum of the second metatarsal (see Fig. 25.11).

Treatment

Conservative treatment is not effective, but the toe can be brought into good position by excising the base of the phalanx and arthrodesing the p.i.p. joint.

As for Keller's operation, the position of the toes can be held with a longitudinal wire.

Subungual exostosis

A small exostosis on the dorsum of the distal phalanx can cause severe pain. The lesion is benign (Fig. 25.16).

Treatment

Excison of the exostosis is the only effective remedy.

Hammer toe

Hammer toe has been described on page 359. Deformities secondary to hallux valgus will recur unless

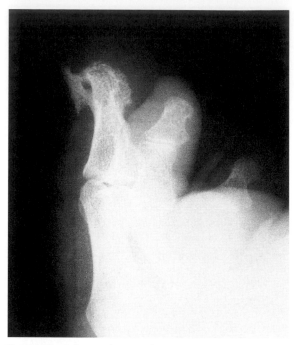

Fig. 25.16 Subungual exostosis.

the hallux valgus is corrected. An untreated hammer toe develops a bursa over the p.i.p. joint and a corn beneath the second metatarsal head.

Treatment

Arthrodesis of the p.i.p. joint will correct the deformity but only if the metatarsophalangeal joint is normal. If this joint is dislocated, as it often is, the base of the phalanx should be excised as well.

Mallet toe

Mallet toe (see Fig. 21.21) is a congenital abnormality of the distal interphalangeal (d.i.p.) joint, and is usually familial. The toe interferes with shoe wear and the terminal phalanx may develop blisters.

Treatment

Unless there are troublesome symptoms from the toe, the deformity should be left alone, but arthrodesis or amputation of the terminal phalanx may be needed if there is excessive pressure on the tip of the toe. Conservative treatment is not effective.

Metatarsalgia

Pain in the forefoot, or metatarsalgia, can be due to many things. A prominent metatarsal head is a common cause of pain and can follow any operation on the forefoot, including Keller's operation (p. 437) or dislocation of the second toe.

Treatment

If soft insoles are not effective, pain from prominent metatarsals may be relieved by a metatarsal osteotomy, which allows the metatarsal head to ride up to a better position and to take a more natural proportion of body weight.

Morton's metatarsalgia

The medial and lateral plantar nerves join in the sole between the third and fourth metatarsal heads (Fig. 25.17). At this point the nerve is subjected to particular pressure and this can produce interneuronal fibrosis within the nerve. A nerve so affected is thickened and the thickening is called a Morton's neuroma.

Patients with a Morton's neuroma characteristically complain of a feeling something 'like a stone in the shoe', often accompanied by tingling in the adjacent sides of the third and fourth toes.

On clinical examination the web space between the third and fourth toes is tender, there may be diminished sensibility of the toes, and sideways compression of the foot will produce a painful click. Similar signs and symptoms result from a ganglion in the web space.

Treatment

A small insole to support the metatarsal shaft is sometimes effective but if the symptoms persist despite this and cause genuine disability then the neuroma must be excised.

Freiberg's disease

The head of the metatarsals may be affected during adolescence by Freiberg's disease, a vascular osteochondritis similar to Perthes' disease (Fig. 25.18). The second and third metatarsals are most often involved.

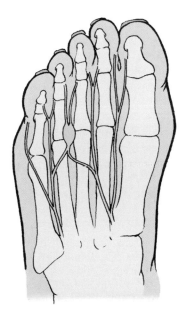

Fig. 25.17 Morton's metatarsalgia.

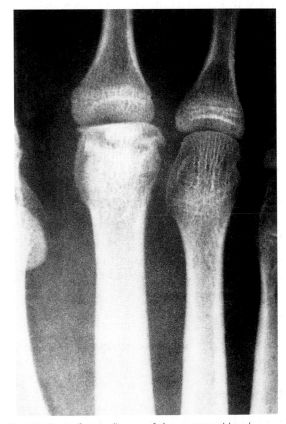

Fig. 25.18 Freiberg's disease of the metatarsal head.

Treatment

Often, no specific treatment is required.

Rheumatoid arthritis

Rheumatoid arthritis attacks small joints and the foot is therefore vulnerable. The changes in the foot are similar to those in the hand, with the added complication that the patient must walk on the painful joints.

Involvement of the metatarsophalangeal joints is a special problem. As the tissues become weaker the phalanges move dorsally, bone is destroyed and the transverse pad of soft weight-bearing tissue which normally lies under the metatarsal heads comes to lie underneath the toes instead (Figs 25.19, 25.20).

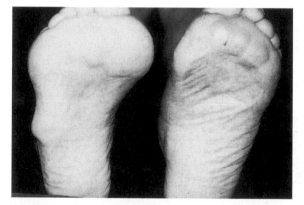

Fig. 25.19 Rheumatoid arthritis of the feet. Note the prominent metatarsal heads and the rheumatoid nodule.

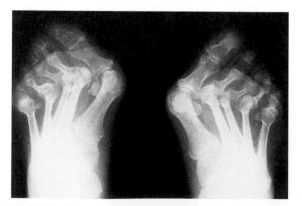

Fig. 25.20 Rheumatoid arthritis of the forefoot with destruction and dislocation of the metatarsophalangeal joints.

The metatarsal heads are then separated from the ground only by atrophic tendons and thin skin. The bones can erode the skin, leading to infection and further bone destruction.

Treatment

Conservative treatment consisting of soft moulded footwear and careful attention to the skin is very important. Prominent exostoses and metatarsal heads cause skin lesions which quickly extend down to bone, particularly if the patient is receiving steroids.

If conservative measures are ineffective a forefoot arthroplasty must be performed to remove all the metatarsal heads and bring the soft pad of weight-bearing skin back under the metatarsal heads. This is a reliable operation giving good long-term results.

Fatigue fractures

The causes and treatment of fatigue fractures have been mentioned on page 100.

Gout

Gout is described on page 305. Traditionally, the first metatarsophalangeal joint is affected but in fact the other joints are affected just as often.

Flat foot (pes planovalgus)

Generalized ligamentous laxity affects the joints of the foot as well as the rest of the body and the arches of patients with this condition flatten when the foot is weight bearing. Children with flat feet that return to normal when standing on tiptoe or lying on the examination couch are described on page 353.

Painful flat feet are a cause of pain in older patients with degenerative osteoarthritis of the subtalar and midtarsal joints. This is often due to a ruptured tibialis posterior tendon.

Although pes planovalgus does cause pain on walking, corns, verrucae and prominent metatarsal heads are more common causes of pain in the forefoot.

Treatment

Apart from comfortable shoes and a support to the medial arch of the foot, no conservative treatment is effective. If the symptoms are disabling, which is very rare, a triple fusion (p. 353) or calcaneal oste-otomy to correct the position of the foot may be required, but most patients manage perfectly well despite their deformed foot. Reconstruction of a ruptured tendon may not be successful and tendon transfers are often needed to restore the arch. In the older patient, a specially made 'surgical' shoe may be required.

Fallen arches

Fallen or dropped arches are part of medical folk-lore. The term is widely used to mean feet that are painful on walking even though the transverse arch probably does not exist and the only arch of any importance is the medial.

Pes cavus

A high arched foot can be due to a congenital bony abnormality but can also be caused by neurological conditions, particularly spasticity of the flexor muscle groups.

Treatment

Provided that there is no underlying neurological abnormality and the foot provides good service, a comfortable shoe is the only treatment required. If the foot is painful or unsatisfactory for any other reason, a corrective osteotomy or soft tissue release may be needed to make the foot plantigrade.

Neurological disorders

One of the pitfalls of orthopaedic surgery is the serious but unusual condition which masquerades as a common problem.

Patients with Friedreich's ataxia, peroneal muscu-lar atrophy and muscular dystrophy may all present to the orthopaedic surgeon with a foot deformity. Wasting of the calf and peroneal muscles should alert the surgeon to the possibility of a neurological condition being present.

Spina bifida occulta and diastematomyelia both cause tethering of the spinal cord and stretching of the nerve roots with growth. Deformity of the feet is often the first clinical sign. Both conditions are usually accompanied by sensory symptoms and this, with the rapid onset, provides a clue to the diagnosis. Beware of feet that develop a deformity after being normal, and deformed feet with sensory symptoms.

Toe-walkers

Children who persistently walk on tiptoe are described on page 350.

Other causes of foot pain

Do not forget that there are many other causes of painful feet that do not reach a doctor. Chiropodists and podiatrists do an excellent job and probably treat more foot conditions than doctors.

Chapter |26|

Disorders of the spine

By the end of this chapter you should be able to:

- Differentiate between mechanical back pain and those patients with a neurological defect.
- Discuss the indications for spinal operations and also be well aware of the risks.
- Investigate the patient with a painful back by taking the history, doing a clinical examination and ordering the appropriate radiology.
- Make a differential diagnosis of a prolapsed disc.
- Remember the cauda equina lesions and resolve never to miss these!
- Be aware of the congenital growth abnormalities and how these present.

Cervical spine

Acute disc prolapse

The cervical spine is very flexible and the intervertebral discs are subjected to considerable strains. The cervical roots cross the discs as they leave the spinal canal, where they are vulnerable to pressure from disc protrusion (Fig. 26.1). Disc protrusions in the neck are usually more lateral than those in the lumbar spine and affect one level only.

As in the lumbar spine, disc protrusions are accompanied by pain, altered sensibility and weakness. The four lowest roots are most often affected and are accompanied by pain and sensory symptoms in the radial side of the forearm and hand, with weakness of grip (C8) and elbow flexion (C5–6).

Movement of the cervical spine is also restricted, particularly flexion and rotation on the affected side.

Treatment

Conservative treatment. Analgesics, rest, a collar and traction will usually produce a remission of symptoms but the pain may be so severe and intractable that disc excision is required as an urgent procedure.

Operative treatment. Disc excision may relieve pain and improve neurological function but it makes the cervical spine more unstable than the corresponding operation on the lumbar spine and the root can still be irritated even when the disc has been excised. To avoid this, operation is sometimes accompanied by a cervical fusion in which a block of bone is inserted

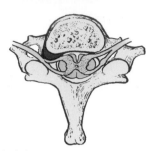

Fig. 26.1 Cervical disc protrusion compressing a cervical root.

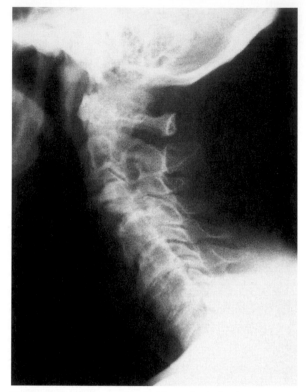

Fig. 26.2 Cervical spondylosis. The patient also has congenital fusion of C2 and C3.

between the adjacent vertebral bodies. The role of cervical fusion, which puts greater strain on the intact discs, is controversial.

Cervical spondylosis

Cervical and lumbar spondylosis are almost universal in patients over the age of 40 but seldom cause symptoms.

Spondylosis is different from osteoarthritis because it occurs around intervertebral discs instead of in synovial joints (Fig. 26.2). The posterior facet joints are synovial joints and may develop osteoarthritis but the cartilage joints between the vertebrae cannot do so because they have no joint space. For practical purposes, however, the two conditions can be considered together and treated as degenerative joint disease.

Patients with cervical spondylosis feel a dull pain in the neck radiating across the shoulders and down the upper part of the arm, worse on movement. The pain can be confused with supraspinatus tendinitis and other shoulder disorders.

Treatment

The standard treatment consists of heat, rest, anti-inflammatory drugs, analgesics and a supporting collar. When the symptoms have subsided, mobilizing exercises to restore movement are important but it must be said that no properly conducted scientific study has ever shown that these exercises influence the natural history of the disease. Voltaire may have been right when he commented that 'The efficient physician is the man who successfully amuses his patients while Nature effects a cure'.

Operation is seldom required for spondylosis but may be necessary if there is severe pain arising from a single identifiable level (Fig. 26.3).

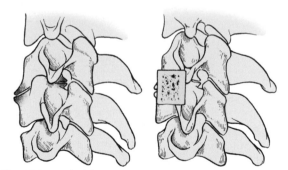

Fig. 26.3 Cervical fusion. A bone block prevents movement and holds the affected vertebrae apart.

Rheumatoid arthritis

Rheumatoid arthritis, which is so destructive to the small joints of the hands and feet, also affects the cervical spine (Fig. 26.4). The atlantoaxial joint is especially at risk because of the complex synovial folds around the transverse ligament of the atlas. If this ligament stretches, the atlas and head can slip forwards and the odontoid process

446

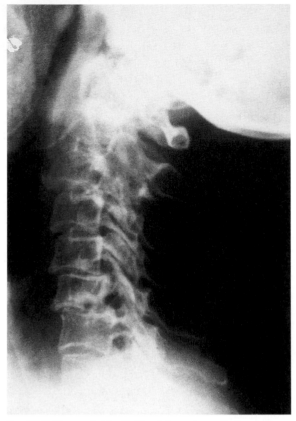

Fig. 26.4 Rheumatoid arthritis of the spine with forward displacement at several levels.

presses against the cervical cord, producing quadriparesis.

This is especially important to anaesthetists. The mouth will not open easily if the temporomandibular joint is affected. If the neck is also stiff, endotracheal intubation is difficult and the manipulation of the neck needed to intubate the patient is hazardous. Accordingly, *patients with rheumatoid arthritis must always have the cervical spine examined radiologically before undergoing anaesthesia.* All staff, particularly those in the recovery room, should be aware of the potential hazards of flexing a rheumatoid neck.

Treatment

A supporting collar is usually sufficient but atlantoaxial fusion may be needed if there is a neurological deficit or unremitting pain.

Acute torticollis

Severe and acute neck pain can be due to many things, including acute disc prolapse, muscle spasm, injury to an osteoarthritic facet joint, inflamed lymph nodes or an undiagnosed cervical dislocation.

Treatment

Treatment depends upon the cause. Most acute stiff necks settle with a collar, warmth and analgesia but serious injuries must be excluded first.

Cervical rib

A vestigial 'rib' of bone or fibrous tissue can run from C7 to the first true rib. When such a rib is present the lowest part of the brachial plexus runs across it and neurological symptoms in the arm may result. Pain down the inner side of the arm in the T1 distribution should raise suspicions of a cervical rib.

Treatment

Excision may be necessary if radiographs demonstrate a complete or incomplete cervical rib; conservative treatment with physiotherapy to improve the power of the shoulder girdle muscles has been ineffective. The operation is straightforward but the root of the neck is 'tiger country' and the operation must only be done by a surgeon who is very familiar with this area.

Congenital short neck (Klippel–Feil syndrome)

Klippel–Feil syndrome consists of a very short neck with fusion of two or more cervical vertebrae and restricted cervical movement (Fig. 26.5). The condition may be familial and is sometimes associated with scoliosis. Richard III ('Deform'd, unfinish'd, sent before my time into this breathing world, scarce half made up') may have had Klippel–Feil syndrome.

Treatment

No specific treatment is required but the scoliosis may need correcting.

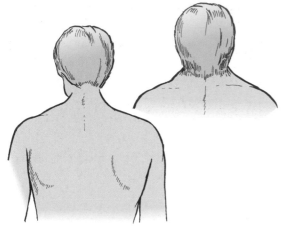

Fig. 26.5 Klippel–Feil syndrome. A short webbed neck with low hairline.

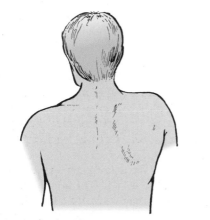

Fig. 26.6 Sprengel's shoulder. A high fixed scapula.

Congenital high scapula (Sprengel's shoulder)

Sprengel's shoulder is a congenital deformity in which the scapula is small and abnormally high (Fig. 26.6). The condition may be bilateral. No cause is known except that there is a failure of development of the shoulder and the muscles attached to it and it is often associated with congenital spinal anomalies.

Treatment

Some improvement in position follows release of the muscles along its upper border if carried out at an early age.

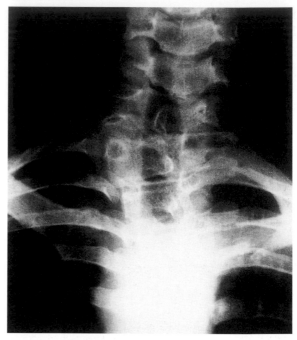

Fig. 26.7 Congenital hemivertebra. There is an extra vertebra and rib on the right side.

Congenital hemivertebra

Congenital hemivertebra (Fig. 26.7) and other anomalies also occur and may be associated with neurological abnormalities.

Neuralgic amyotrophy

Neuralgic amyotrophy is an odd condition which is probably due to a patchy demyelination of the brachial plexus. The symptoms may follow vaccination. Like meralgia paraesthetica, this condition is important because it has neurological features that may be confused with a spinal disorder.

Characteristic features are:

1. Sudden severe pain down the arm, similar to that of a disc protrusion.
2. Paralysis of parts of the shoulder girdle as the pain eases. The nerve to serratus anterior is said to be involved most frequently, producing a true winged scapula.
3. Muscle wasting is seen in the affected area.

Treatment

The pain usually resolves without treatment over a period of weeks, but the weakness may take up to 2 years to recover. Apart from reassurance and excluding other disorders, no treatment is required.

Acute stiff neck

Not all pain in the neck is due to a disc protrusion or cervical spondylosis. An acute stiff neck, perhaps due to a small muscle tear or a derangement of the facet joints, can occur for no apparent reason.

Treatment

The symptoms usually resolve spontaneously over a period of days or weeks. A supporting collar eases the pain and manipulation is sometimes helpful.

Torticollis in children

See page 363.

Lumbar spine

Back pain

In any one year, more working hours are lost from back pain than from any other medical condition. Back problems therefore take up much of the medical profession's time. As many as 25% of referrals to some orthopaedic clinics are for back pain.

It is a bad principle to operate on a painful back unless a definite mechanical cause has been identified. In the past, painful backs were operated upon far too often and the results were poor. Many patients were no better and some were made worse by operation. Spinal surgery, particularly spinal fusion, earned a bad name, richly deserved because operation was often followed by severe pain and stiffness which disabled the patient more than the original condition.

Back pain alone is not an orthopaedic problem. It is best managed conservatively by departments of physical medicine and rheumatology, and to refer every patient with back pain to an orthopaedic surgeon is a little like referring every patient with headache to a dentist. Unfortunately, patients with backache are frequently referred to orthopaedic clinics for historical reasons.

Spinal surgery, however, is definitely an orthopaedic problem and many surgeons with a specialist interest in the spine also treat the painful spine. The spine should only undergo operation for anatomical

lesions proven beyond doubt, which limits the common indications to the following conditions:

Indications for spinal operations

- Disc excision for proven disc protrusions with neurological signs.
- Instability caused by spondylolisthesis or unstable discs.
- Scoliosis, kyphosis and other spinal deformities.
- Some tumours and infections.

Note: Backache is not included!

Acute back strain

Acute pain in the back radiating down to the knee but not beyond and without neurological abnormality is usually due to an acute muscle or ligament strain in the lumbar spine. The symptoms can be precipitated by a sudden violent movement or by a comparatively trivial movement following a period of hard work when the muscles are stiff.

Tall slim people with willowy backs and weak muscles are said to be especially prone to acute back strains, as are those in sedentary occupations, such as medicine, who live a life of ease during the week and punish themselves at the weekend with excessive gardening.

Those who sit for a long time and then have to lift heavy weights without an adequate 'warm-up', e.g. carriers who may drive for more than an hour with the spine flexed in a bumpy vehicle and then leap out of their seat to lift a heavy weight from the back of the van, are also very vulnerable.

The sacroiliac joints are also said to be subject to acute strains, but without conclusive proof. The joints have a large surface area, they have poor mechanical cohesion and violent twisting strains can cause severe pain around them.

Prevention

The 'strain' is usually the result of incorrect lifting and most can be avoided. Workers who have to lift heavy weights, including nurses who lift patients, should be taught correct lifting techniques (Fig. 26.8). Four principles are important:

Correct lifting technique

1. Do not lift with the spine flexed; in this position, the weight is hanging on taut ligaments and

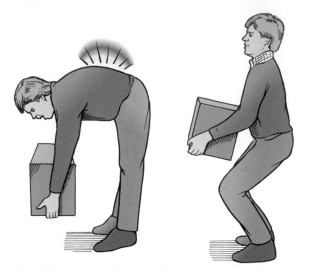

Fig. 26.8 Incorrect and correct lifting. Keep the weight close to the body and the back straight. Lift with the knees.

stretched muscles, which makes them vulnerable to additional load. Instead, lift with the lumbar spine extended.

2. Keep the weight to be lifted as near to the body as possible. The further the weight is from the body, the more effort that has to be expended in lifting it.

3. Lift with the knees, not the back muscles.

4. Make the job as easy as possible. Ensure that there is good access to the load, if possible split it into lighter loads but, if it cannot be split, share the job with two or more people.

In the workplace, lifting can be made easier by storing goods at waist height and avoiding the need for a twisting motion while lifting or carrying or by using lifting equipment and conveyor belts.

Treatment

The following measures form the standard treatment for acute back injuries and are reliable; rest, analgesics and gradual mobilization are the most important:

1. Rest.
2. Analgesics.
3. Heat.
4. Gradual mobilization.
5. Lumbosacral brace.
6. Manipulation.

Rest. The patient should rest in the most comfortable position possible, which is usually on the back or side with the knees flexed. If lying in bed is painful it is perfectly acceptable to rest in a comfortable chair.

Analgesics. Any analgesic or NSAID can be used. Narcotics such as pethidine should not be needed.

Heat, either from a hot water bottle or a heat pad, is very comforting for pains arising from muscles and ligaments and the diagnosis should be reconsidered if heat does not help. The mechanism of relief is obscure, but is probably nothing more than old-fashioned counterirritation. Even if unscientific, patients find warmth helpful.

Gradual mobilization. As the pain subsides, gradual mobilization can be started, but the patient must be prevented from lifting weights and risking further injury for at least 6 weeks. This may be difficult if the patient is a hardworking self-employed worker who needs to get back to work to earn a living. It is nevertheless essential if recurrent strains are to be avoided.

Mobilization of the spine is important. If a full range of spinal movement can be achieved, it is likely that the muscle or ligament has healed and the presence of a full range of movement ensures that loads can be borne equally throughout the spine.

If movement is limited, further injury is probable. The stiff areas of the spine are more likely to be injured by sudden stress and the mobile areas will be taking more strain than normal. A good range of movement should therefore be achieved before the patient returns to work, and the range of movement maintained by an exercise routine.

Lumbosacral brace. If the patient insists on returning to work before full movement has returned, a lumbosacral support will lessen the risk of recurrence. A brace will support the back when the patient is lifting and, perhaps more important, will 'remind' patients of their condition so that they lift correctly.

Spinal supports should be worn only for pain relief or to protect the back when it is at greatest risk. If they are worn permanently the spine will become stiff, the muscles will take less strain, and further injury becomes more likely.

Manipulation. Manipulating an acutely painful back is occasionally harmful if there is some underlying undiagnosed pathology but is sometimes dramatically successful, particularly if the sacroiliac joint is affected. Manipulation is a skill which takes much training and should not be attempted by the inexperienced. Both osteopaths and chiropractors are skilled manipulators.

Differential diagnosis

There are two serious conditions that can masquerade as an acute back strain:

1. A lumbar disc protrusion. This can be easily distinguished from a back strain because the pain extends below the knee and is accompanied by neurological symptoms such as numbness, weakness or altered sensibility below the knee (p. 16). Always check sensibility, power and reflexes distal to the knee.

2. Spinal tumours, particularly metastases. Radiographs are essential to exclude tumours in the vertebrae if there is any doubt.

Recurrent back strains

Patients suffering recurrent back strains should seek the help of a rheumatologist or specialist in rehabilitation rather than an orthopaedic surgeon.

Treatment

Operations have no place in the management of recurrent back strain. All the measures described for the management of acute back strains should be used, with special attention to prevention. Spinal fusion will make matters worse unless the disc is also unstable.

Prolapsed intervertebral disc

Anatomy

The discs are not solid lumps of inert gristle resembling rubber pads, as patients often think, but living structures which flatten slightly during the day and re-expand at night. They consist of a firm nucleus pulposus surrounded by the annulus fibrosus, a ring of fibrocartilage and fibrous tissue which links the two vertebrae together. The disc is a symphysis between each pair of vertebrae and, with the two posterior facet joints, allows movement between the vertebrae.

The tension within the disc is maintained by fluid imbibition at the cellular level. If imbibition fails for any reason, the pressure within the disc falls, the disc collapses, increased movement occurs between the adjacent vertebrae, the annulus fibrosus is exposed to increased stress and this is accompanied

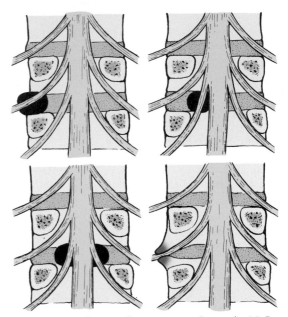

Fig. 26.9 Disc prolapse and root compression at the L4–5 junction. A laterally placed prolapse may compress the L4 root, a more central prolapse will compress L5 and a central prolapse the cauda equina. Osteophytes in the lateral canal will also produce root compression.

by vague low back pain. CT scans can demonstrate the lesion, and injection of saline or contrast medium may reproduce the back pain.

As degeneration proceeds, the annulus fibrosus softens and the degenerate disc bulges the annular ligament backwards, usually just lateral to the midline (Fig. 26.9). If this occurs in a tight spinal canal opposite a nerve root, the function of the root is affected.

Ninety per cent of lumbar disc protrusions involve the lowest two spaces, L4–5 or L5–S1. Lesions which press on the L5 root cause altered sensibility on the outer side of the calf and weakness of the peronei and ankle extensors, while those affecting the S1 root produce altered sensibility on the foot or back of the calf, weak ankle flexors and a depressed ankle jerk. The resting muscle tone of the glutei, hamstrings, calf muscles and other posterior muscle groups may also be reduced and these muscles may waste.

Clinical features

Unless there are neurological symptoms and signs below the knee, the patient probably does not have a true prolapsed intervertebral disc. Disc lesions seldom cause severe back pain and it is quite wrong to use the term as a synonym for acute back strain.

If the disc presses on a nerve root, the postural reflexes diminish pressure on the root by holding the spine curved to produce a 'sciatic scoliosis'.

Straight leg raising, which stretches the nerve, is restricted by pain. Other tests which stretch the nerve are also positive (p. 17).

Be wary of patients with no straight leg raising; the nerve root is not stretched until the leg is lifted 30°, and pain before this level is reached is more likely to be caused by apprehension, hysteria, malingering, or one of the conditions listed below. Beware also of the patient who can lean forward and touch the toes on the couch yet has restricted straight leg raising. These features are not compatible with a simple organic disorder.

Investigations

It is helpful to know the exact site of the lesion if operation is planned. MRI (Fig. 26.10) is the mainstay of treatment, but radiculography (Fig. 26.11) or CT (Fig. 26.12) can be used.

Differential diagnosis

Any condition that causes root irritation or pain in the leg can be mistaken for a disc prolapse, including the following conditions:

> ### Differential diagnosis of prolapsed discs
> (Fig. 26.13)
>
> 1. Tumours within the spinal canal.
> 2. Neurofibromas in the root canal.
> 3. Ependymoma and other tumours.
> 4. Intracranial tumour.
> 5. Ankylosing spondylitis.
> 6. Intrapelvic mass.
> 7. Osteoarthritis of the hip.
> 8. Spondylosis.
> 9. Malingering.
> 10. Vertebral tumours.
> 11. Tuberculosis.
> 12. Infective discitis.
> 13. Intermittent claudication.

Treatment

Left untreated, the symptoms disappear spontaneously even if the protrusion remains. In other patients, the annulus fibrosis will rupture and disc material will be extruded into the spinal canal. This may make the symptoms either dramatically better or dramatically worse.

In patients over the age of 40 a plain radiograph should always be obtained and routine investiga-

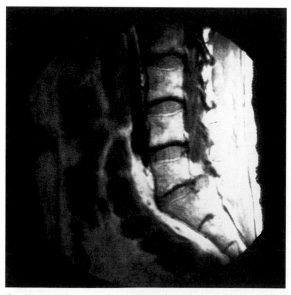

Fig. 26.10 MRI scan of a prolapsed intervertebral disc at L5–S1. By kind permission of the MRIS Unit, Addenbrooke's Hospital, Cambridge.

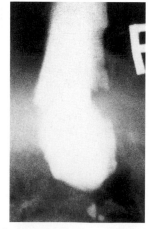

Fig. 26.11 Radiculogram showing a disc prolapse on the right side.

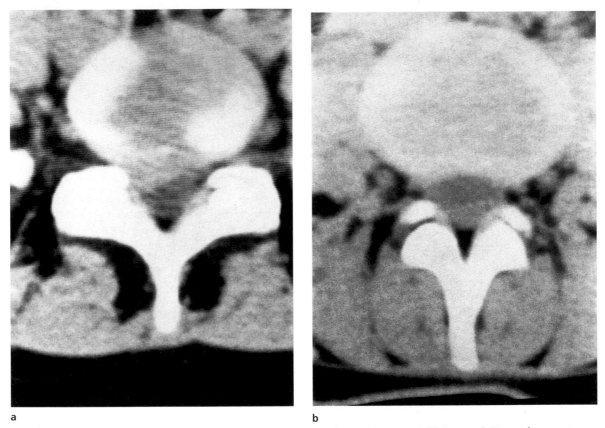

a   b

Fig. 26.12 (a) CT scan showing prolapsed disc material compressing the spinal contents. (b) A normal CT scan for comparison.

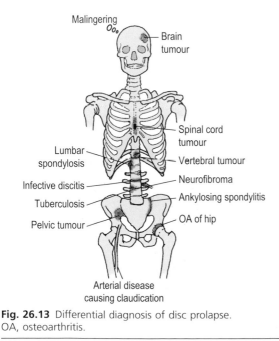

Fig. 26.13 Differential diagnosis of disc prolapse. OA, osteoarthritis.

tions carried out to exclude a spinal tumour and systemic disease before any treatment is started. The incidence of positive findings in patients between the ages of 20 and 40 is so low that some radiologists believe a preliminary radiograph is unnecessary until conservative treatment has failed, but most cautious doctors will wish to see a radiograph at some stage.

Conservative treatment. Because some natural recovery is likely, it is wrong to operate without a fair trial of conservative treatment unless there is a cauda equina lesion (p. 455). Treatment consists of two main measures:

1. Rest, analgesics and muscle relaxants.

2. Traction.

Rest. The patient should stay in bed in the most comfortable position with adequate analgesia and, if necessary, muscle relaxants such as diazepam 5 mg twice daily. Bed rest should be total, in hospital if possible. Total bed rest at home is a formidable undertaking that places a great strain on the family.

Most patients defy instructions and get up for meals and toilet purposes.

Traction helps to keep the patient in bed and some say that is all it does. It may also relieve muscle spasm and pain but it does not 'replace the disc'.

'Putting the disc back'. Manipulation of spines with acute disc prolapse is very dangerous. While osteopathic and chiropractic manipulations are excellent for chronic back problems, manipulation in the presence of neurological symptoms and signs can rupture the annulus fibrosus, extrude disc material and cause severe neurological damage. The concept of 'putting the disc back' by manipulation, as if it were a piece of jigsaw, is firmly rooted in the public mind and is quite wrong; a prolapsed disc is not a firm, rounded lump of gristle shaped like a 'Smartie', but looks more like a piece of soggy string (Fig. 26.14). Discs do not pop in and out like the cuckoo on a cuckoo clock (Fig. 26.15).

At operation, the disc will usually extrude itself from the disc space under pressure when the annulus fibrosus is excised, and to imagine that these discs can be replaced by manipulation is a fallacy.

Operative treatment. There are four indications for considering operation on prolapsed discs:

1. No improvement in the symptoms and signs after 6 weeks of rest.
2. An increase in the neurological deficit.
3. Bladder or bowel involvement suggesting a cauda equina lesion.
4. Intractable pain.

If operation is considered, a CT or MRI scan is needed to demonstrate spinal nerve roots and identify the disc protrusion. If the site of the disc protrusion matches the clinical signs, the disc can either be softened by chymopapain injection or excised surgically.

Chymopapain injection (chemonucleolysis). Injection with chymopapain, a proteolytic enzyme found in pawpaws and used commercially as a meat tenderizer, is suitable for discs that are also ideal for surgical excision. It is not helpful for patients with chronic disc lesions and no neurological signs. If the indications are correct, chymopapain injection is effective in about 70% of patients and in some centres has replaced surgical excision of the disc.

The injection must be done under image intensifier control on an inpatient basis and is accompanied by quite severe back pain. There is also a small incidence of anaphylactic reaction. Chymopapain injection is successful in the short term but there is some evidence that the long-term results are less

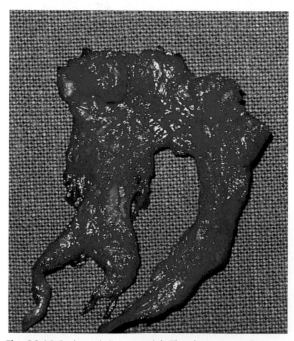

Fig. 26.14 Prolapsed disc material. The degenerate disc material is soft and soggy.

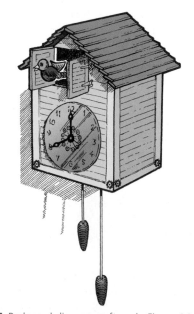

Fig. 26.15 Prolapsed discs are soft, as in Figure 26.14. They do not pop in and out of place like a cuckoo in a clock.

satisfactory than surgical treatment; however, the morbidity is still less than that of disc excision.

Disc excision is done either by neurosurgeons or by orthopaedic surgeons. The disc is approached from behind after excising the ligamentum flavum and, if necessary, the inferior portion of the lamina overlying the root. This procedure is called fenestration (from the Latin *fenestra*, a window). All disc material should be removed, including any that has sequestrated into the spinal canal.

Disc excision relieves neurological symptoms in about 75% of patients, provided that it is done in the right patients and for the right indications; i.e. neurological symptoms that match the neurological signs and a radiologically proven disc protrusion. The physical signs of muscle weakness and loss of reflexes do not always return to normal after laminectomy and disc excision.

The operation disturbs the 'triple joint' between neighbouring vertebrae and their facet joints. Without a complete disc, the bodies move towards each other and put unnatural stresses upon the posterior facet joints, which then degenerate. This is an unavoidable problem and some degree of stiffness and back pain can be expected in 30–60% of patients after a disc prolapse, whether it is treated conservatively, surgically or by chemonucleolysis with chymopapain.

Microdiscectomy. Discs can be excised through small skin incisions or under endoscopic control. The technique is new and difficult but the results are encouraging. The recovery period is shorter and surgical trauma is minimized.

Cauda equina lesions

A very small proportion of discs rupture in the midline of the annulus fibrosus instead of in the lateral recesses and produce a cauda equina lesion with the following clinical features:

- Painless retention of urine.
- Perianal anaesthesia.
- Bilateral sciatica.

If these signs are present, there is no place for conservative management and the disc must be removed surgically as an emergency. Failure to do this can result in a disabling and permanent cauda equina lesion.

High lumbar discs

Disc protrusions at levels above L4 are uncommon and produce unusual physical signs. Any patient with back pain and a neurological deficit higher than L5 should be investigated by a neurologist in case a spinal tumour is present.

Treatment

The treatment and indications for operation are the same as those for protrusions at lower levels, although excision is needed more often because the canal is relatively narrow in the upper part of the lumbar spine.

Ankylosing spondylitis

Ankylosing spondylitis is an inflammatory disease of joints which involves the sacroiliac and spinal joints before others. The HLAb27 gene is commonly found. The disease is commonest in young men and should be considered in any man between 15 and 30 years of age with the following features:

- Diffuse low back pain or pain in a root distribution without neurological signs.
- Stiffness of the back worst in the morning.
- Chest expansion less than 5 cm.
- Raised ESR.
- Erosions of the sacroiliac joints.
- A rapid response to anti-inflammatory drugs.
- A family history of ankylosing spondylitis.
- Painless effusions in a large joint.

Treatment

Untreated, the whole of the spine from coccyx to occiput can become a single rigid bar and it is important to maintain motion. Ankylosing spondylitis is best managed by a rheumatologist. Treatment of the acute attack is similar to rheumatoid arthritis, with rest and anti-inflammatory drugs followed by mobilization. In the longer term, regular physiotherapy to maintain motion is essential.

Lumbar spondylosis

Lumbar spondylosis is present to some extent in everybody over the age of 40. Few have symptoms

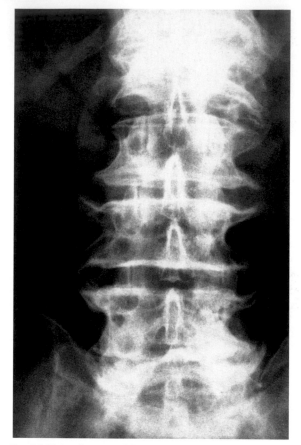
Fig. 26.16 Lumbar spondylosis.

even when the radiographs show the characteristic changes of an osteophyte on the anterior lip of the vertebral body and disc space narrowing (Fig. 26.16).

In advanced spondylosis, the lumbar spine is grossly abnormal, with large osteophytes, narrowed disc spaces and sclerotic vertebral bodies.

The symptoms of spondylosis are like those of degenerative joint disease elsewhere: pain or aching after activity, and loss of movement.

Treatment

Unless there is a neurological deficit due to nerve root compression, surgery has no place in the management of lumbar spondylosis, which is best treated in a department of physical medicine.

Operation is not needed unless there is root entrapment. The following conservative measures are usually sufficient to relieve symptoms:

1. Analgesics and anti-inflammatory drugs.
2. Physiotherapy to restore as much mobility as possible.
3. A lumbosacral brace to support the spine, just as a wrist support will help an osteoarthritic wrist.
4. Encouraging the patient to maintain the range of movement that they have and to learn to accept their disability.

Root entrapment

Osteophytes can encroach upon the root canal and cause root compression. The symptoms and signs are similar to those of an acute disc prolapse but less acute and less well localized. Investigation requires MRI or a CT scan (Fig. 26.17).

Treatment

If the nerve root lesion can be localized, the root can be unroofed to decompress the nerve, but the osteophytes are likely to recur and decompression does not improve the underlying spondylosis and osteoarthritis of the facet joints.

Spinal stenosis

The width of the spinal canal in normal individuals varies greatly. Some patients have narrow canals which can be made still narrower by osteophytes, disc prolapses or other space occupying lesions. A narrow spinal canal is also present in achondroplasia.

If the spinal canal is very narrow, congestion of the cord and roots can occur with exercise and this can cause pain in the buttocks and legs. The symptoms are usually brought on by extension of the spine when standing or walking and are eased by flexing the spine or sitting. The symptoms have much similarity with intermittent claudication, and the condition is sometimes known as 'spinal claudication'.

Investigation

CT scans and MRI demonstrate the constriction in the spinal canal very clearly.

Treatment

Conservative treatment is often helpful and consists of weight reduction, a spinal support and

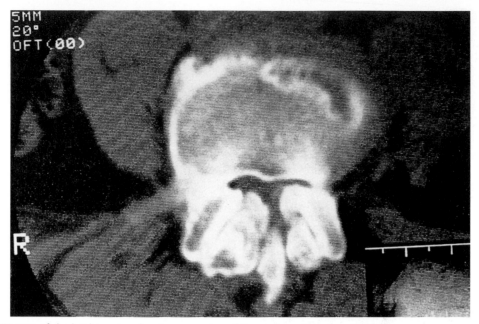

Fig. 26.17 CT scan of the lumbar spine showing narrowing of the root canal due to osteophytes.

physiotherapy to reduce hyperextension of the lumbar spine.

If these measures fail, operation to decompress the spinal cord is usually needed. A wide laminectomy will produce relief but symptoms can recur if soft tissue forms around the site of laminectomy.

Spondylolisthesis and spondylolysis

Spondylolisthesis is such a wonderful word that there is a temptation to use it whenever possible. In fact, it means only 'vertebral slipping' and must be distinguished from spondylolysis which means a 'broken vertebra'. There are several causes of spondylolisthesis (Fig. 26.18). The different types are classified as follows, using Roman numerals:

I Dysplastic – a developmental anomaly at the lumbosacral junction.

II Isthmic – a fatigue fracture of the pars interarticularis.

III Degenerative – degenerative osteoarthrosis.

IV Traumatic – acute trauma.

V Pathological – weakening of the pars interarticularis by a tumour, osteoporosis, tuberculosis or Paget's disease.

Dysplastic. A congenital deficiency of the lumbosacral facets allows the L5 vertebra to slip forwards off

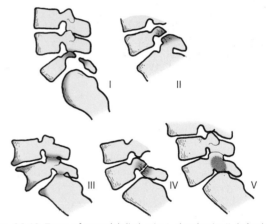

Fig. 26.18 Types of spondylolisthesis: I, dysplastic; II, isthmic; III, degenerative; IV, traumatic; V, pathological.

S1 (Fig. 26.19). The pars interarticularis becomes attenuated and may break. This is a rare condition, commoner in girls than boys, and causes severe hamstring spasm (p. 351).

Isthmic. The most common type of spondylolisthesis is slipping at a spondylolysis of the pars interarticularis caused by a fatigue fracture (Fig. 26.20). The condition is common in young vigorous patients, particularly athletes who hyperextend the spine, e.g. javelin throwers and fast bowlers, and

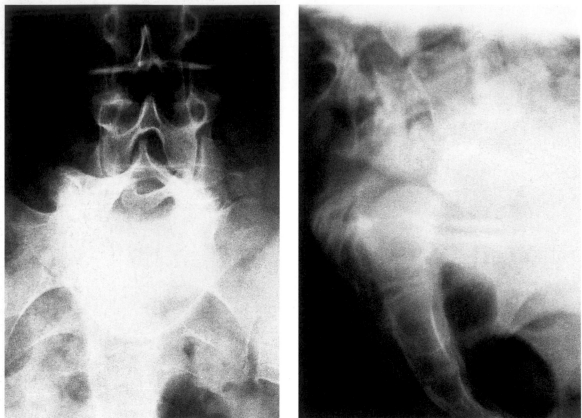

a   b

Fig. 26.19 Anteroposterior (a) and lateral (b) radiographs of a dysplastic spondylolisthesis. On the anteroposterior view, the fifth lumbar vertebra looks as if it was viewed from above. Upside down, it looks like Napoleon's hat on a totem pole.

presents with a dull low back pain radiating to the buttocks. The cause is obscure. Five per cent of the normal population have a spondylolysis by the age of 5 but this figure rises to 6% in adults so it cannot all be the result of hyperextension or violence on the sportsfield.

The midline of the spine is tender at the lumbosacral junction and a step can usually be felt at the affected level. Neurological signs are absent unless there is root compression at the site of the lesion.

Radiographs show a defect (spondylolysis) in the pars interarticularis which separates the back and front halves of the vertebra and allows the vertebral body to slip forwards, producing a spondylolisthesis. The defect is most easily seen on oblique films.

Degenerative. Vertebral slipping can result from mechanical wear of the posterior facet joints, but in this condition there is no spondylolysis and the main problem is degenerative joint disease. It is commonest in women over the age of 55.

Traumatic. In exceptional cases, the slip can be due to an acute traumatic fracture (see Fig. 10.32).

Pathological. Both tumours and osteoporosis can weaken the pars interarticularis enough to allow the upper vertebra to slip forwards.

Treatment

Restriction of activity, a lumbosacral support for use when the back is painful and exercises to build up the extensor muscles of the spine are all helpful.

This is one of the few spinal conditions that may be helped by operation. Operation is indicated if conservative measures are not effective or there is progression of the slip in a growing child. An intertransverse fusion to link the two separated halves of the affected vertebra is simple and reliable.

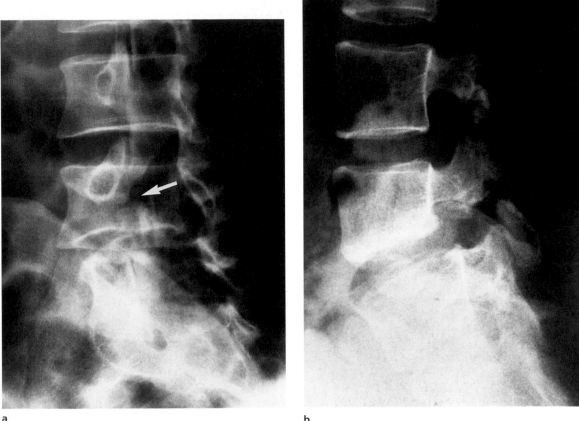

a   b

Fig. 26.20 (a) Isthmic spondylolisthesis. Note the defect (*arrowed*) in the pars articularis. (b) Isthmic spondylolisthesis of L5–S1 and spondylolysis of L4.

Osteochondritis

Scheuermann's disease

Scheuermann's disease is described on page 331. The ring apophyses of the vertebrae are affected and growth at the front of each vertebra is arrested. The condition affects children, usually boys, between the ages of 13 and 16 and produces a smooth rounded kyphosis. The condition is usually painless even while it is active.

Treatment

If the kyphosis is severe, bracing may be effective, and in very severe cases a spinal fusion may be needed. It is not kind to keep urging the children to 'stand up straight' because they are unable to do so.

Calvé's disease

Calvé's disease (p. 331) probably does not exist but it was described as a collapse of the immature vertebral body and assumed to be an osteochondritis. Some cases may perhaps be due to osteochondritis, but tuberculosis and spinal tumours cause the same appearance and are more serious.

Congenital anomalies

Minor congenital anomalies of the vertebrae are exceedingly common but seldom have serious consequences.

Lumbarization and sacralization

The boundary between the lumbar spine and sacrum is not always precise. In some patients L5 may have a large transverse process either articulating with or fused to the sacrum (partial sacralization) or S1 may be separate from the sacrum (sacralization). Some patients with these abnormalities have back pain but there is no hard evidence that the abnormalities themselves cause pain. Nevertheless, the presence of pain at the site of a congenital anomaly is often regarded as strong circumstantial evidence.

Treatment

Patients with transitional lumbosacral vertebrae should be treated as if their radiographs were normal, using anti-inflammatory drugs and physiotherapy. Operation on the anomaly should be avoided.

Congenital hemivertebra

A hemivertebra leaves the patient with a lateral kink in the spine, which causes a compensatory scoliosis above and below. This may itself cause root irritation and throw greater strain on the small joints of the spine (Fig. 26.21).

Treatment

Physiotherapy and analgesics are usually sufficient, but the hemivertebra may need to be excised if the deformity or the symptoms are severe.

Spina bifida

As many as 20% of the population have radiological spina bifida occulta without serious symptoms (Fig. 26.22), perhaps accompanied by a small hairy patch or lipoma at the lumbosacral junction or a minor neurological deficit (Fig. 26.23). Others have myelocoele, meningocoele or meningomyelocoele with exposed spinal nerve roots due to a failure of tubulation of the spinal cord, and these patients have serious problems in the neonatal period and early childhood (p. 356). Between these two extremes there is a spectrum of pathology.

Treatment

The management of severe spina bifida in children is described on page 356.

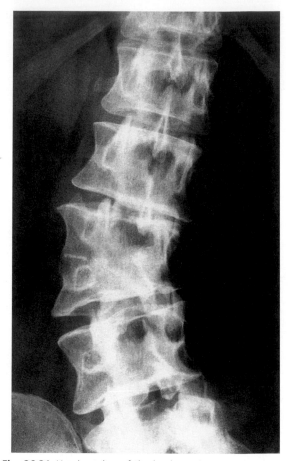

Fig. 26.21 Hemivertebra of the lumbar spine.

Diastematomyelia

Some congenital abnormalities of the lumbar spine include a fibrous band or bony bar which tethers the spinal cord. As growth proceeds, the spinal cord is stretched and neurological signs appear (Fig. 26.24). Children between 5 and 10 years are most often affected. The sacral roots are the first to be involved, causing pain in the foot and a high arch to the foot. Later, numbness develops and the foot becomes flat as the sacral roots are more seriously damaged.

Any child with unexplained pain in the feet or legs, particularly with a progressive foot deformity, should be suspected of having a diastematomyelia. A plain radiograph may demonstrate a bony abnormality and a CT scan or MRI may show a fibrous tether. The opinion of a neurological surgeon is helpful.

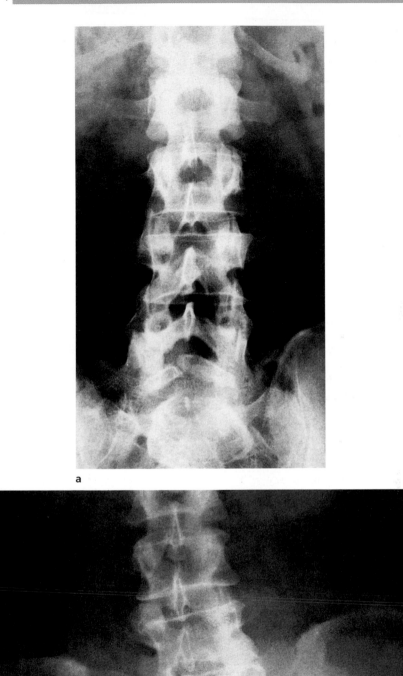

Fig. 26.22 Spina bifida occulta: (a) affecting the fifth lumbar vertebra; (b) with a hemivertebra at the lumbosacral junction.

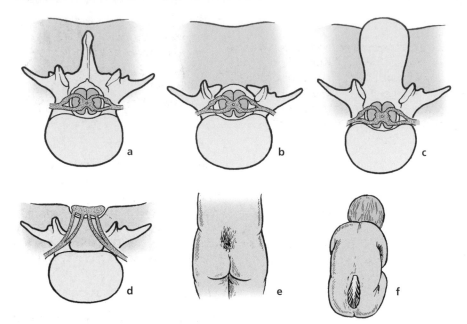

Fig. 26.23 Types of spina bifida: (a) normal; (b) spinal bifida occulta; (c) meningocoele; (d) meningomyelocoele with exposed nerve roots; (e) hairy patch at lumbosacral junction; (f) neonate with meningomyelocoele.

Treatment

Less severe manifestations are best treated conservatively unless there is evidence of tethering of the roots by bony bars or fibrous bands, which should be divided or excised by a neurological surgeon.

Other conditions

Spinal tumours

Metastases

The commonest spinal tumour is a metastasis and the possibility of a tumour must always be remembered when treating any patient with back pain, even if the history is long. A history of back pain from other causes does not bring immunity to spinal tumours and it is quite possible for a patient with established back pain of many years standing to develop a bone tumour in addition to the original problem. Any painful back should be examined radiologically if a metastasis is suspected, even though making the diagnosis of a spinal tumour does not always help the patient. An ESR is useful: if normal, a metastasis is unlikely.

The commonest tumours to metastasize to the spine are those which usually spread to bone:

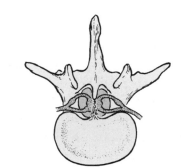

Fig. 26.24 Diastematomyelia. A fibrous or bony bar splits the spinal cord.

1. Prostate.
2. Breast.
3. Kidney.
4. Bronchus.

Metastatic tumours commonly go to the pedicles, which are destroyed. This can easily be recognized radiologically by looking for an owl in each vertebra on the anteroposterior view. The pedicles correspond to the eyes and the spinous process to the beak. If a pedicle is destroyed, its outline cannot be seen. *Beware the winking owl!*

Primary tumours

Other bone tumours are seen in the spine, including osteoblastoma and giant cell tumour, but osteogenic sarcoma, which occurs typically around the growing end of long bones, is very rare. Tumours of the nervous system, such as neurofibroma and meningioma, also occur and multiple myeloma may cause vertebral collapse.

Osteoporosis

Osteoporosis is a very common condition, particularly in women after the menopause, and causes a dull low back pain with a gradually increasing kyphosis (p. 320). Pathological fractures and sudden collapse of a vertebral body can follow a trivial injury, or even just coughing.

Treatment

Apart from diagnosis and a spinal support, there is little to offer; the osteoporosis is usually too far advanced to be treatable by the time the patient is seen (p. 320).

Tuberculosis

Spinal tuberculosis is now rare in developed countries but still a scourge elsewhere. The characteristic features of the disease are as follows (Fig. 26.25):

1. The patient is unwell and has lost weight.
2. The affected vertebrae are tender.
3. The disease involves the vertebral body and crosses the disc space.
4. The infection causes abscesses within the psoas sheath which point at the psoas insertion in the groin.
5. Radiologically, there is destruction of the anterior vertebral margin with wedging of one or more vertebrae and widening of the psoas sheath.
6. The vertebral collapse produces a sharp angled gibbus, which may be the first physical sign. In late cases, the gibbus may be very marked.

Complications

Complications may be serious, with the formation of sinuses, which may become secondarily infected, and paraplegia (Pott's paraplegia), which has three common causes: (1) pus and intracellular pressure; (2) mechanical injury to the cord from bony pressure; and (3) vascular embarrassment to the spinal cord where it crosses the gibbus.

Treatment

Treatment is by oral antibacterials (p. 315), which are only effective if the patient actually takes them. The treatment must be continued for months or years. Alternatively, operation is needed to drain the pus, remove dead bone and fuse the affected vertebrae to prevent future bone collapse. If bone collapse has already occurred and the spinal cord is threatened, bone grafting and fusion is required.

Infective discitis

The intervertebral discs can become infected, often by obscure bacteria or fungi. Spread can occur directly from bone infection in adjacent vertebrae. The patients have diffuse back pain, often severe, and a raised ESR. The radiographs show erosion of bone on both sides of the intervertebral disc. Disc infections are more common in drug addicts and immunosuppressed patients.

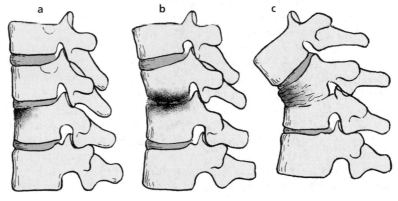

Fig. 26.25 Tuberculosis of the spine: (a) early involvement of a vertebral body; (b) erosion of both vertebrae and narrowing of the disc space; (c) collapse of the vertebrae with sharp gibbus.

The infecting organism can sometimes be identified by blood or urine culture or by needle biopsy of the disc. If these measures do not succeed in identifying the organism, open biopsy will be needed.

In children, discitis can occur without any apparent infection and usually leads to painless fusion of adjacent vertebrae.

Treatment

If the organism can be identified, systemic antibiotics are effective, but exploration of the disc is sometimes necessary.

Meralgia paraesthetica

The lateral cutaneous nerve of the thigh enters the thigh just medial to the anterior superior iliac spine and may be trapped either at this point or within the abdomen (Fig. 26.26). Meralgia paraesthetica is Greek for 'pain in the thigh with altered sensibility' and this is an excellent description of the symptoms.

The condition is not serious but it is important to know of it because, like disseminated sclerosis, peripheral neuritis, tabes dorsalis, subacute combined degeneration of the cord and a host of other peripheral neuropathies, it can cause neurological symptoms and signs in the leg without involvement of the spine and must be considered in the differential diagnosis of a prolapsed disc.

Treatment

The condition usually resolves spontaneously and seldom requires decompression of the nerve.

Coccydynia

The coccyx is a richly innervated structure, supposedly because it is the vestige of the tail. Whether this is true or not, there is no doubt that it is extremely sensitive to injury and that pain in the coccyx can be very difficult to eradicate.

The symptoms often begin after a fall onto the coccyx through missing a chair or falling onto the ice, but more often in accidents at work. The pain is severe and persistent and the position of the coccyx makes sitting difficult. Coccydynia can also be caused by disc prolapses and pelvic disorders, including carcinoma of the rectum and uterus, which should always be considered.

Coccydynia is more common in women than men and is more difficult to treat in neurotic and litigious individuals, who seem particularly susceptible to the condition.

Treatment

Injection with hydrocortisone is often effective but if the pain is still present after three injections, denervation of the coccyx with ultrasound or a radiofrequency probe in a pain clinic should be considered.

Coccygectomy is sometimes done but should only be considered as the last resort. It may succeed in a few patients but in many the pain remains after the coccyx has been removed.

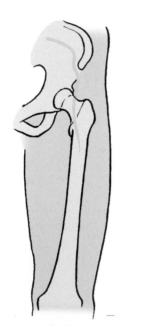

Fig. 26.26 Meralgia paraesthetica. Abnormal sensibility in the distribution of the lateral cutaneous nerve of the thigh.

Manipulative medicine

Osteopaths and chiropractors are skilled in manipulation and can produce remarkably good results in patients with severe pain in the neck and back. Anybody who can relieve pain is a friend of the medical profession but problems can arise if the practitioner does not look beyond the spine for the cause of symptoms, or believes that spinal manipulation can cure diseases in other structures.

Patients attending manipulative therapists without medical assessment are therefore the cause of some concern. Provided serious organic disease has been excluded, it is hard to find a reason why a patient should not be treated by an osteopath or chiroprac-tor rather than a physiotherapist, if that is their preference.

It must be remembered that most of the conditions treated successfully by manipulation are self-limiting disorders, and experienced manipulators readily refer patients with persistent problems to orthopaedic surgeons or rheumatologists.

Glossary

Many of the words used in orthopaedics can be difficult to understand, particularly those describing a deformity, and a few minutes self-testing to check that you know the correct meaning of the terms in the following glossary will be well spent.

Most of the words are explained in detail the first time they appear in the text. Those that the reader might be expected to know without explanation are printed in bold type the first time they are used. A few obsolescent or obscure words that are occasionally used in orthopaedic conversation but which do not appear in the text are also included in the Glossary.

Abduction means moving a limb away from the midline of the body, or a digit away from the midline of the hand or foot (Fig. 2.3). Beware of confusion: the abductor hallucis moves the big toe away from the midline of the foot, but towards the midline of the body, and the adductor hallucis is an adductor because it moves the big toe towards the midline of the foot, even though this is away from the midline of the body.

Adduction is the opposite of abduction. If a leg is adducted so that it crosses the midline, the movement is still called adduction, even though the limb is actually moving away from the midline of the body.

Angulation is a term applied to the deformity at fracture sites, and is confusing. Does 'backward angulation' mean that the convexity of the bone points backwards, or that the distal end of the limb is angled backwards?

Ankylosis. A fibrous link, e.g. the replacement of a joint by fibrous tissue following infection (Fig. 18.7).

AO Arbeitsgemeinschaft für Osteosynthesefragen. The Working Party for Questions Relating to the Joining of Bone Fragments – the German for 'ASIF' – see below. Both AO and ASIF are used, but AO is more common.

Apparent shortening. If the patient has a stiff hip and the leg is held adducted, it will appear to the patient that the leg is shorter than the other side, even though the limb itself is in fact of full length (see page 24 and Fig. 2.29).

Arthritis means any inflammation of any joint. A vague term of no real medical significance, often misinterpreted by patients to mean a crippling disease. See 'Rheumatism'.

Arthro-. A prefix meaning 'relating to a joint'.

Arthrodesis is an operation to produce bony fusion across a joint (Figs 6.21, 6.22, 6.23).

Arthrography is a radiological examination that demonstrates the non-calcified structures in a joint, usually using double-contrast techniques.

Arthroplasty. Any operation to fashion a new joint. See page 299 and Fig. 6.24 for an explanation of excision arthroplasty, interposition arthroplasty and replacement arthroplasty.

Arthroscopy. An operation to look inside a joint with an arthroscope.

Arthrotomy. Any operation in which a joint is opened surgically.

Aseptic necrosis. Bone death without infection, as opposed to septic necrosis. See also 'Avascular necrosis'.

ASIF. Association for the Study of Internal Fixation (the English for AO). An organization based in

Switzerland which develops instruments and implants for the fixation of fractures.

Astragalus is an old word for the talus, perpetuated in 'astragalectomy', the operation to remove the talus.

Avascular necrosis. A bad term (all necrosis is avascular) but still used to mean 'aseptic necrosis'.

Back knee. A deformity in which the knee bends backwards.

Backward angulation. See 'Angulation'.

Bone cement. Any material, but usually acrylic cement, for fixing prostheses into bone.

Bone lever. A surgical instrument used for holding soft tissues away from bone and for manipulating bones.

Bone wax. A wax applied to bleeding cancellous bone surfaces to stop the bleeding.

Brace. Any splint or support that can be removed or replaced. See 'Orthosis'.

Break. A fracture. A fracture and a break are the same thing, but patients often believe that one is worse than the other.

Butterfly fragment. When a long bone such as the tibia is broken by a twisting movement, a spiral fracture results. If the tip of one of the bone ends breaks off, it produces a curved triangular fragment that bears a fanciful resemblance to a butterfly on some radiological views.

Calcaneovalgus. A deformity in which the foot points upwards and outwards (Fig. 21.5c).

Cancellous screw. A type of screw used for fixing cancellous bone. See 'Screw' and Fig. 9.22.

Chisel. A carpenter's instrument bearing a superficial resemblance to an osteotome. The chisel has one flat side and one bevelled side; an osteotome is curved on both sides. See 'Osteotome'.

Circumduction. Moving the upper or lower limb around in a circular movement.

Closed fracture. A fracture in which the skin remains intact. See 'Simple fracture'.

Club foot. A popular term for talipes equinovarus (Fig. 21.5), but sometimes applied to any foot deformity. If left untreated, the foot of a patient with talipes equinovarus resembles a club.

Comminuted fracture. A fracture in which there are many small fragments of bone.

Complicated fracture. A difficult fracture to treat, or one in which complications have occurred. It is not the opposite of a simple fracture.

Compound fracture. A fracture in which the skin is broken. This term is now becoming obsolete and has been replaced by 'open fracture'. See 'Simple fracture'.

Contralateral. The limb on the opposite side of the body, as opposed to ipsilateral, which means 'on the same side of the body'.

Cortical screw. A type of bone screw used for fixing cortical bone. See 'Screw'.

Coxarthrosis. Another word for osteoarthritis of the hip, often used by European surgeons.

CTEV. Congenital talipes equinovarus. See 'Club foot'.

DDH. Developmental dysplasia of the hip.

Debridement. The removal of debris from a wound, a very important but often neglected procedure. In French, *débridement* means incision and drainage of a wound. French surgeons refer to the operation of debridement as *parage*.

Delayed union is a complication of a fracture in which the bone ends join, but very slowly.

-desis. A suffix meaning fixation, e.g. 'arthrodesis', 'tenodesis'.

Diplegia. A neurological condition involving both lower limbs, usually applied to the spastic diplegia of cerebral palsy.

Dislocation. The injury in which the components of a joint become completely separated without a fracture. See also 'Fracture dislocation' and 'Subluxation'.

Dorsal. The side of the forearm on the same side as the back of the hand. Used to describe the extensor muscles.

Equinovarus. A deformity in which the foot is pointing downwards and inwards. This is the common deformity of a club foot, often known as congenital talipes equinovarus (CTEV). See 'Club foot'.

Equinus. A deformity in which the foot points downwards. The deformity derives its name from the position of a horse's foot; the horse runs on its toes, the hooves being the equivalent of the nails on human digits (Fig. 2.47b).

Eversion is the movement of the subtalar joint in which the foot is turned upwards and outwards. The opposite is inversion. See also 'Pronation' and 'Supination'.

Excision arthroplasty. An arthroplasty in which the joint is excised. See page 299 and Figure 6.24.

Extensor lag. If a joint, e.g. the knee, will go straight passively but the muscles will not extend it actively, the resulting droop of the joint is known as an extensor (or flexor, abductor, etc.) lag. It has nothing to do with a 'lag' screw.

Extra-articular. Outside the joint, as opposed to intra-articular.

Fatigue fracture. A fracture resulting from repeated minor stress (see page 100, Figs 15.2, 15.3). These fractures are also known as stress fractures, which is misleading because all fractures result from stress of one kind or another.

Fixed deformity. A deformity that cannot be corrected by manipulation.

Flaccid. The condition of muscles which have no tone, usually the result of damage to the lower motor neurone. The opposite is 'spastic'.

Forward angulation. A deformity which occurs at fracture sites. See 'Angulation'.

Fracture. The same as a break. See also Simple, Open, Closed, Compound, Complicated, Comminuted and Fatigue.

Fracture dislocation. A dislocation accompanied by a fracture involving the dislocated joint.

Gonarthrosis. Another name for osteoarthritis of the knee, favoured by European surgeons.

Hemiplegia. A neurological disorder involving one side of the body, e.g. right arm and right leg, usually the result of a cerebrovascular accident.

Hyperextension. Movement in the opposite direction to flexion in joints where this does not normally occur, e.g. the knee.

IDK. Acronym for 'internal derangement of the knee' – as well as 'I don't know'.

Interposition. The state of affairs when soft tissue is interposed between the ends of bones. This can occur accidentally in fractures or as an interposition arthroplasty (p. 299).

Intra-articular. Within the synovial cavity of a joint. The opposite is extra-articular.

Intramedullary. Within the medullary cavity of a long bone.

Inversion is downwards and inwards movement of the foot occurring at the subtalar joint. See 'Eversion'.

Involucrum. The expanded bony tube that contains the sequestrum in chronic osteomyelitis.

K-nail is short for Küntscher nail, an intramedullary fixation device. Commonly, but incorrectly, applied to any intramedullary nail. See page 134 and Figure 9.24.

K-wire. Kirschner wire. A narrow wire used to hold the position of healing bones after fractures or operations. The wire was originally passed through the upper end of the tibia and held on a 'traction bow' to apply traction to the femur.

Kirschner wire. See K-wire.

Küntscher nail. See K-nail.

Kyphosis. Curvature of the spine in which the concavity faces forwards. The thoracic spine has a normal kyphosis (Fig. 2.8).

Kyphoscoliosis. Deformity of the spine in which there is kyphosis and scoliosis (Fig. 2.7).

Lag screw. A bone screw which has threads at its end only, so that it will apply compression across the fracture site (see page 132, Fig. 9.22).

LFA. Low friction arthroplasty, or Charnley total hip replacement, one type of total hip replacement.

Lordosis. Curvature of the spine in which the concavity faces backwards. There is a normal cervical and lumbar lordosis (Fig. 2.8).

Luxation. Another word for dislocation, now rarely used. See 'Subluxation'.

Malleolar screw. Bone screw originally used to fix malleoli but also useful in other situations (Fig. 9.22).

Malunion. A complication of a fracture in which the bones join solidly, but are in an unacceptable position.

Neurolysis. Releasing a nerve from adhesions (not destroying it, as '-lysis' sometimes means).

Non-union. A complication of a fracture in which the bones do not join.

Open fracture. A fracture in which the skin has been breached either from within (e.g. bone) or without. See 'Compound'.

Opposition is the movement in which the thumb is brought across to meet the little finger (Fig. 2.24).

Orthosis. An appliance, splint, caliper or brace to correct deformity or provide support.

Osteosynthesis. An operation to join bones, usually fractures, by internal fixation.

Osteotome. An instrument used for cutting bone. It differs from a chisel by being bevelled on both flat surfaces. See 'Chisel'.

Osteotomy. An operation to cut across a bone.

-otomy. Suffix indicating the surgical division of something, e.g. osteotomy (to cut a bone) or tenotomy (to cut a tendon).

Overdrilling. Drilling a large enough hole through a bone fragment to prevent the screw gripping so that a lag effect can be produced. See 'Lag screw'.

Paraplegia. A motor abnormality of the lower half of the body, usually the result of damage to the spinal cord.

-plasty. Suffix indicating an operation in which something is shaped or formed, such as arthroplasty.

Pronation. Movement of the forearm so that the hand faces downwards. Also applied to the comparable movement in the foot in which the sole faces downwards.

Prosthesis. An appliance used to replace an absent part of the body, e.g. a lower limb prosthesis or an artificial leg, or a total hip prosthesis which is implanted during the operation of total hip replacement. A removable prosthesis is an 'exoprosthesis'; one that is implanted is an 'endoprosthesis'.

Pseudarthrosis. A false joint, usually resulting from the non-union of a fracture. Sometimes also applied to the result of an excision arthroplasty (see page 97, Fig. 7.7).

Pyarthrosis. A joint filled with pus.

Radial. Towards the same side of the forearm as the radius. This is the same as 'lateral' in the anatomical position, but not when the forearm is pronated.

Real shortening. Shortening of a limb, usually the lower limb, in which there is real loss of bone. To be distinguished from apparent shortening (Fig. 2.29).

Recurvatum. Abnormal hyperextension, generally applied to the elbow or knee. See 'Back knee'.

Reduction. Putting a fracture or dislocation back in its correct position.

Rheumatism. An old term, but still used by patients. 'Rheum' is an ancient word for watery secretions of the body, such as tears, saliva or synovial fluid. Rheumatism means different things to different patients, but usually implies pain around joints. See 'Arthritis'.

Rotation. Movement about the long axis of a limb, usually resulting from movement of the shoulder or hip.

RTA. Road traffic accident.

Scoliosis. Deformity of the spine in which the concavity faces sideways (see page 15, Fig. 2.7).

Screw. Device used for fixing fractures (Fig. 9.22).

Self-tapping screw. A type of screw that cuts its own thread (Fig. 9.22).

Sequestrum. The dead piece of bone inside the involucrum in chronic osteomyelitis.

Sesamoid bones are small bones, shaped like a sesame seed, lying within a tendon at points of great pressure. The patella is the largest sesamoid in the body.

Shin splints. Pain in front of the tibia, usually due to a fatigue fracture of the tibia, not a brace or cast.

Shortening. Loss of length in a long bone.

Simple fracture. An old term applied to a fracture in which the skin remains intact. 'Simple' fractures are not always easy to treat. The term derives from ancient military surgery and indicated that amputation was not necessary. The opposite was a compound fracture, i.e. a fracture with an open wound, which was treated by amputation because of the risk of tetanus and deep infection. See 'Compound fracture' and page 97.

Spastic. A muscle that has excessive tone, often due to cerebral palsy. The opposite is flaccid.

Splint. Any device to prevent movement at a fracture or joint. See 'Orthosis'.

Spondylitis. Inflammation of the spine, e.g. ankylosing spondylitis.

Spondylo-. Prefix that means 'pertaining to a vertebra'.

Spondylolisthesis. Slipping of one vertebra upon another (see page 457).

Spondylolysis. A condition in which there is a defect in a vertebra, often the result of a fatigue fracture (see page 457).

Spondylosis. Degenerative change in the spine.

Sprain. A partial tear of a ligament.

Stress fracture. See 'Fatigue fracture'.

Stress riser. A mechanical term indicating the point at which stress is concentrated, as at the junction of the fixed and mobile part of the lumbar spine, or where the stiffness of a bone changes markedly, e.g. at the lower end of a prosthesis (see page 46).

Subluxation. A partial dislocation.

Supination. Movement of the forearm so that the hand faces upwards. Also applied to the comparable movement in the foot in which the sole faces the inside edge of the opposite foot.

Symphysis. A joint with a disc of fibrocartilage at its centre and no cavity (see page 35, Fig. 3.6).

Talipes. Club foot. See also 'CTEV'.

Tenotome. A knife with a very short blade used for cutting a tendon.

Tenotomy. The operation of cutting a tendon.

THR. Total hip replacement.

TKR. Total knee replacement.

Ulnar. Towards the same side of the forearm as the ulna. See 'Radial'.

Valgus. A limb deformity in which the extremity is moved away from the midline. The point of reference is always proximal; a patient with knock knee has genu valgum. Valgus deformities always relate to the midline of the body, unlike abduction and adduction, which can relate to the midline of a hand or foot. The adductor hallucis, for example, can accentuate a valgus deformity of the big toe. The opposite of valgus is varus. See 'Abduction'.

Varus. The opposite of valgus.

Ventral. The side of forearm on the same side as the palm – used particularly to describe the ventral musculature and the flexor compartment of the forearm.

Volar. On the same side of the hand as the palm.

Index

Note: Page numbers in **bold** refer to figures, page numbers in *italic* refer to tables.

BRITISH MEDICAL ASSOCIATION
BMA Library